Manual of Anesthesia and the Medically Compromised Patient

J.B. LIPPINCOTT COMPANY
Philadelphia

Grand Rapids • New York • St. Louis • San Francisco
London • Sydney • Tokyo

Manual of

ANESTHESIA
and the Medically Compromised Patient

Edited by

Eugene Y. Cheng, MD
Assistant Professor of Anesthesiology and Internal Medicine
Director, Critical Care Medicine
Department of Anesthesiology
Medical College of Wisconsin
Milwaukee, Wisconsin

Jonathan Kay, MD
Attending Anesthesiologist
St. Luke's Medical Center
Milwaukee, Wisconsin

21 CONTRIBUTORS

Acquisitions Editor: Nancy L. Mullins
Copy Editor: Judith Bronson
Project Editor: Kathy Crown
Indexer: Maria Coughlin
Design Coordinator: Ellen C. Dawson
Production Manager: Caren Erlichman
Production Coordinator: Kevin P. Johnson
Compositor: Circle Graphics
Text Printer/Binder: R.R. Donnelley & Sons Company

6 5 4 3 2 1

Library of Congress Cataloging-in-Publication Data

Manual of anesthesia and the medically compromised patient / edited by
  Eugene Y. Cheng, Jonathan Kay.
      p.   cm.
  Includes bibliographical references.
  ISBN 0-397-50901-4
  1. Anesthesia. I. Cheng, Eugene Y. II. Kay, Jonathan.
  [DNLM: 1. Anesthesia.   WO 200 M294]
  RD81.M335   1990
  617.9'6—dc20
  DNLM/DLC   90-5629
  for Library of Congress   CIP

The authors and publisher have exerted every effort to ensure that drug selection and dosage set forth in this text are in accord with current recommendations and practice at the time of publication. However, in view of ongoing research, changes in government regulations, and the constant flow of information relating to drug therapy and drug reactions, the reader is urged to check the package insert for each drug for any change in indications and dosage and for added warnings and precautions. This is particularly important when the recommended agent is a new or infrequently employed drug.

CONTRIBUTORS

Eugene Y. Cheng, MD
Assistant Professor of Anesthesiology and Internal Medicine
Director, Critical Care Medicine
Department of Anesthesiology
Medical College of Wisconsin
Milwaukee, Wisconsin

Douglas B. Coursin, MD
Associate Professor of Anesthesiology and Internal Medicine
University of Wisconsin—Madison
Madison, Wisconsin

Steven Croy, MD
Former Fellow, Anesthesia and Critical Care
University of Wisconsin—Madison;
Staff Anesthesiologist
Rockford Memorial Hospital
Rockford, Illinois

Orlando G. Florete, Jr, MD
Fellow, Critical Care Medicine
Department of Anesthesiology
University of Florida College of Medicine
Gainesville, Florida

Thomas J. Gallagher, MD
Professor of Anesthesiology and Surgery
Chief, Critical Care Medicine
Department of Anesthesiology
University of Florida College of Medicine
Gainesville, Florida

Susan L. Goelzer, MD
Assistant Professor
Anesthesiology and Internal Medicine
University of Wisconsin—Madison
Madison, Wisconsin

J. David Haddox, DDS, MD
Assistant Professor
Departments of Anesthesiology, Psychiatry and Mental Health
  Sciences
Associate Director, Pain Management Center
Medical College of Wisconsin
Milwaukee, Wisconsin

Jonathan Kay, MD
Attending Anesthesiologist
St. Luke's Medical Center
Milwaukee, Wisconsin

Lee A. Kearse, Jr, MD, PhD
Director, Intraoperative Neurophysiology
Assistant in Anesthesia in Neurology and Neurosurgery
Massachusetts General Hospital;
Instructor in Anesthesia
Harvard Medical School
Boston, Massachusetts

Brian J. McGrath, MD
Assistant Professor
Co-Director, Intensive Care Unit
Department of Anesthesiology
George Washington University Medical Center
Washington, D.C.

John Morley, MD
Assistant Professor
Department of Anesthesiology
Medical College of Wisconsin
Froedtert Memorial Lutheran Hospital
Milwaukee, Wisconsin

Peter John Papadakos, MD
Department of Anesthesiology—Critical Care Division
Senior Instructor, Surgical Intensive Care Unit
University of Rochester Medical Center
Strong Memorial Hospital
Rochester, New York

Patricia H. Petrozza, MD
Assistant Professor
Department of Anesthesiology
Bowman Gray School of Medicine
Winston-Salem, North Carolina

Richard Prielipp, MD
Assistant Professor
Anesthesia and Critical Care Medicine
Bowman Gray School of Medicine
Winston-Salem, North Carolina

Donald S. Prough, MD
Associate Professor
Anesthesia and Neurology
Head, Critical Care Section
Bowman Gray School of Medicine
Winston-Salem, North Carolina

Raymond L. Sabon, MD
Associate Staff, Department of Anesthesiology
Butterworth Hospital
Grand Rapids, Michigan

Robert N. Sladen, MB, MRCP (UK), FRCP (C)
Associate Professor of Anesthesiology and Surgery
Duke University Medical Center;
Chief, Anesthesiology Service
Veterans Affairs Medical Center
Durham, North Carolina

Rebekah Wang-Cheng, MD
Assistant Professor
Departments of Medicine and Psychiatry
Medical College of Wisconsin
Milwaukee, Wisconsin

Anne B. Wong, MD
Associate Clinical Professor
Department of Anesthesiology
University of California
Irvine Medical Center
Orange, California

David Wong, MD
Acting Chief of Anesthesiology
Associate Clinical Professor
Department of Anesthesiology
University of California
Irvine Medical Center
Orange, California

John F. Williams, MD
Assistant Professor
Department of Anesthesiology
George Washington University Medical Center
Washington, District of Columbia

PREFACE

The anesthesiologist is often considered the "internist" of the operating room. Many patients coming for surgery are older, more ill, and have had less preoperative evaluation and treatment than in the past, yet the anesthesiologist must be able to design an anesthetic regimen that will preserve the patient's physiologic homeostasis. This can best be accomplished with proper understanding of the underlying medical problems.

In the last several years, a new type of anesthesiologist has evolved: the anesthesiologist-intensivist. These anesthesiologists not only provide intraoperative anesthesia but often are involved with the preoperative and postoperative care of patients with multisystem organ dysfunction. By necessity, these anesthesiologists must be familiar with the standard of care required for many of the illnesses patients have prior to surgery. With this in mind, our contributors are primarily anesthesiologists with training in critical care medicine. We believe they provide a unique perspective on medical problems and their relation to anesthetic care.

This manual is more than a simple quick reference but is not as extensive as a major textbook. Our goal is to provide current information on the incidence, etiology, and pathogenesis of the more commonly encountered medical illnesses and important anesthetic perioperative concerns. At the end of each section, we summarized the principal anesthetic considerations for each medical problem for quick reference. The outline format was chosen to help organize the information in a rapidly accessible form. We hope this book will provide information that is current, straightforward, and practical for all involved in providing anesthesia for medically ill patients.

Eugene Y. Cheng, MD
Jonathan Kay, MD

ACKNOWLEDGMENTS

We appreciate the time and effort all the contributors spent on their sections, knowing how busy they can be without the additional obligation of writing book chapters. Special thanks to Debbie Schmidling, Nordeana Nimphius, Kim Stommel, and Carole Panaro for their tireless efforts in manuscript preparations, management of correspondence, and other tasks needed for the completion of this book.

Foremost is our thanks and gratitude to our wives, Rebekah Wang-Cheng and Marilyn Kay, for their support and understanding and willingness to sacrifice many hours of family life while we were involved in this project.

CONTENTS

Manual of Anesthesia and the Medically Compromised Patient

CHAPTER
1

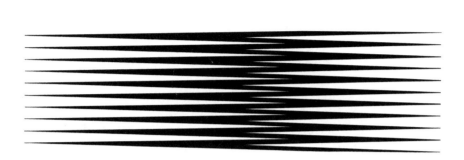

Cardiovascular Disorders

≡ Cardiac Disease: Congestive Heart Failure, Coronary Artery Disease, and Valvular Disease

Orlando G. Florete, Jr.
T. James Gallagher

Cardiovascular diseases remain the primary cause of morbidity and account for half of all reported deaths in the United States. The anesthesiologist must recognize their presence and assess their severity, because inadequate preoperative diagnosis, incomplete preparation for surgery, lack of understanding of cardiac pathophysiology, and improper or unduly delayed treatment of perioperative complications can contribute to anesthetic-related complications and death.

Once disease is diagnosed, its severity must be evaluated and a determination made about whether medical treatment can improve cardiac function. Optimal anesthetic management and use of invasive monitoring depend on making the correct diagnosis and understanding the burden the disease imposes on the patient's hemodynamic state. A patient with compensated heart disease preoperatively may be unable to meet the increased demands during the perioperative period. Myocardial pump failure, with or without myocardial ischemia and cardiac dysrhythmias, most often occurs at this time. A thorough history and physical examination supplemented by laboratory tests such as the electrocardiogram (ECG), chest radiograph, and, in certain cases, echocardiography, radionuclide studies, or cardiac catheterization form the basis of assessment prior to surgery.

The present-day anesthesiologist deals daily with the problem of how to approach a cardiac patient undergoing surgery. With the improvements in anesthetic techniques and the availability of intensive care facilities, many cardiac patients who in the past would have been considered at too great a risk are now being considered for noncardiac surgery. This chapter describes common cardiovascular diseases and their concomitant risks, defines the pathophysiological processes, and describes basic approaches to therapy.

Congestive Heart Failure

Congestive heart failure results from the inability of the heart to pump blood in a quantity commensurate with the body's metabolic requirements. Heart failure is an increasing medical problem despite advances in therapy and the overall reduction of cardiovascular mortality rates.

I. INCIDENCE AND OUTCOME

Heart failure afflicts an estimated four million Americans. Annually, approximately two million physician office visits, 2% of all hospital admissions, and 200,000 deaths are attributed to myocardial failure.

    A. The prognosis remains dismal and worsens with the extent of myocardial dysfunction. In the Framingham study, the probability of death within 4 years after the initial injury was 52% for men and 43% for women. For patients who are severely symptomatic, the outlook is even worse. Class III (moderately compromised) or IV (severely compromised) congestive heart failure, as defined by the New York Heart Association (NYHA), has a 48% mortality rate at 1 year that increases to 68% at 2 years. Sudden death and progressive lethal cardiac failure are equally common.

    B. With the geriatric population growing, congestive heart failure has become the leading cause of in-hospital death in patients with cardiac disease. It is the most important single preoperative abnormality contributing to postoperative cardiac complications and death.

II. ETIOLOGY

    A. Primary Causation

Abnormality of the myocardium is the primary causative factor for heart failure. Myocardial pump dysfunction can occur acutely after massive myocardial infarction (MI), with severe valvular insufficiency, or after infection or exposure to toxins. Dysrhythmias, restriction of ventricular filling, or abnormal preload conditions also can cause pump failure despite normal myocardial muscle function. Table 1-1 summarizes the causative factors and provides examples of each category.

    B. Risk Factors

Chronic heart failure may be secondary to progressive dysfunction that is associated with several risk factors and aggravating conditions.

        1. Hypertension, a primary stress factor, causes further deterioration of otherwise-compromised heart function. Inappropriate reduction of therapy is the principal cause of decompensation in a previously stable patient.

        2. Other risk factors are increasing age, diabetes

Table 1–1. Causes of Congestive Heart Failure

Failing Myocardium

Coronary artery disease (most common cause)
  Failure secondary to acute myocardial infarction or ischemia
  Chronic failure attributable to one or more infarctions, scar formation,
    or long-standing myocardial ischemia
Cardiomyopathy
  Dilated
  Hypertrophic
  Restrictive and infiltrative
Myocarditis
Valvular heart disease
Congenital heart disease

Normal Myocardium

Rhythm disturbance (heart block, bradycardia, supraventricular
  dysrhythmias)
Restricted ventricular filling (cardiac tamponade, pericarditis)
Circulatory failure
  Acute volume overload (excessive fluid resuscitation)
  High-output states (anemia, thyrotoxicosis, beri-beri, Paget's disease,
    arteriovenous fistula)

mellitus, and the development of other cardiac problems.

3. An unrelated illness or infection; the administration of cardiac depressant or salt-retaining drugs; excessive physical, environmental, or emotional stress; pregnancy; febrile states; or surgery may precipitate or aggravate heart failure.

4. Pain that increases arterial blood pressure or fluid overload postoperatively may cause heart failure in a patient with borderline myocardial function.

III. PATHOPHYSIOLOGY

A. Determinants of Cardiac Output
Four major factors determine the adequacy of cardiac output: preload or venous return, afterload, contractility, and heart rate. These factors interact to maintain normal pump activity. Derangement of any one of them leads to a decrease in cardiac output and the manifestation of heart failure.

B. Adaptive Physiological Mechanisms
The heart utilizes adaptive mechanisms to maintain a normal output. Compensation may be central (i.e., mechanisms inherent to the heart—the Frank–Starling reflex, myocardial hypertrophy, and increased heart rate)—or

peripheral (e.g., activation of neurohumoral mechanisms, redistribution of blood flow, salt and water retention).

1. Central compensatory mechanisms
   a. Frank–Starling reflex
      The Frank–Starling mechanism acts immediately after acute heart failure. Left ventricular stroke volume increases following an elevation of left ventricular end-diastolic pressure (preload). The ejection fraction improves secondary to an increasing length of the ventricular muscle fibers. However, this mechanism applies only when preload is within normal range (see Appendix B). Once the left ventricular filling pressure exceeds 18 to 22 mmHg, the left ventricular function curve levels off, and an increase in left ventricular end-diastolic volume increases the left ventricular filling pressure without producing an appreciable change in cardiac output.
   b. Cardiac hypertrophy
      Hypertrophy is a compensatory response of the heart to chronic stress. The pattern differs with the time course and the type of stress imposed on the ventricle. With *pressure* overload, the increase in wall stress during systole results in concentric hypertrophy. The ventricular wall increases in thickness secondary to replication of sarcomeres in parallel, whereas the chamber either remains the same size or shrinks. Isolated aortic valvular stenosis causes this pattern. *Volume* overload increases wall stress during diastole, leading to replication of sarcomeres in series. This causes eccentric hypertrophy, whereby the thickness of the left ventricular wall and the internal diameter of the ventricle increase proportionately. Mitral regurgitation exemplifies this pattern. Both forms of hypertrophy maintain myocardial contractility despite the external stress. Heart failure results when hypertrophy can no longer compensate for the stress.
   c. Increased heart rate and contractility
      The autonomic nervous system modulates the heart rate. Normally, tachycardia is accom-

panied by an increase in the inotropic state (rate-treppe phenomenon or the Bowditch effect). In heart failure, stroke volume is relatively fixed, and cardiac output increases in proportion to the increase in the heart rate. As the failure worsens, however, further increases in the heart rate cannot match the need for cardiac output.

2.   Peripheral compensatory mechanisms
Central compensating mechanisms eventually fail because of progressive intrinsic myocardial changes. In order to maintain a normal output, several neurohumoral mechanisms are then activated (Fig. 1-1).

   a.   The afferent signals initiating these mechanisms include various neural receptors sensitive to local stretch and transmural thoracic receptors, particularly in the atria, ventricles, and pulmonary capillaries. Additionally, peripheral receptors such as the carotid sinus

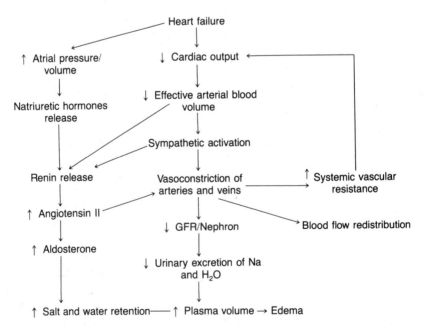

Figure 1-1 Pathophysiological changes and neurohumoral compensations in congestive heart failure.

baroreceptor and those in the juxtaglomerular apparatus monitor the relation between arterial pressure and vascular capacity. Other sensing sites are found in the central nervous system and the liver.

b. Once activated, neurohumoral mechanisms operate to maintain arterial pressure by vasoconstriction and expansion of extracellular volume. Alteration in intracardiac filling pressure and redistribution of regional blood flow also occur. These neurohumoral compensatory mechanisms include:

1) Autonomic nervous system activation

Activation of the nervous system increases the plasma norepinephrine concentration (to more than three times the normal amount), as well as the epinephrine and dopamine levels. These changes occur both at rest and during exercise and are secondary to increased release from adrenergic nerve endings and cardiac stores. Cardiac norepinephrine depletion is observed, which reduces inotropic capability. The elevated plasma norepinephrine concentration correlates directly with the degree of left ventricular dysfunction and the cardiac mortality rate.

Several vascular presynaptic and postsynaptic receptors modulate norepinephrine release (Fig. 1-2). Presynaptic beta-2 and angiotensin II receptors stimulate the release of norepinephrine, whereas stimulation of presynaptic alpha-2, dopaminergic (DA_2), prostaglandin E (PGE), opiate, and muscarinic receptors inhibit its release. Six putative postsynaptic vascular receptors have been identified. Postsynaptic alpha-1 receptors respond by vasoconstriction to neuronally released norepinephrine. The postsynaptic alpha-2 receptors are responsive to epinephrine and norepinephrine released directly into the

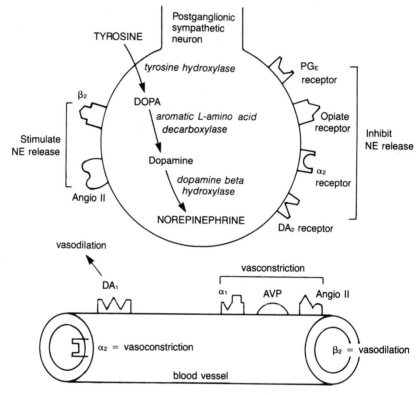

Figure 1-2 Synthesis of norepinephrine (NE) and its interaction with the sympathetic presynaptic and postsynaptic receptors.

systemic circulation, whereas neuronally released catecholamines cause vasoconstriction. Beta adrenoreceptors are likewise more sensitive to circulatory than to neuronally released catecholamine and modulate vasodilation rather than vasoconstriction. Postsynaptic dopaminergic (DA_1) receptors in the renal, mesenteric, coronary, and cerebral circulations modulate vasodilation. Smooth-muscle arteriolar vasculature also contains postsynaptic angiotensin II and arginine vasopressin (AVP) receptors, which interact with those substances to promote vasoconstriction and salt and water retention. With chronic stimulation, lymphocytic and ventricular beta receptors, as well as platelet alpha-2 adrenoreceptors, are downregulated. Downregulation indicates both a decrease in the number of adrenergic receptors and a decrease in their sensitivity to adrenergic stimulation. Reduction in platelet alpha-2 receptors reflects a diminished presynaptic neuron inhibition of norepinephrine release. This contributes to catecholamine elevation in heart failure and stimulates inotropism, increases the heart rate, redistributes blood flow from nonvital beds, and maintains arterial pressure despite the limited cardiac output. However, sympathetic overcompensation may become deleterious in the later stage of heart failure.

Complications include increased afterload and dysrhythmias. A vicious cycle develops. Sympathetic overdrive (as well as activation of other neurohumoral mechanisms) persists and causes increased preload and afterload, which intensifies heart failure.

Heart failure also impairs the parasympathetic system. Parasympathetic restraint on the inherent pacemaker's automaticity markedly decreases. At any arterial pressure, patients exhibit less slowing of the heart rate. Additionally, the impairment of baroreflex control blunts the response of the heart rate, arterial pressure, and vascular resistance to upright tilt, with accompanying hypotension.

2) Stimulation of the renin–angiotensin–aldosterone system
Reduction in cardiac output in a patient with heart failure results in renal hypoperfusion. This stimulates the juxtaglomerular apparatus to secrete renin, which converts angiotensinogen to angiotensin I. An enzyme produced predom-

inantly by the lungs acts on angiotensin I, converting it to angiotensin II. Angiotensin II constricts peripheral arterioles, elevates vascular resistance, and decreases the glomerular filtration rate. Other renal effects include increased tubular sodium reabsorption and redistribution of renal blood flow. Angiotensin II also stimulates norepinephrine release, blocks its neuronal uptake, and enhances its biosynthesis in the nerve terminal. Angiotensin II will stimulate the release of epinephrine from the adrenal medulla, of AVP from the pituitary, and of aldosterone from the adrenal cortex.

3) Arginine vasopressin release
Another neurohumoral compensation important in heart failure is the twofold increase in circulating AVP. A low arterial pressure and reduced atrial stretch receptor sensitivity stimulate its release. AVP is a potent vasoconstrictor and facilitates water reabsorption from the collecting ducts. It may account for the dilutional hypo-osmolality secondary to the inability of patients in heart failure to excrete a water load.

4) Release of atrial natriuretic factor
Plasma volume expansion and elevation of the left atrial pressure or volume induce the release of atrial natriuretic hormone (ANH) from atrial myocyte granules. This hormone causes water and sodium loss. The kidneys exhibit refractoriness to the effects of ANH in heart failure that may reflect a downregulation of receptors. The hormone's inhibition of sympathetic and renin activity causes vasodilation. In severe heart failure, these effects are far outweighed by sodium retention and vasoconstriction attributable to various neurohumoral compensating forces.

IV. CLINICAL FEATURES

   A. The cardinal manifestation of left ventricular failure is progressive respiratory distress. Accumulation of fluid within the lungs increases their rigidity and decreases compliance. The work of breathing therefore increases, leading to dyspnea. This symptom can progress to dyspnea on mild exertion, paroxysmal nocturnal dyspnea, orthopnea, dyspnea at rest, and, finally, pulmonary edema. The patient may wheeze and cough. Involvement of the right ventricle worsens the symptoms.

   B. As the glomerular filtration rate decreases, so does urinary output. The accumulation of salt and water causes peripheral edema and increases weight and body girth secondary to ascites.

   C. Cerebral symptoms such as confusion, memory impairment, anxiety, headache, insomnia, delirium, and even hallucinations are observed.

   D. The patient often complains of anorexia, nausea, vomiting, abdominal distention and pain, and constipation, all of which are caused by venous engorgement and congestion in the gastrointestinal tract.

   E. Inadequate blood flow to the muscles results in weakness and rapid fatigue.

V. PREOPERATIVE ASSESSMENT

   A. Physical Examination

      1. The patient in acute failure may be pale, diaphoretic, and, in some instances, cyanotic.

      2. Breathing is usually shallow and rapid, particularly during physical exertion or when lying supine. Pleural effusions may muffle or obliterate breath sounds. Bilateral moist rales on inspiration are usually present, initially at the most dependent region of the lungs. As the failure worsens, rales may be heard in nonbasilar areas. Copious secretions and rhonchi, with or without wheezing, may be noted.

      3. Cardiac examination may show abnormal pulsations and displacement of the apical impulse, which indicates cardiomegaly. Neck vein distention indicates elevated central venous pressure. Valvular lesions may cause palpable thrills. On ausculation, the first heart sound usually is soft except in mitral stenosis or hypertensive cardiovascular disease. A gallop (third heart sound), the cardiac hallmark of ventricular failure, is best heard when the patient assumes a left recumbent position and often is accompanied by pulsus alternans. Heart murmurs may or may not be present, depending on the underlying lesion. Abdominal distention secondary to ascites and congestive hepatosplenomegaly may be found. Peripheral pitting edema tends to accumulate at the most dependent portion of the body.

B. Diagnostic Tests

1. The chest roentgenogram helps in screening for heart failure. The size and shape of the cardiac silhouette provides certain information regarding the underlying disease. The earliest radiographic sign of left ventricular failure is pulmonary vascular distention. Progressive interstitial fluid accumulation results in pulmonary edema, and a large homogenous butterfly-shaped density may be seen. However, these features may lag as much as 12 hours behind acute elevation of the ventricular filling pressure. Also, the pattern of pulmonary congestion may persist as long as 4 days after normalization of the filling pressure.

2. The 12-lead ECG may show nonspecific changes but is usually abnormal as a consequence of the underlying cardiac disease.

3. Doppler and two-dimensional echocardiography may establish the primary cardiac etiology and determine the severity of myocardial dysfunction. Serial studies can monitor left ventricular function during therapy or reveal a change in clinical course.

4. Other special studies include radionuclide ventriculography and treadmill exercise testing. Pulmonary artery catheterization may help in assessing the degree of functional impairment and determining the underlying cause of the cardiovascular dysfunction.

C. Operative Risk

1. Operating on NYHA Class III and IV patients carries an extremely high risk. The presence of a third heart sound or elevated jugular venous pressure implies the same weighted risk of postoperative cardiac complications as in a patient within 6 months of MI.

2. Patients with NYHA Class I and II heart failure have

only a slight risk of developing postoperative pulmonary edema.

3. More than 50% of patients who suffer postoperative pulmonary edema secondary to acute left ventricular decompensation have had no previous symptoms of heart failure.

4. Patients in heart failure should have elective surgery postponed pending adequate control and stabilization.

5. Emergency surgery necessitates the transfer of the patient to a major medical center, where careful invasive monitoring should be done to optimize preload, afterload, and left and right ventricular stroke work.

VI. PERIOPERATIVE MANAGEMENT

The basic principles of heart failure management are listed in Table 1-2. Pharmacotherapy remains the cornerstone. The goals are to optimize cardiac output, improve the quality of life, and prolong survival. The heart's pumping performance

---

Table 1–2. Basic Principles in the Treatment of Congestive Heart Failure

Reduction of Cardiac Workload

Decreased physical activity and emotional stress
Weight control
Vasodilator therapy
Assisted circulation

Improvement of Myocardial Pump Function

Digitalis
Sympathomimetics
Inotropic agents other than glycosides and catecholamines
Pacemakers

Control of Excessive Salt and Water Retention

Dietary restriction
Diuretics
Mechanical removal of fluids
    Thoracentesis
    Paracentesis
    Phlebotomy
    Dialysis/continuous arteriovenous hemofiltration

Heart Transplantation

may improve with the use of inotropic agents or drugs that
reduce preload or afterload. Pacemakers may correct any
atrial or ventricular asynchrony. In severe cases, mechanical
circulatory support may be required. Salt and water restriction and diuretic therapy prevent excessive fluid accumulation. Sometimes, mechanical removal of fluids by phlebotomy,
dialysis, or thoracentesis alleviates symptoms. End-stage disease may necessitate heart transplantation if the patient has
severe heart failure with a life expectancy of less than 1 year.
Patients less than 55 years old who are psychologically stable
and compliant with medical therapy should be considered for
this procedure.

A. Pharmacotherapy

    1. Inotropic agents

        Inotropic drugs are used on the premise that suffi-
cient reserve cardiac contractility remains and can
be stimulated in order to increase cardiac output.
Inotropic drugs increase intracellular calcium
availability to cardiac contractile elements. They
improve exercise performance within hours to days,
but their use can increase myocardial oxygen consumption and induce tachycardia or other dysrhythmias. Table 1-3 lists the available inotropic
drugs, their recommended dosages, and the significant side effects.

        a. Digitalis

            Digitalis, the drug most commonly used for
long-term management of heart failure, exerts
its positive inotropic effect by inhibition of the
Na^+, K^+-ATPase enzyme system. The resultant
increase in intracellular Na^+ fosters an exchange of extracellular calcium for intracellular sodium, which makes more calcium available for myocardial activation. Digitalis also
slows the heart rate by vagal stimulation and
decreases AV node conduction. Unfortunately,
digitalis has a low toxic-to-therapeutic ratio,
and toxicity occurs in 15% to 20% of patients.
Hypoxia, renal failure, and electrolyte abnormalities such as hypokalemia and hypomagnesemia predispose to digitalis toxicity.

            Digitalis is best continued until the time
of surgery, especially if the patient has atrial
fibrillation with a ventricular rate more than

Table 1–3. Positive Inotropic Agents

Drug	Dose	Comments
Digitalis Glycosides		
Digoxin	Total digitalizing 1.25–1.5 mg PO *or* 1.0–1.5 mg IV Daily maintenance 0.125–0.5 mg PO	Narrow toxic-to-therapeutic ratio; dysrhythmias, nausea, vomiting, anorexia, headache, insomnia, disorientation
Cathecholamines and Sympathomimetic Agents		
Epinephrine	0.1–1.0 µg/kg per min IV	Increases myocardial O_2 consumption; may cause hypertension and dysrhythmias
Norepinephrine	0.05–0.5 µg/kg per min IV	Can cause significant vasoconstriction
Dopamine	2–20 µg/kg per min IV	Significant vasoconstriction and tachycardia at high doses
Dobutamine	5–15 µg/kg per min IV	No renal vasodilation or significant increase in heart rate or blood pressure
Nonglycoside, Noncatecholamine Agents		
Amrinone	0.75 mg/kg loading dose; then 5–10 µg/kg per min	Causes thrombocytopenia, hepatic and gastrointestinal disturbance, fever, and dysrhythmias

80 per minute. In the absence of heart failure, preoperative digitalization is not recommended for counteracting the cardiac depression caused by anesthetic agents.

    b.   Dopamine and dobutamine
Patients with severe heart failure may require parenteral inotropic agents for stabilization before or during surgery. Dopamine and dobutamine are the two most commonly employed drugs. Dopamine, a norepinephrine precursor, has both alpha- and beta-agonist properties; it not only increases contractility but also stimulates specific dopaminergic receptors in the renal, mesenteric, coronary, and

intracerebral arterial beds, resulting in vasodilation. At higher doses (>10 μg/kg per min), the alpha-adrenergic effects predominate, causing vasoconstriction and elevation of arterial pressure and peripheral resistance. Dobutamine, on the other hand, has a predominant cardiac beta-1-receptor agonist effect but does have some beta-2 effect, especially at high doses (>10 μg/kg per min). At infusion rates below 10 μg/kg per minute, cardiac performance usually improves without undue raising of the heart rate. At higher doses, hypotension and dysrhythmias may occur with increased beta-2 activity. Unlike dopamine, dobutamine does not have specific dopaminergic receptor activity. The combination of either drug with a vasodilator such as nitroprusside that has afterload-releasing effects produces a greater increase in cardiac output. The inotropic effects of dopamine and dobutamine complement each other, and the drugs can be used concurrently.

c. Amrinone
Amrinone and its derivative milrinone (not approved for use in the US) belong to a new class of nonglycoside, noncatecholamine inotropic drugs that exert their effects by selective inhibition of phosphodiesterase FIII, leading to an increase in cAMP and intracellular calcium. In addition, these drugs have vasodilator properties and produce hemodynamic changes similar to those of dobutamine. Oral amrinone often caused gastrointestinal side effects and is no longer available in the US, but the intravenous form may play a role in the treatment of patients with moderate to severe failure. Milrinone appears to be 10 to 40 times more potent and better tolerated, having lesser side effects than amrinone.

2. Diuretics
Diuretics relieve the symptoms of systemic and pulmonary congestion caused by excessive salt and water retention. They also decrease vascular wall stiffness and vasoconstriction by reducing the sodium

content of the walls, thereby indirectly decreasing afterload. The endpoint of diuresis is a left ventricular filling pressure that maximizes cardiac output without causing orthostatic hypotension. Continuing diuresis below the optimal filling pressure could lead to decreased cardiac output. Several types of diuretics may be used alone or in combination.

   a.   Thiazides

Thiazides act primarily by inhibiting sodium and chloride reabsorption in the distal convoluted tubules. When used in combination with the longer-acting derivative metolazone or with a loop diuretic, they produce greater diuresis.

   b.   Potassium-sparing agents

Potassium-sparing drugs such as spironolactone, triamterene, and amiloride are relatively weak and are usually added to another diuretic for their potassium-sparing effect. Spironolactone antagonizes the effects of aldosterone, and triamterene and amiloride inhibit the electrogenic entry of sodium.

   c.   Loop diuretics

The loop diuretics (furosemide, bumetanide, and ethacrynic acid) are the most potent diuretics and act by inhibiting chloride transport in the ascending limb of Henle's loop. They act rapidly but relatively briefly. Their greatest utility is in the treatment of acute pulmonary edema or severe congestive heart failure.

3.   Vasodilators

The increased preload and afterload in heart failure impedes left ventricular ejection and contributes to low cardiac output. Vasodilators do not improve cardiac performance by direct cardiac stimulation. Rather, they reduce impedance to left ventricular ejection (afterload), increase venous capacitance (preload), or both. The effects of the various vasodilating drugs on the Frank–Starling mechanism are shown in Figure 1-3.

   a.   Vasodilators may be classified according to their site of action. Some (e.g., nitroglycerin and nitrates) act predominantly by dilating systemic veins. Others exert their effect by ar-

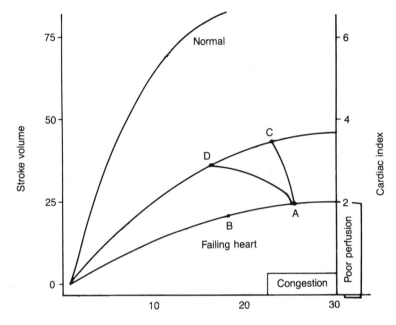

Figure 1-3 Effect of vasodilator therapy on Frank-Starling mechanism in a failing heart. A to B shows the effect of venodilators, which lower preload with minimal change in cardiac output. A to C indicates the effect of arterial vasodilators, where an improvement in stroke volume is observed without a significant change in preload. A to D demonstrates the effect of a balanced dilator, where both a decrease in preload and an increase in stroke volume are observed.

teriolar dilation. Hydralazine, the calcium channel blockers, and minoxidil belong to this category. A third group exerts a more balanced effect on both arteries and veins and includes nitroprusside, prazosin, and, presumably, the angiotensin-coverting enzyme (ACE) inhibitors. Table 1-4 lists the various vasodilators and their recommended dosages.

b. During the perioperative period, the two most commonly used vasodilators are nitroglycerin and sodium nitroprusside.

1) Nitroglycerin significantly reduces systemic and pulmonary venous pressures, reduces congestion, and alleviates myocardial ischemia. Nitroglycerin is effec-

Table 1–4. Effects and Dosages of Various Vasodilator Drugs

Drug	Venous Dilating Effect	Arteriolar Dilating Effect	Dosage
Nitroglycerin	Marked	Mild	0.5–6.0 µg/kg per min IV 5–50 mg transdermal
Isosorbide Dinitrate	Marked	Mild	5–20 mg/2 hours sublingual 10–60 mg/4 hours PO
Nitroprusside	Marked	Marked	0.5–8 µg/kg per min IV
Hydralazine	–	Marked	50–100 mg/6 hours PO
Captopril	Moderate	Moderate	6.25–25 mg/6–8 hours PO
Enalapril	Moderate	Moderate	2.5–5.0 mg/24 hours
Prazosin	Marked	Moderate	2.5 mg/6 hours PO
Trimazosin	Marked	Moderate	50–300 mg BID PO
Nifedipine	Mild	Moderate	10–40 mg/6 hours PO or sublingual

tive in severe heart failure in reducing preload but has modest clinical effects compared with other vasodilators. It thus serves as an adjunct to other vasodilators and inotropic agents.

2) Sodium nitroprusside has a balanced effect on circulation: it secondarily increases cardiac output as it decreases systemic and pulmonary venous pressures. Nitroprusside relaxes arterial and venous smooth muscles to approximately equal degrees. Its popularity results from its rapid onset of action, short half-life, and linear dose–response relation. In combination with dopamine or dobutamine, nitroprusside produces a greater increase in cardiac output. Acute toxicity develops because of accumulation of the metabolic byproducts thiocyanate and cyanide. Because the drug is available only in intravenous form, alternative vasodilator therapy should be initiated once tapering of nitroprusside begins.

VII. SUMMARY OF ANESTHETIC CONSIDERATIONS

The patient with stable, well-compensated congestive heart failure does not require an extensive cardiac workup prior to surgery. The patient who presents with shortness of breath on minimal exertion or lying supine and with S3, distended neck veins, peripheral edema, and moist rales has moderate to severe heart failure, and in these cases, additional tests such as echocardiography or radionuclide ventriculography should be performed. If severe failure is documented and medical therapy does not normalize myocardial function, intraoperative monitoring with intra-arterial cannulation and pulmonary artery catheterization is necessary.

Prior to surgery, patients with congestive heart failure should have their pharmacotherapy optimized. Digoxin and afterload-reducing agents such as ACE inhibitors and hydralazine should be given. Diuretics may be omitted the day of surgery without adverse effects.

Management of perioperative changes in cardiovascular condition should be guided by information from the pulmonary artery catheter. Acute changes are best treated with short-acting intravenous agents.

Coronary Artery Disease

I. INCIDENCE, OUTCOME, AND ETIOLOGY

    A. Coronary artery disease affects 2.5% of Americans, 42% of whom are as a result limited in their activity. The disease causes about 800,000 new MIs each year and 450,000 recurring ones. The extent of coronary artery disease and the degree of left ventricular dysfunction determine the prognosis. Patients with normal myocardial function and significant single-vessel disease have a mortality rate of 2% per year, compared with 8% and 11% per year, respectively, in patients with two- and three-vessel disease. If the left main coronary artery is involved, the mortality rate averages 15%. The mortality rate increases if the patient has concomitant left ventricular dysfunction. Coronary patients who undergo anesthesia for noncardiac surgery are at greater risk of complications and death: they have a twofold to threefold increase in the perioperative mortality rate and a tenfold increase in coronary occlusion.

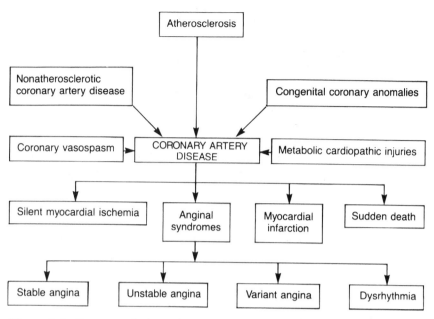

Figure 1-4 Causes and clinical spectrum of coronary artery disease.

Coronary artery disease may be asymptomatic. Almost one in five MIs remains undetected, and as many as half of postoperative reinfarctions are silent or have atypical manifestations. The symptomatic phase most commonly presents as anginal syndromes, MI, or sudden death, the last presumably caused by ventricular dysrhythmia (Fig. 1-4). Less commonly, it shows itself as dysrhythmias of sufficient severity to cause symptoms, even in the absence of angina or infarction. Once the patient is symptomatic, the clinical course is variable. The patient may remain symptomatic with either a stable or a progressive course, become asymptomatic, or die suddenly.

B. More than 90% of coronary artery disease results from atherosclerosis, which is precipitated by mechanical, immunologic, toxic, infectious, or metabolic injury of the endothelial wall. Formation of the atherosclerotic lesion involves the interplay of three biologic processes: proliferation of internal smooth-muscle cells and macrophages, formation of connective tissue matrix, and accumulation of lipid within the walls and in the surrounding connective tissues. Less common causes of coronary artery disease include vasospasm, nonatherosclerotic arteriopathy, congenital anomalies, and various metabolic cardiopathic injuries.

C.   Certain conditions increase the susceptibility of an individual to the development of coronary artery disease. These factors interact, stimulating the progression of atherosclerosis, and their alteration may prevent or retard the formation of atherosclerotic plaque or reduce its size, thus improving outcome. The primary risk factors for coronary artery disease are hypercholesterolemia, hypertension, and cigarette smoking. Less important factors include a low level of high-density lipoprotein cholesterol, obesity, type A personality, little physical activity, and a high serum triglyceride level. Advancing age and male gender are important but unmodifiable risk factors.

II. PATHOPHYSIOLOGY

A.   The basic defect in coronary artery disease is an imbalance between the myocardial oxygen supply and the demand (Fig. 1-5). Under basal conditions, the energy requirement of the heart accounts for less than 5% of oxygen demand. However, the oxygen requirement rises with increases in heart rate, contractility, and intramyocardial wall tension. The sympathetic nervous system modulates these factors. Because the heart extracts a high and relatively fixed percentage of oxygen from the coronary arterial blood for basal metabolism, an increase in oxygen need is met by increases in coronary blood flow. Additionally, oxygen delivery depends on the oxygen content of arterial blood, which, in turn, is determined primarily by the amount of hemoglobin and the oxygen saturation.

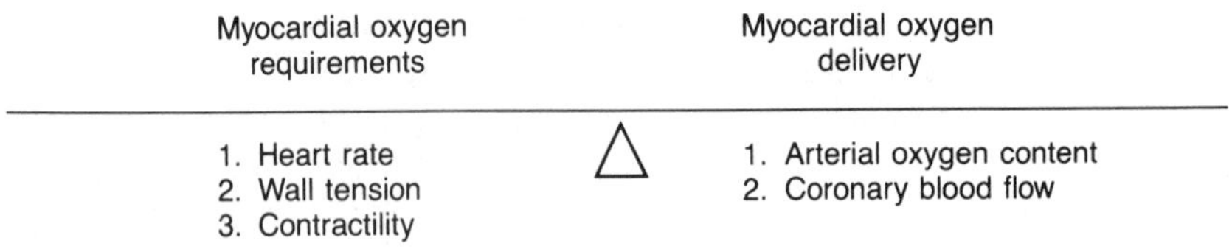

Myocardial oxygen requirements		Myocardial oxygen delivery
1. Heart rate 2. Wall tension 3. Contractility	△	1. Arterial oxygen content 2. Coronary blood flow

Figure 1-5   The myocardial oxygen balance and its determinants.

B. As in other vascular beds, coronary blood flow relates directly to the perfusion pressure and inversely to vascular resistance. Because of the increased myocardial pressure in systole, blood flow to the left ventricle and subendocardium occurs primarily during diastole. The coronary circulation has an immense dilatory reserve. Autoregulation of blood flow occurs by changes in coronary vascular resistance secondary to changes in local metabolic requirements. Patients with normal coronary arteries readily match an increased oxygen demand by vasodilation, thereby increasing coronary blood flow and oxygen supply.

C. Patients with coronary artery disease have a deranged autoregulation, so that a deficit in the oxygen supply may develop. Obstruction to coronary blood flow, either by a fixed stenotic lesion or by vasospasm, causes dilation of the vessel distal to the block. As the obstruction worsens, the dilatory reserve also diminishes to the point that the coronary vessel is maximally dilated. When the stenosis becomes critical and the maximum dilatory reserve is reached, the patient cannot augment coronary flow appropriately in response to stress. Once this happens, myocardial ischemia develops.

D. Various biochemical, electrical, and mechanical abnormalities occur secondary to myocardial ischemia. Accumulation of lactate indicates impaired oxygenation and a shift to an anaerobic pattern of metabolism. T-wave inversion and ST-segment displacement indicate alteration in cardiac electrophysiology. Electrical instability is another important consequence. Ventricular tachycardia and fibrillation can develop.

E. The contractility of the ischemic myocardium may be markedly impaired. Transient ischemia, as in angina, can cause reversible depression of myocardial pump function, whereas prolonged ischemia results in necrosis and irreversible myocardial damage. Because ischemia may be focal or regional, an asymmetric distribution of myocardial hypokinesia and akinesia occurs. This causes asynchrony of ventricular contraction and reduces the efficiency of myocardial performance. Heart failure develops late in the disease process. Ischemia of the papillary muscle and mitral valve leaflets may lead to mitral regurgitation. Figure 1-6 shows the pathophysiologic consequences of myocardial ischemia.

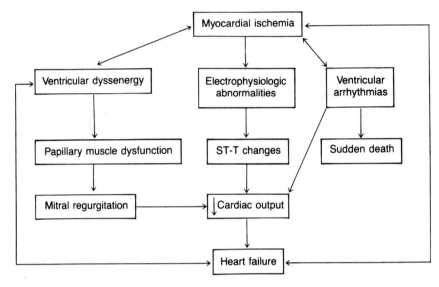

Figure 1-6   Pathophysiological consequences of myocardial ischemia.

III.   ANGINAL SYNDROMES

A.   Angina Pectoris

Surgical stress stimulates the sympathetic nervous system and increases adrenergic activity and myocardial oxygen consumption. The presence of angina pectoris modifies the management of the surgical patient and necessitates additional preoperative evaluation and preparation. Five components of preoperative cardiac evaluation are essential before the anesthesiologist can proceed: history, physical examination, current treatment, ECG, chest radiograph, and simple laboratory tests (hematocrit, K^+, BUN, creatine, glucose). This initial evaluation identifies patients in whom angina pectoris is likely to represent a manifestation of coronary artery disease. Further investigation, such as radionuclide studies and cardiac catheterization, depends on the initial findings (Table 1-5).

1.   History

    a.   Angina pectoris is a symptom complex that reflects transient inadequacy of myocardial blood flow. It is the most common manifestation of coronary artery disease, commonly affecting more men than women. Ischemia oc-

Table 1–5. Diagnostic Evaluation of Patients with Coronary Artery Disease

Medical history
Physical examination
Chest radiograph and fluoroscopy
Resting ECG
Treadmill test (exercise ECG)
   ECG changes
   Functional capacity (endurance time)
   Blood pressure and heart rate response
   Symptomatic response
Radionuclide imaging (rest and exercise)
   Myocardial perfusion
   Ventricular function
Cardiac catheterization and coronary angiography
   Coronary anatomy
      Presence, location, and extent of stenosis
      Presence and extent of collateral circulation
   Ejection fraction
   Wall motion

curs because of an increased myocardial oxygen demand in the presence of fixed coronary obstruction, an increase in coronary vascular tone, or both.

b. Typically, a middle-aged or elderly patient complains of chest pain described as "heavy," "squeezing," "constricting," "suffocating," or "crushing." It may radiate to the shoulder, jaw, or arms. In some, the sensation is a vague, nonlocalized, mild pressure-like discomfort or an uncomfortable numb sensation (Levine sign). The most important diagnostic feature of angina pectoris is its relation to provocative factors, the most common being physical exertion. Other precipitating factors include emotion and excitement, eating, exposure to cold, and sexual activity. The pain usually begins gradually and lasts only a few minutes. Characteristically, it stops when the provocative factors are stopped or after sublingual administration of nitrates. The frequency of anginal attacks varies from individual to individual.

They occur daily in some, once a week in others. Sometimes, symptoms wax or wane. A change in the character, quality, frequency, duration, or severity of the pain implies a more severe ischemic episode or vasospasm or possibly heralds an acute MI.

c. Inability to climb two flights of stairs and dyspnea during anginal attacks suggest left ventricular dysfunction secondary to ischemia. The added stress of anesthesia, fluid replacement, and surgery may push such a patient into frank heart failure, another important risk factor in perioperative morbidity and death. The presence of another disease (e.g., valvular heart disease or chronic obstructive lung disease [COLD]) further increases the risk of surgery. Commonly, patients with coronary artery disease have concomitant peripheral or cerebral vascular disease.

d. Ninety percent of patients complaining of classic anginal pain have hemodynamically significant coronary stenosis diagnosed by arteriography. Fifty percent of patients with atypical angina-like pain have significant coronary stenosis. Sixteen percent of patients judged to have nonanginal pain actually have significant coronary disease.

2. Physical examination

a. Angina pectoris demonstrates no pathognomonic sign on physical examination. Cardiac examination provides information with regard to chamber size, seen as a displacement of the apical impulse. Transient auscultatory evidence of left ventricular dysfunction may be heard. These findings include the presence of third and fourth heart sounds and, rarely, paradoxical splitting of the second sound. A systolic murmur of mitral regurgitation indicates papillary muscle dysfunction. The physical examination may pinpoint a systemic disease, an abnormal metabolic state, or risk factors that can be treated preoperatively.

b. It is important to identify preoperatively the heart rate and systolic pressure at which angina develops, as attacks often occur at a predictable heart rate and blood pressure. Specifically, anginal pains occur at a constant rate–pressure product (heart rate times systolic blood pressure). Preventing the rate–pressure product from exceeding the product that is associated with angina may decrease the incidence of intraoperative ischemia.

3. Diagnostic tests
   a. Resting ECG
      Between angina attacks, the ECG may not show any abnormality. However, ST-T changes may develop during a pain episode. The ECG may demonstrate two types of ischemic patterns: ST-segment depression greater than 1 mm, which denotes subendocardial ischemia, and ST-segment elevation, which is characteristic of transmural ventricular wall ischemia. ST-segment elevation suggests significant coronary artery occlusion that is a prelude to transmural MI. The ECG may help localize the ischemic area. Ischemic changes in leads II, III, and aVF suggest right coronary artery involvement. This includes the posteroinferior portion of the left ventricle and the right ventricle and atrium. Involvement of the left anterior descending coronary artery will cause changes in leads V_1–V_4. This suggests anterior septal ischemia. ST-T changes in leads I, aVL, V_5, and V_6 involve the circumflex artery, which includes the lateral aspects of the left ventricle. Additionally, nonspecific abnormalities such as left ventricular hypertrophy, bundle branch blocks, AV conduction disorders, and previous MI must be considered evidence of myocardial or coronary artery disease.
   b. Chest radiography and fluoroscopy
      Generally, no specific finding of coronary artery disease is observable on the chest radiograph. The film may demonstrate cardiac enlargement or pulmonary edema suggestive of the congestive heart failure often associated with long-standing myocardial ischemia.

c. Exercise electrocardiography
When the medical history strongly suggests
coronary artery disease or the presence of predisposing factors, but the resting ECG does not
show ischemia, exercise testing may confirm
the diagnosis. A positive test has ST-segment
depression greater than 1 mm. However, 10%
of the adult population may have a false-posi-
tive test. Therefore, exercise testing should be
combined with other diagnostic modalities.
Paients who can achieve a moderate workload
or an adequate heart rate response (160 beats
per minute or greater than 85% of the predicted maximal rate) without ischemic ECG
changes are excellent candidates for major surgery. Those who develop ischemic changes
within 3 minutes of exercise, have prolonged
(>8 min) ST-segment depression, or develop
exercise-induced hypotension are likely to have
a more severe form of coronary artery disease.
To localize the area of ischemia, thallium
stress testing may be performed. These patients belong to the high-risk category and
must be well evaluated and treated prior to
surgery.

d. Radionuclide studies
Isotope imaging greatly increases the accuracy
of diagnosing coronary artery disease. When
the interpretation of the exercise ECG is unreliable (as when the resting ECG is abnormal,
such as in Wolff–Parkinson–White syndrome,
left ventricular hypertrophy, use of digitalis, or
ST-segment changes with signs or symptoms),
radionuclide imaging can provide useful information, including insight into ventricular
function and myocardial perfusion. After
thallium injection, an area of hypoperfusion
(cold spot) that presents only during exercise
indicates ischemia. If the patient is incapacitated, a dipyridamole (Persantine)–thallium
stress test can be used to demonstrate areas of
hypoperfusion. A persistent perfusion defect
suggests an old MI. In addition, radionuclide
scanning has been utilized for the assessment,

after coronary surgery, of ventricular function during exercise and at rest.

e. Cardiac catheterizaton and coronary angiography

Cardiac catheterization and coronary angiography remain the gold standard in the diagnosis of coronary artery disease. Generally, they are not performed before noncardiac surgery; however, patients identified as having a poor prognosis, those with disabling symptoms despite intensive medical therapy, or those belonging to the high-risk group according to the exercise ECG should undergo cardiac catheterization and angiography. Data obtained from these studies provide unequivocal evidence of the presence or absence of significant coronary artery stenosis as well as the location and severity of the lesion and the extent of collateral circulation. Imaging of spontaneous or induced vasospasm is possible, and the response to various medications can be assessed. The left ventriculogram provides data for estimating ejection fraction and segmental wall motion. Generally, an ejection fraction above 0.55, cardiac filling pressure below 12 mmHg, a cardiac index above 2.5 L/min per m², and no areas of dyskinesia or akinesia suggest good ventricular function. Additionally, these procedures provide information about the probability of survival and of future coronary events. The findings may thus guide future therapeutic intervention.

4. Medications

Preoperative drug therapy of patients with angina pectoris includes nitrates, beta-blockers, and calcium antagonists. They are continued up to the time of surgery and may be used during the intraoperative period.

a. Nitrates

Since 1867, when amyl nitrite was first tried by Brunton for the treatment of angina, nitrates have become the mainstay of the treatment of coronary artery disease. These drugs cause widespread nonspecific relaxation of smooth muscle, particularly vascular smooth muscle. The most striking responses are in the venous capacitance vessels, where marked dilation results in reduction of venous return and an immediate decrease in left ventricular volume. Large doses of the drug cause arteriolar relaxation, which produces a modest decrease in systemic vascular resistance. The reduction in ventricular volume and peripheral resistance causes wall tension and myocardial oxygen consumption to decrease in a failing or ischemic heart. Furthermore, the coronary arteries dilate, and flow to the collateral circulation increases, thus improving regional blood flow to ischemic areas and the subendocardium. These hemodynamic effects result in an improvement of the oxygen supply-to-demand ratio.

Nitrates are available in oral, sublingual, transdermal, and parenteral forms. They should be continued during the perioperative period, because they have no significant adverse interaction with the drugs used during anesthesia. Intravenous nitroglycerin is not only effective for the relief of angina but also can be used to control high blood pressure and to treat congestive heart failure. In some instances, its combination with a beta-blocker proves valuable in the treatment of angina. This combination allows the nitrates to be taken in higher doses without reflex tachycardia or increased contractility. Nitrates, by decreasing venous return, offset the tendency of beta-blockers to increase left ventricular diastolic volume.

b. Beta-blockers
The various beta-adrenergic blockers have been used with increasing frequency in the treatment of coronary artery disease. They reduce myocardial oxygen requirements by reducing the heart rate, arterial pressure, and myocardial contractility. They also protect the heart against dysrhythmias and improve the survival rate after acute MI. Besides pro-

pranolol, drugs such as metoprolol, labetalol, and esmolol are available for parenteral administration and can be used perioperatively. Major medical centers recommend the maintenance of beta-blockade until immediately before operation, the administration of beta-blockers during premedication, and their further use during surgery when anesthetic drugs fail to control tachycardia. Patients who are abruptly withdrawn from beta-blockers show significant adverse effects, with increased hypertension, angina pectoris, or MI. This rebound phenomenon reflects an increased beta-adrenergic receptor density, which becomes apparent within 24 hours and persists up to 2 weeks after drug withdrawal.

Beta-blockers have undesirable side effects, especially when used injudiciously. The drugs induce increases in end-diastolic volume and decreases in myocardial pump function. Congestive heart failure may be precipitated in patients with impaired left ventricular function. Likewise, AV heart block, significant bradycardia, and bronchospasm have been reported. Occasionally, when beta-blockers are used in patients with high sympathetic tone, hypertension occurs because of unopposed stimulation of alpha-1 receptors. Although beta-blockers have an additional myocardial depressant effect when combined with anesthetic agents, the depression is not considered significant except with methoxyflurane. The various beta-blockers, along with their dosages and peculiar characteristics, are listed in Table 1-6.

c. Calcium antagonists

Calcium channel blockers are a new group of chemically heterogeneous drugs that interfere with the entry of calcium into cells through the slow channel of the sarcolemma and inhibit the release of calcium from various intracellular pools. These drugs reduce the vascular smooth-muscle tone and the contractile state of the myocardium, although each calcium

Table 1–6. Dosage and Effects of Available Beta-Adrenergic Blocking Drugs

Drug	Dose	Comments
Propranolol	60 mg QID PO or 0.25–0.5 mg up to 2–5 mg IV	Prototype drug; nonselective with membrane-stabilizing activity; eliminated through hepatic metabolism
Metoprolol	50–100 mg q 12 hours	Cardioselective; eliminated through hepatic metabolism
Labetalol	100–600 mg BID PO 5–50 mg IV	Nonselective; eliminated through hepatic metabolism; partial agonist activity
Esmolol	Loading: 250–500 μg/kg over 1 min IV Maintenance: 50–300 μg/kg per min IV	Cardioselective; shortest half-life and duration of action; metabolized by RBC esterases; available in parenteral form only
Atenolol	50–100 mg QD PO	Cardioselective; renal excretion
Nadolol	40–80 mg QD PO	Nonselective; renal excretion
Pindolol	5–20 mg TID PO	Nonselective; (+) intrinsic sympathetic and membrane-stabilizing activities; hepatic excretion
Timolol	20 mg BID PO	Noncardioselective; renal and hepatic excretion
Acebutolol	200–600 mg BID PO	Cardioselective; (+) intrinsic sympathetic and membrane-stabilizing activities; hepatic excretion

channel blocker has significantly different actions with respect to coronary vasodilation, venomotor tone, antiarrhythmic properties, systemic vascular resistance, and cardiac inotropy (Table 1-7).

Calcium channel blockers are used in the treatment of coronary artery disease, dysrhythmias, and hypertension. They also protect the heart, brain, and kidneys from ischemic damage. They are effective, either alone or in combination with nitrates and betablockers, in chronic stable angina. Calcium antagonists provide symptomatic relief of angina and improve exercise performance in patients

Table 1–7. *Pharmacologic and Hemodynamic Properties of Available Calcium Antagonists and Their Dosages*

	Nifedipine	Verapamil	Diltiazem
Dosage	10–30 mg/ 6 hours PO or sub- lingual	80–160 mg/ 8 hours PO or 5–10 mg/ 4–6 hours IV	30–90 mg/ 6–8 hours
Onset of Action (min)	30–60 (oral) immediate (sublingual)	30–60 (oral) immediate (IV)	30–60 (oral)
Elimination Half-Life (hours)	1.5–5.0	3–7	2–6
Excretion	80% renal, 20% fecal	70% renal, 15% fecal	40% renal, 60% fecal
Heart Rate	Increase	Decrease	Decrease or no change
Coronary Vasodilation	Mild to mod- erate	Mild to mod- erate	Mild to mod- erate
Peripheral Vasodilation	Marked	Mild to mod- erate	Mild to mod- erate
Myocardial Depression	May or may not occur	Yes	Yes
Decreased AV Conduction	No	Yes	Yes

with stable angina pectoris, variant angina, and unstable angina. Because these drugs alter calcium flux across the cell membrane, negative chronotropic, inotropic, and dromotropic effects and vasodilation occur. Calcium antagonists prevent and relieve vasospasm, dilate epicardial coronary vessels, and dilate systemic and pulmonary arterioles, thereby decreasing blood pressure and afterload with relatively little change in venous return and preload. Nifedipine has minimal antiarrhythmic properties and is less likely to produce AV block than is verapamil. Verapamil has a more negative inotropic effect than does nifedipine, and diltiazem is intermediate between these two drugs in its hemodynamic effects. The use of calcium channel blockers during the perioperative period may introduce adverse interaction with anesthetic drugs, as the negative inotropic effect of calcium antagonists may exaggerate the myocardial depression produced by most anesthetic agents.

The hemodynamic effects of adenosine, an endogenous vasodilator, have been reported recently. During continuous intravenous infusion, adenosine increases myocardial blood flow in normal coronary arteries. It causes bradycardia by direct suppression of the pacemaker activity of the sinoatrial node, thus decreasing myocardial oxygen demand. Adenosine also acts directly on systemic vascular smooth muscle, causing a reduction in peripheral vascular resistance. However, its role in the management of coronary artery disease in the perioperative period needs further study.

If the symptoms of angina persist in spite of intensive medical therapy and treatment of any precipitating factors, elective surgery must be postponed, and the patient must undergo cardiac catheterization. Depending on the angiographic result, coronary artery bypass grafting or angioplasty should be considered. Asymptomatic patients who develop angina shortly before surgery should have their operation delayed for at least 4 hours while treatment for angina is instituted and the ischemic myocardium is allowed to recover.

B. Unstable Angina

Unstable angina is a manifestation of coronary artery disease that falls between angina pectoris and MI. Coronary atherosclerosis remains the principal cause of the underlying myocardial ischemia. In addition, a sudden reduction of coronary blood flow may follow hemorrhage into an atherosclerotic plaque or increased platelet aggregation and plugging of stenotic blood vessels, such as during transient coronary vasospasm. The condition presents with a crescendo pattern of anginal discomfort that often occurs at rest. Nitroglycerin seldom relieves the pain. Unstable angina often precedes MI and sudden death.

A subset of patients believed to have unstable angina develop chest pain at rest with reversible ST-segment elevation during the episode. Such angina appears attributable to coronary vasospasm, usually superimposed on a stenotic major coronary artery. Prinzmetal called this entity "variant angina," and it accounts for approximately 25% of all cases of unstable angina.

1. History and physical examination
   a. Patients often complain of a severe chest pain that is increasing in frequency and duration.
   b. Angina often occurs at rest as well as with minimal exertion.
   c. A new onset of angina of increased severity over the past 1 to 3 months is considered to be unstable angina.
   d. As in angina pectoris, no pathognomonic sign can be elicited.
2. Laboratory investigations
   a. The ECG may show transient ST changes, often associated with T-wave inversion during pain, that usually disappear with relief of pain.
   b. Cardiac enzymes (e.g., CPK-MB) are normal. Patients with variant angina may require Holter monitoring for demonstration of the characteristic ECG changes.
   c. Definitive diagnosis with angiography is necessary for complete evaluation. If angiography does not demonstrate any significant stenosis of the coronary arteries, maneuvers to provoke vasospasm, such as ergonovine infusion, cold pressor test, and exercise, may be used. Ten to fifteen per cent of these patients have significant left main coronary artery disease that necessitates revascularization. Approximately 10% have normal coronary arteries, and presumably, coronary vasospasm plays an important role in this group of patients. The remaining 75% usually have multivessel disease.
3. Treatment
   a. Once significant coronary artery disease is diagnosed, elective surgery should be postponed,

and the patient should be medically stabilized. If necessary, angioplasty or bypass grafting may be performed to relieve angina and protect the myocardium before noncardiac surgery.

 b. The mainstay of medical therapy is nitrates and beta-adrenergic blocking agents. Maintenance of the systolic blood pressure between 100 and 120 mmHg and a heart rate of 50 to 60 per minute can markedly lower the myocardial oxygen requirement.

 c. Calcium antagonists (nifedipine, verapamil, or diltiazem) may help control the pain, especially if coronary vasospasm plays a significant part in its production. Beta-blockers should be added only with extreme caution in variant angina, as beta-2-receptor blockade may allow unopposed alpha-receptor mediated coronary vasoconstriction.

 d. If the angina remains refractory to medical therapy, intraaortic balloon counterpulsation can be very effective. This technique provides a period of relative stability during which cardiac catheterization and angiography, and possibly coronary artery bypass surgery, can be performed.

 e. In some instances, emergency surgery cannot be avoided, even if the patient has unstable angina. In this case, the patient should be transferred to a large center with critical-care facilities. Aggressive medical therapy with intravenous nitroglycerin, beta-blockers, calcium blockers, or all three is begun. Adequate sedation and analgesia must be provided, as well as vigorous treatment of underlying risk factors such as hypertension, infection, heart failure, or dysrhythmias. Pulmonary artery catheterization must be part of the management.

IV. MYOCARDIAL INFARCTION

 A. General Characteristics

  1. Myocardial necrosis resulting from ischemia secondary to total or near-total coronary artery obstruction is the most common cause of hospitalization in the critical care environment. Myocardial infarction affects more than one million Americans each year, and an average male in North America has approximately a 20% chance of suffering either an MI or sudden death before reaching 65 years of age.

2. A mortality rate of 10% to 15% during the initial hospitalization and an additional 10% during the first year after infarction has been reported. Approximately half of the posthospitalization deaths occur suddenly.

3. In the general surgical population, 3000 MIs will occur annually in the 7-day period after an operation. The highest incidence appears to be during the first 3 days (Fig. 1-7). Forty percent of these infarctions occur in patients without a history of MI. Half of all affected patients die within 48 hours.

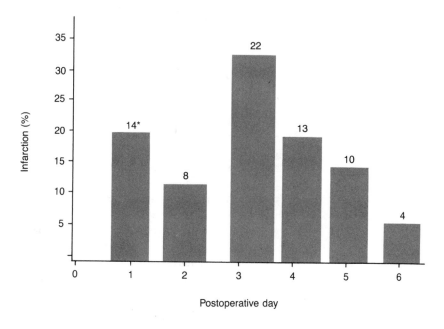

* Number of patients

Figure 1-7 Distribution of myocardial infarction occurrence by time since operation. *(From Tarhan S, Moffit EA, Taylor WF, Giuliani ER. Myocardial infarction after general anesthesia. JAMA 1972; 220:1451.)*

B. Pathogenesis and Pathophysiology

1. Myocardial infarction represents the end point of the imbalance between myocardial oxygen demand and supply, which results from some degree of coronary obstruction secondary to atherosclerosis or vasospasm. Recent studies showed fresh thrombotic plugs in coronary arteries supplying an infarcted area. Postmortem angiography and autopsy revealed thrombosis in 90% of cases.

2. Three percent of patients sustaining MIs have angiographically normal coronary arteries, and coronary spasm may be involved in these cases. The following events trigger vasospasm: exercise, alkalosis, cool pressure testing, mechanical stimulation, and use of drugs such as alpha-adrenergic agonists, calcium chloride, and ergotamine.

3. The mechanisms of vasospasm include neurohumoral, vascular, and platelet-related factors.

   a. Platelets aggregate on damaged or modified coronary endothelium and may initiate the event that leads to MI. Adherent platelets release ADP, which causes further platelet aggregation and initiates the thrombotic process. Also, degranulation of platelets causes the release of coagulation factors and vasoactive substances such as serotonin, ADP, and thromboxane A_2; the latter can induce or aggravate vasospasm.

   b. Damaged endothelium loses its ability to secrete prostacyclin, which is both an inhibitor of platelet aggregation and a vasodilator.

   c. The combination of these events leads to an acute reduction in oxygen delivery; the resultant cellular hypoxia causes a shift to anaerobic metabolism, with production of lactic acid. The myocardial cells lose their contractile properties, and myocardial dysfunction appears.

   d. The ischemic insult can be reversible during the first 20 minutes; however, irreversible cellular damage occurs once this limit is exceeded. After 60 minutes, irreversible damage becomes extensive, with cellular edema and loss of myocardial function. The central area of necrosis is surrounded by a penumbra of ischemic cells, which are potentially salvageable.

    e.   Within the first 4 hours, leukocytes infiltrate the necrotic area, and tissue edema sets in. The edema peaks by the 36th hour and begins to be resorbed at about the 48th hour. On the 11th day, collagen fibers replace necrotic cells, and, by the third week, scarring is well defined. Fibrosis is complete 5 to 6 weeks after infarction.

C. Detection and Diagnosis

    1.   Perioperative MI can be difficult to diagnose, as a high percentage of postoperative reinfarctions (up to 50%) are silent. Various degrees of AV block and cardiac dysrhythmias often accompany an MI. Chest pain occurs in only 25% of patients and may be masked by postoperative pain. Nonspecific signs such as pallor, diaphoresis, dyspnea, and bradycardia should make one suspect the diagnosis.

    2.   Patients with perioperative MI show characteristic serial ECG changes. ST elevation and high-voltage T waves usually appear first. Persistent T-wave elevation (beyond 4 days) suggests a ventricular aneurysm. As the ST-T wave begins to return to the isoelectric point, the T wave becomes symmetrically inverted. The deep Q wave of necrosis, lasting more than 0.04 seconds, may not appear until the second or third day.

    3.   Irreversibly injured myocardial cells release a variety of enzymes into the blood stream. Traditionally, three of these enzymes (AST [SGOT], LDH, and CPK) were measured, but new enzyme assessments are replacing these traditional tests. Elevation of the CPK-MB isoenzyme serves as the primary confirmatory test of MI: the serum concentration begins to increase within 3 hours, peaks at about 12 hours, and returns to near-normal levels between 24 and 36 hours after the MI. It also is helpful to analyze LDH for the cardiac-specific isoenzyme. Its level increases above normal 8 to 12 hours after infarction, peaks at 18 to 36 hours, and gradually returns to normal after 10 to 14 days.

D. Perioperative Risk and Mortality Rate After Noncardiac Surgery

1. Knapp et al. found that the reinfarction and mortality rates were 6% and 59%, respectively, among patients with a history of MI. With no history of infarction, the chance of postoperative infarction averaged 0.7% and the mortality rate 19%.

2. In 1964, Topkins and Artusio showed a postoperative infarction rate of 0.66% and a mortality rate of 26.5% in patients without previous MI. If there had been an infarction preoperatively, the postoperative reinfarction rate was 6.5% and the mortality rate 70%.

3. These authors observed that the type of anesthetic agent, surgical procedure, and duration of surgery appeared to have no significant role in determining the risk of postoperative MI. They concluded that if the infarction had occurred less than 6 months before the current surgery, the reinfarction rate was unacceptably high (54%). If the infarction had occurred 6 to 24 months previously, the reinfarction rate was 20% to 25%, and if the infarction had occurred more than 2 years previously, the reinfarction rate was 5.9%.

4. Tarhan et al. reported a postoperative reinfarction rate of 37% when surgery was performed during the 3-month period after MI, 16% in the 3- to 6-month period, and 6% beyond 6 months. Their overall mortality rate after MI was 50%. In patients with no previous infarction, a 0.13% incidence of infarction 1 week postoperatively was reported.

5. A follow-up study by Steen et al. in 1970 did not show any significant improvement in reinfarction or mortality rates despite new developments in anesthesia and monitoring. They reported an average reinfarction rate of 6%, with a mortality rate of 69%.

6. In 1983, Rao et al. showed a more favorable perioperative reinfarction rate of 1.9% and concluded that preoperative optimization of patient status, aggressive invasive hemodynamic monitoring, and prompt treatment of any hemodynamic aberration had influenced outcome (Table 1-8).

Table 1–8. Relation of Incidence of Reinfarction to Interval from Previous Myocardial Infarction and Overall Mortality Rate

Interval (months)	Incidence of Reinfarction (%)			
	Tarhan (1967–1968)	*Steen (1974–1975)*	*Rao (1973–1976)*	*Rao (1977–1982)*
0–3	37	27	36	5.7
4–6	16	11	26	2.3
7–12	5	6	5	1
13–18	4	3	5	1.56
19–24	5	6	5	1.56
>25	5	4	5	1.7
Mortality rate (%)	54	69	57	36

7. Other observations emerged from these studies.
   a. The reinfarction rate did not differ between men and women.
   b. Preoperative hypertension added significantly to morbidity (reinfarction rates were 9.4% for hypertensive and 4.7% for normotensive patients).
   c. Patients with intraoperative hypotension or hypertension and tachycardia had a higher incidence of reinfarction.
   d. The presence of stable angina pectoris or diabetes mellitus and the location of the previous infarction played no role in the incidence of reinfarction.
   e. The type of anesthetic did not significantly affect postoperative reinfarction or mortality rates.
   f. Intrathoracic and upper abdominal procedures were associated with an increase in the incidence of postoperative infarction.
   g. The duration of surgery was important: procedures less than 3 hours carried reinfarction rates of 5.9% versus 15.9% for procedures longer than 3 hours (Fig. 1-8).

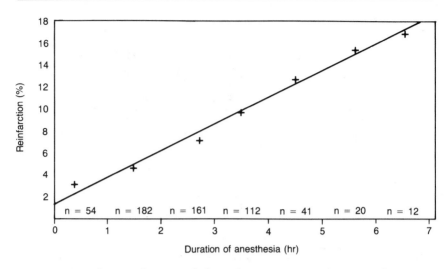

Figure 1-8 Relation of myocardial reinfarction rate to duration of anesthesia. *(From Steen PA, Tinker JH, Tarhan S. Myocardial reinfarction after anesthesia and surgery. JAMA 1978; 239:2566.)*

      h.   Most (85%) of postoperative MIs occurred within the first 3 days.

      i.   Congestive heart failure or dysrhythmia increased the risk of perioperative MI.

  8. On the basis of the above information, many anesthesiologists recommend postponement of elective surgery for at least 6 months after MI. If surgery is required sooner, aggressive invasive monitoring is recommended. Careful monitoring must be maintained for the first several days postoperatively.

E. Management

  1. The therapeutic goals in the management of MI include reduction of the myocardial workload to decrease ischemia, limitation of infarct size, and prevention or elimination of life-threatening dysrhythmias. Critical care facilities allow continuous monitoring and prompt treatment of such dysrhythmias. The in-hospital mortality rate after MI has decreased from 30% to 20%, and most deaths now are attributable to the complications associated with left ventricular failure. The prognosis relates to the quantity of surviving, functional myocardium. Cardiogenic shock develops with infarction of 40% or more of the left ventricule.

2. Certain general measures are utilized in the management of all patients. Sedation, control of pain, bed rest for the initial 48 hours, and low-flow oxygen constitute the initial therapy.

3. Antiarrhythmic prophylaxis with lidocaine decreases the incidence of ventricular fibrillation and is used routinely.

4. Invasive hemodynamic monitoring can be done safely at the bedside in complicated cases. Indications for invasive monitoring include hypotension not responsive to volume repletion, moderate to severe heart failure, recurrent chest pain, clinical evidence of cardiac tamponade, acute ventricular septal defect, or mitral regurgitation.

5. Beta-blockers and nitrates diminish oxygen consumption and thus may reduce infarct size; beta-blockers improve the long-term survival rate.

6. Calcium antagonists may be added if angina persists.

7. In patients with left ventricular failure, inotropic agents and vasodilators can be used.

8. Antithrombotic agents such as aspirin or minidose heparin seem to improve survival rates and prevent reinfarction.

9. Coronary thrombolysis with either streptokinase or tissue plasminogen activator shows encouraging results if given early.

F. Complications

1. Myocardial infarction may develop suddenly without prodromal symptoms or signs. Thirty percent of patients experiencing MIs die before hospital admission, and another 15% die in the hospital. Two thirds of the deaths occur suddenly, and half of these deaths happen within 1 hour of the onset of symptoms.

2. Seventy-five percent of the deaths are attributable to ventricular fibrillation, whereas 10% to 25% are secondary to myocardial failure.

3. Cardiac dysrhythmias and conduction defects can occur even in the later phase of MI, necessitating close monitoring and ECG surveillance.

4. Twenty to thirty-five percent of post-MI patients develop left ventricular insufficiency, which can be life threatening. The reduction in cardiac output

further decreases coronary blood flow, worsens ischemia, and extends the area of necrosis.

5. Rupture of the ventricular septum occurs in 0.5% to 1.0% of MIs and produces a septal defect with a left-to-right shunt. Myocardial rupture typically occurs 3 to 10 days after MI and causes immediate death by hemopericardium and acute tamponade. Incomplete rupture can lead to pseudoaneurysm formation.

6. Papillary muscle necrosis may cause acute mitral regurgitation and manifests itself by the sudden appearance of a new holosystolic apical murmur and hypotension. This problem requires surgical treatment, best undertaken after medical stabilization and intra-aortic balloon counterpulsation.

7. Left ventricular aneurysm may develop as a late complication months or even years after MI.

8. Pericarditis often accompanies an infarction and is usually benign. In 3% to 4% of cases, the patient develops pericardial and pleural inflammation with recurrent fever (Dresler's syndrome). Antimyocardial antibodies are implicated as a causative factor.

V. SUMMARY OF ANESTHETIC CONSIDERATIONS

Patients with significant coronary artery disease may not have severe symptoms or a history of MI. Patients with risk factors such as smoking, hypercholesterolemia, hypertension, advanced age, and male sex should be questioned closely for any indicators of myocardial ischemia. A history of a "heavy," "squeezing," or "crushing" pain with excitement, physical exertion, or cold accompanied by dyspnea, fatigue, nausea, or diaphoresis is consistent with significant coronary artery disease.

All patients suspected of having coronary artery disease should have a preoperative ECG. New changes of the ECG such as ST–T-wave depression or elevation or the new development of Q waves warrant further cardiac workup. Patients who have a history of coronary artery disease but normal ECG who have not had diagnostic tests also require further cardiac workup. An exercise stress test should be done to confirm the diagnosis. To localize the area of ischemia, thallium stress testing may be performed. If the patient is incapacitated, a dipyridamole–thallium stress test may be used. With documentation of severe disease, most patients will undergo cardiac catheterization. This will help identify those who will benefit from surgical or medical therapy.

All medications such as beta-blockers, nitrates, and calcium antagonists prescribed for angina or post-MI should be given preoperatively.

Patients within 6 months of an MI who need surgery should be aggressively monitored intraoperatively and postoperatively with invasive blood pressure monitoring and pulmonary artery catheterization. If patients have a perioperative MI, invasive monitors should be closely watched and prompt treatment provided for decreased blood pressure or cardiac output. Thrombolytic or antithrombolytic agents, when used early, have helped increase survival, but bleeding must be watched for, and patients should not be allowed to become significantly anemic.

Valvular Disease

The most common valvular diseases encountered by the anesthesiologist are those associated with stenotic or insufficient aortic and mitral valves. Less common are tricuspid or pulmonary valvular problems. Perioperative management depends on the severity and pathophysiology of the valvular defect.

I.   AORTIC STENOSIS
   A.   Etiology
        Aortic stenosis usually results from a congenital, degenerative, or inflammatory (rheumatic) process. Congenitally bicuspid aortic valves may function normally for decades. However, altered left ventricular outflow patterns cause cusp trauma and eventually produce fibrous changes, calcifications, and stenosis. Rheumatic aortic stenosis almost always accompanies mitral valve disease. Senile calcification of the aortic valve may also cause significant outflow obstruction.
   B.   Pathophysiology
        1.   Narrowing of the left ventricular outflow tract limits cardiac output and increases left ventricular pressures. Anatomic restriction of the orifice or reduction of the mobility of the valve cusps by calcification progressively increases the resistance to left ventricular ejection. As this process worsens, the heart responds to the pressure overload by compen-

satory concentric hypertrophy. The pressure gradient across the aortic valve serves as an estimate of the severity of the stenosis. When the degree of aortic stenosis becomes significant (pressure gradient >50 mmHg), symptoms ensue. As the disease worsens, left ventricular systolic dysfunction develops. Concomitant increases in afterload further depress left ventricular function and trigger a cycle leading to rapid deterioration and imminent cardiac failure. Correction of stenosis may reverse the hypertrophy and restore left ventricular function to normal.

2.   Valvular aortic stenosis has a long asymptomatic stage, as much as 30 years or more. The normal adult aortic orifice measures 3 to 4 cm^2; when the orifice decreases to 1.0 to 1.5 cm^2 (mild stenosis), flow resistance occurs. A systolic ejection murmur at the second right interspace and a fourth heart sound are heard.

C. Signs and Symptoms

1.   Symptoms develop when the stenosis becomes moderately severe (<1 cm^2). Angina is the earliest symptom in 34% of patients, and syncope is an initial symptom in 15%. Anginal pain may occur in the absence of an obstructive coronary lesion and is probably attributable to underperfusion of the subendocardial portion of the left ventricle. Myocardial hypertrophy, left ventricular pressure higher than coronary perfusion pressure, and prolongation of systole at the expense of diastole contribute to a reduced oxygen supply relative to demand. Syncope and increased risk of sudden death are unique features of aortic stenosis. Hypersensitivity of the carotid sinus reflex, malfunction of the baroreceptor mechanism, cerebral ischemia because of inability to increase cardiac output through a stenotic aortic orifice, or dysrhythmia may explain the syncopal episodes. Once symptoms appear, the estimated life expectancy is 3 years.

2.   Dyspnea is a late finding of aortic stenosis. When heart failure develops, the estimated survival time decreases to 1.5 to 2 years.

3.   Other complications include infective endocarditis (1.8 cases per 1000 patient years), dysrhythmias, and systemic embolization.

D. Preoperative Assessment and Management

1. Asymptomatic aortic stenosis with normal heart size usually does not cause problems during anesthesia and surgery.

2. Before an elective noncardiac operation, symptomatic patients require assessment for possible valve replacement. Noninvasive studies such as chest radiography, ECG, and an echocardiogram may show the severity of valvular obstruction but do not identify patients at increased risk for death or morbidity. Cardiac catheterization and angiography are needed to identify patients at risk for sudden preoperative death and in urgent need of valve replacement (those with aortic valve orifices <1.0 cm^2). Markers for sudden preoperative death include angiographic evidence of left ventricular failure, an elevated pulmonary artery occlusion pressure, and severe pulmonary hypertension.

3. For patients with significant aortic stenosis who are not candidates for valve replacement, management goals during the perioperative period include maintenance of normal sinus rhythm and avoidance of wide swings in heart rate, systemic vascular resistance, and intravascular fluid volume. Myocardial depression secondary to anesthetic agents and a sudden decrease in peripheral vascular resistance will reduce coronary perfusion and cause myocardial ischemia. Because of the relatively fixed stroke volume, bradycardia reduces cardiac output. Tachycardia can compromise coronary blood flow because of the decreased diastolic filling time. Preoperative antibiotic administration provides prophylaxis against infective endocarditis (Table 1-9).

II. AORTIC REGURGITATION

A. Etiology

Aortic regurgitation has a more diverse range of etiologies than aortic stenosis. These include congenital abnormality, myxomatous degeneration, systemic arterial hypertension, rheumatic heart disease, trauma, and infective endocarditis.

B. Diagnosis

1. An early diastolic heart murmur heard maximally down the left sternal edge, a collapsing pulse, and

Table 1–9. Prophylaxis of Infective Endocarditis in Adults

Regimen A: Dental Procedures and Upper Airway Surgery

1. Oral penicillin. Penicillin V (2.0 g) 60 min before procedure followed by 1.0 g six hours later
2. Patients allergic to penicillin. Erythromycin (1.0 g orally) 60 min before procedure followed by 500 mg six hours later

Regimen B: Recommended for Patients with Prosthetic Valves

1. Ampicillin plus gentamicin. Ampicillin (1.0–2.0 g IM or IV) plus gentamicin (1.5 mg/kg IM or IV) both given 30 min before procedure. Penicillin V (1.0 g) six hours later.
2. Patients allergic to penicillin. Vancomycin (1.0 g IV over 60 min) started 60 min before procedure. No repeat dose is necessary.

Regimen C: Gastrointestinal and Genitourinary Surgery and Instrumentation

1. Ampicillin plus gentamicin. Ampicillin (2.0 g IM or IV) plus gentamicin (1.5 mg/kg IM or IV) both given 30 min before procedure. May repeat once eight hours later.
2. Patients allergic to penicillin. Vancomycin plus gentamicin. Vancomycin (1.0 g IV given over 60 min) plus gentamicin (1.5 mg/kg IM or IV) each given 60 min before procedure. May be repeated once 8–12 hours later.

wide pulse pressure classically characterize this condition.

2. The chest radiograph and ECG evidence the left ventricular enlargement typical of aortic regurgitation. Exercise testing may be used as an index of cardiac function. Echocardiography provides useful information about the severity of the lesion and the state of myocardial function. Cardiac catheterization confirms the diagnosis and detects associated valvular diseases.

3. The patient may tolerate chronic aortic regurgitation for years with symptoms not in evidence until the fourth or fifth decade. After the onset of congestive failure, orthopnea, and paroxysmal nocturnal dyspnea, the average life expectancy is about 1 year.

C. Pathophysiology

In aortic insufficiency, a large volume load fills the left ventricle as the regurgitant flow from the aorta adds to normal ventricular filling from the left atrium. This increased load contributes to an eccentric ventricular hypertrophy and a more compliant left ventricle. Because of the slow progression of the lesion, the left ventricle has time to dilate and can handle large regurgitant volumes at normal filling pressures. The patient thus remains symptom free for many years with excellent exercise tolerance, even with significant regurgitation. Eventually, however, mechanical changes in the left ventricular muscle lead to irreversible depression of pump function, with development of dyspnea, congestive heart failure, and angina. Syncope and sudden death are uncommon, however.

    D. Perioperative Management

        1. Elective valvular replacement should be performed in the minimally symptomatic or asymptomatic patient before left ventricular failure supervenes. However, in an emergency when valve replacement cannot be done, stabilization of the patient with vasodilator therapy, intravenous nitroprusside, or other afterload-reducing drugs can significantly reduce the impedance to left ventricular ejection and substantially increase the forward cardiac output.

        2. Preoperative antibiotic administration protects the patient from infective endocarditis (Table 1-9). Myocardial depressants must be avoided.

III. MITRAL STENOSIS

    A. Etiology

    Mitral stenosis is usually the result of rheumatic fever. Less commonly, in the elderly, mitral anulus calcification causes inflow obstruction. The progressive increase in the left atrial pressure and reduction in the size of the valve orifice produce the typical signs and symptoms. These usually appear 20 or more years after the initial episode of rheumatic fever and indicate reduction of the valve orifice by 50% (normal = 4–6 cm^2). When the valve orifice is reduced to 1 cm^2, a gradient of approximately 20 mmHg is required to maintain normal flow across the valve.

    B. The signs and symptoms depend on the speed with which the left atrial pressure increases. The classic physical signs include a sharp opening snap, a rumbling diastolic murmur, a sharp and loud first heart sound, and, rarely, a single second sound with late P2 accentuation. The opening snap is caused by vibrations of the mobile, but stenotic, mitral valve, and once the valve becomes calcified, the opening snap may disappear. The diastolic murmur results from the turbulent flow through the restricted mitral orifice. With the onset of pulmonary hypertension, the pulmonary component of the second sound (P2) becomes louder, and other manifestations of right ventricular hypertrophy appear.

C. Diagnostic Tests

Chest radiographs may show left atrial and right ventricular enlargement. The ECG confirms atrial hypertrophy (P-mitrale). Echocardiography reinforces the diagnosis and provides information about the severity of the decrease in the function of the left ventricle.

D. The basic pathophysiologic abnormality in mitral stenosis involves progressive mechanical obstruction to left ventricular diastolic filling.

1. The obstruction causes chronic increases in left atrial pressure. This increase affects the pulmonary circulation, which produces pulmonary venous congestion and edema. Pulmonary artery pressure increases, causing the right ventricle to hypertrophy. Eventually, the right ventricle fails, which results in passive systemic venous pressure, hepatomegaly, and generalized edema.

2. In severe mitral stenosis, the stroke volume is relatively fixed. Bradycardia will adversely affect cardiac output, and atrial fibrillation can exacerbate the situation. Tachycardia reduces the diastolic filling time and increases the left atrial pressure, which promotes pulmonary edema.

E. Perioperative Management

1. In patients over 40 years old having noncardiac surgery, significant mitral stenosis results in a 7% perioperative mortality rate.

2. Symptomatic patients with gross changes on the ECG and chest radiograph should have valvotomy before elective surgery.

3. Because mitral stenosis is the most common form of valvular disease associated with thromboembolism, anticoagulant medication should be reduced gradually in the preoperative period to maintain coagulation values at high normal levels. Resumption of anticoagulation in the postoperative period decreases the incidence of thromboembolism.

4. Because most patients take diuretics, serum potassium should be monitored.

5. The anesthesiologist should avoid drugs that increase the heart rate or cause sudden reduction in systemic vascular resistance.

6. Preoperative relief of anxiety considerably reduces the likelihood of the adverse circulatory responses produced by sympathetic stimulation.

7. Arterial hypoxemia, acidosis, or injudicious fluid loading all increase pulmonary artery pressure and so should be avoided. As in other valvular heart diseases, prophylactic antibiotics should be given for protection against infective endocarditis (see Table 1-9).

IV. MITRAL REGURGITATION
   A. Etiology
   Mitral regurgitation is usually the result of rheumatic fever and often is associated with mitral stenosis. Dysfunction of the valve leaflets, chordae tendinae, or papillary muscle may cause mitral regurgitation. In the elderly, coronary artery disease, myxomatous degeneration of the valve cusps with valve prolapse, and annulus calcification result in an insufficient valve.
   B. Pathophysiology
      1. A decrease in forward left ventricular stroke volume is the basic hemodynamic problem in mitral regurgitation. During systole, a large regurgitant flow occurs in the direction of the left atrium. The heart enlarges to accommodate the volume load, and both atrial and ventricular compliance increase. The regurgitant fraction depends on the size of the mitral valve orifice, the duration of ventricular ejection, and the pressure gradient across the mitral valve.
      2. Bradycardia, which increases the duration of ventricular ejection, may worsen the regurgitation.
      3. An increase in systemic vascular resistance and impedance to forward flow reduce the forward left ventricular stroke volume. With a greatly distended left atrium, large regurgitant flows are accommodated with little change in atrial pressure. Pulmonary hypertension tends to be mild until relatively late in the disease.

4. In some instances, arterial hypertension increases regurgitant flow and precipitates cardiac failure. The distended left atrium may fibrillate, but adequate forward output is usually maintained until late in the disease. However, if acute mitral regurgitation results from papillary muscle dysfunction or chordal rupture, pulmonary hypertension and right ventricular overload develop rapidly.

5. The combination of mitral regurgitation and mitral stenosis causes volume and pressure overload. The flow across the stenotic valve significantly increases the left atrial pressure. The patient develops heart failure, atrial fibrillation, and pulmonary hypertension earlier than do patients with mitral regurgitation only.

C. Clinical Findings
1. The physical findings include a faint first heart sound and a blowing pansystolic apical murmur radiating to the axilla and left parasternal border.
2. The ECG and chest radiograph confirm left-sided cardiac enlargement. Echocardiography and cardiac catheterization provide information about the severity of regurgitation and the functional state of the myocardium.

D. Perioperative Management
1. Asymptomatic mitral regurgitation is the best tolerated of all valvular lesions.
2. Indications for mitral valve replacement include less than stable NYHA Class II heart failure, severe valvular regurgitation, and adequate left ventricular function as defined by cardiac cineangiography. If required, mitral valve replacement should be performed before any noncardiac operation.
3. Preoperative medication is usually not critical in asymptomatic patients. Patients in NYHA Class III or IV heart failure may need intravenous vasodilators to reduce arterial resistance to left ventricular ejection.
4. Preoperative antibiotics are given to prevent infective endocarditis (see Table 1-9).

V. MITRAL VALVE PROLAPSE
A. Etiology
Mitral valve prolapse is the most common valvular cardiac abnormality, with a prevalence of 5% to 20%. The

disorder afflicts women more than men. Its etiology remains unclear, but, in some, it follows an autosomal dominant pattern of inheritance. Other associated congenital diseases include Marfan's syndrome, Ehlers–Danlos syndrome, Wolff–Parkinson–White syndrome, hypertrophic cardiomyopathy, ostium secondum atrial septal defect, and Ebstein anomaly. Poor left ventricular contraction secondary to muscular dystrophy, coronary artery disease, or cardiomyopathy may cause prolapse.

B. Pathophysiology

    1. The primary pathologic defects are redundant and myxomatous degeneration of the valve leaflets, dilation of the valve anulus, and chordal abnormalities. Because of these anatomic aberrations, the valve protrudes or balloons into the left atrium during left ventricular contraction. This subjects the valve leaflets, the chordae, the papillary muscles, and the underlying ventricular wall to destructive stresses. Typically, the abnormality involves the posterior valve leaflet or both leaflets. Uncommonly, the anterior leaflet becomes redundant. Because the valvular apparatus seems to be too big for the ventricle, increased left ventricular volume lessens the prolapse. Maneuvers that elevate afterload or decrease contractility diminish the prolapse.

    2. Clinically, the pathognomonic feature of the disorder is a mid-to-late systolic click. Auscultation reveals either a holosystolic or late systolic murmur beginning with the click. Although asymptomatic patients are predominant, a small portion complain of palpitations, atypical chest pain, syncope, or fatigue. Potentially serious complications have been reported, including mitral regurgitation, various cardiac dysrhythmias, infective endocarditis, thromboembolism, and sudden death.

C. Perioperative Management

    1. Once suspected, the diagnosis can be confirmed by echocardiography. Beta-blockers are the preferred treatment and should be continued through the day of surgery.

    2. The presence of mitral prolapse does not necessitate invasive perioperative monitoring. Antibiotic prophylaxis for infective endocarditis is recommended.

3.   Perioperative management includes fluid loading to maintain a large left ventricular end-diastolic volume. Sudden afterload reduction should be avoided. Acidosis, hypercarbia, hypoxemia, and electrolyte disturbances should be prevented and potentially dysrhythmic agents (e.g., epinephrine and atropine) avoided.

VI. TRICUSPID REGURGITATION

A. Etiology
Normal closure of the tricuspid valve depends on the complex integrated functions of the leaflets, chordae tendinae, papillary muscles, and adjacent right ventricular myocardium. Malfunction of any one of these components results in tricuspid regurgitation. Primary regurgitation is caused by intrinsic abnormality in the valve apparatus. Secondary (functional) regurgitation develops when right ventricular pressure or volume overload results in an insufficient tricuspid valve. If this condition is accompanied by tricuspid stenosis or other valvular involvement, rheumatic fever is usually the underlying etiology.

B. Pathophysiology
The basic pathophysiological change in tricuspid regurgitation is right atrial volume overload. The vena cava and the right atrium have high compliance; thus, no significant increase in right atrial pressure is noted, even in the presence of a large regurgitant volume. Although in itself benign, the association of tricuspid regurgitation with pulmonary hypertension or right ventricular failure increases the regurgitant flow, and left ventricular stroke volume may decline secondary to reduced pulmonary blood flow.

C. Perioperative Management
Perioperative management of patients with tricuspid regurgitation is aimed at maintaining a high normal intravascular fluid volume and central venous pressure in order to assure adequate left ventricular filling. Vasodilators must be used carefully, because reduction in venous return may compromise stroke volume. Positive-pressure ventilation should be minimized or avoided.

VII. PROSTHETIC HEART VALVES

A. Replacement of diseased valves causes subjective improvement in 90% of survivors. Radiologic signs of cardiomegaly and pulmonary hypertension gradually decrease. The replacement valve may undergo mild stenosis or dysfunction, and thromboembolism and mild hemolysis may occur.

B. The preoperative management of patients with a mechanical valve prosthesis involves temporary discontinuation of anticoagulation. Warfarin is usually discontinued 4 to 5 days before the operation; dipyridamole (400 mg/day) may be continued to the day of surgery.

C. Heparin infusion should be started when the warfarin effect diminishes in order to maintain an activated partial thromboplastin time at one and one-half times the control value. Heparin infusion is continued until 4 to 5 hours before surgery; subcutaneous heparin (5000 units/12 hours) can be given during and early after surgery except in patients undergoing brain or eye operations. Warfarin should be restarted soon after the operation.

VIII. SUMMARY OF ANESTHETIC CONSIDERATIONS

Valvular heart disease is usually asymptomatic. A history of rheumatic fever, infective endocarditis, or heart murmur should help identify patients with possible valvular disease. Noninvasive studies such as a chest radiograph and echocardiogram will help determine the severity of valvular disease. If the disease is very symptomatic or the echocardiogram demonstrates significant valvular compromise, elective surgery should be postponed. Cardiac catheterization and angiography is needed to define clearly the extent of valvular disease and help determine if valvular surgery is necessary.

Patients with significant valvular disease who are not candidates for valve replacement will require an anesthetic that will not cause myocardial depression or disturbances in cardiac rhythm or intravascular volume. Tachycardia and decreases in peripheral vascular resistance are especially dangerous to patients with aortic or mitral stenosis. Decreasing afterload in patients with aortic or mitral regurgitation will help maintain or even increase forward cardiac output. Tachycardia is better tolerated than bradycardia.

Patients with prosthetic valves are often receiving oral anticoagulation. Warfarin in most cases can be discontinued safely 3 to 4 days before surgery. If patients are at high risk for clotting, warfarin effects can be reversed rapidly with fresh frozen plasma and heparin infusion used for anticoagulation. Stopping heparin infusion approximately 6 hours before surgery will allow coagulation to normalize. Anticoagulation can be restarted 24 to 48 hours after surgery except in patients at high risk of bleeding (i.e., intracerebral or intraocular surgery). Aspirin should be discontinued 2 weeks before surgery. Dipyridamole can be continued to the day of surgery.

Patients with Cardiac Disease Needing Noncardiac Surgery

I.   DETERMINING THE RISK OF SURGERY
Regardless of the underlying heart disease, the surgical risk increases with age, emergency surgery, and thoracic, upper abdominal, or vascular surgery.
   A.   The earlier classification of heart disease according to the NYHA and the Dripp's American Society of Anesthesiologists system for perioperative assessment of surgical risk do not predict perioperative cardiac problems adequately.
   B.   In 1977, Goldman et al. identified nine significant contributors to the development of life-threatening and fatal complications after major noncardiac surgery (Table 1-10). Each variable was given a point value, and four classes were identified, with Class I having the lowest value and Class IV the highest value and percentage of life-threatening complications and cardiac death. Using this multifactorial index, Goldman's group predicted 80% of the cardiac outcomes. However, this index appears to underestimate risk by about 40% in patients who undergo resection of abdominal aortic aneurysms and those who are selected on the basis of any high-risk status.
   C.   Waters et al., in a prospective evaluation of this index, found that the scoring system did not predict cardiac events any better than did the subjective physical status rating developed by the American Society of Anesthesiologists. Although the multifactorial index may be useful for the overall assessment of risk in unselected general surgical patients, its use should be viewed as adjunctive. It should never replace clinical judgment and a thorough preoperative preparation and evaluation.
II.   PATIENTS WITH PREVIOUS CORONARY ARTERY BYPASS SURGERY
   A.   Coronary artery bypass surgery is an important treatment for coronary artery disease. Data suggest it improves the quality of life in 80% to 90% of patients with

Table 1–10. Cardiac Risk Index Score in Noncardiac Surgery

Factors	Points
History	
Age >70 years	5
Myocardial infarction <6 months	10
Physical Examination	
S_3 or jugular venous distention	11
Electrocardiogram	
Any rhythm other than sinus	7
≥5 PVC/min[†]	7
General Information	
PO_2 <60 mmHg	3
PCO_2 >50 mmHg	3
Potassium <3 mEq/L	3
BUN >50 or creatinine >3 mg/dl	3
Bedridden from noncardiac causes	3
Operation	
Emergency	4
Intraperitoneal, intrathoracic, or aortic	3
Total points possible	**50**

Interpretation:
  Class 1 = 0–5 points
  Class 2 = 6–12 points
  Class 3 = 13–25 points
  Class 4 = ≥26 points

[†]PVC = premature ventricular contraction.
(Modified from Goldman L, Caldera DL, Nussbaum SR. Multifactorial index of cardiac risk in noncardiac surgical procedures. N Engl J Med 1977;297:845.)

angina pectoris refractory to medical therapy. Bypass surgery prevents premature death in patients who have left main coronary artery stenosis and decreases the incidence of infarction in patients with variant angina or those with previous MI. The operative mortality rate is low (<1%), which makes it possible to recommend surgical treatment in certain patients. The overall 5-year survival rate has been reported to exceed 90%.

B. Bypass patients who later require elective noncardiac surgery do well. The bypass lessens the risk of perioperative myocardial ischemia and decreases ischemic morbidity and mortality rates. For example, Mahar et al. examined the incidence of perioperative MI in patients with known triple-vessel coronary artery disease. In 226 noncardiac operations done in 99 postbypass patients, no perioperative MIs occurred. In contrast, the 49 patients without prior MI, who underwent 58 noncardiac operations, had a 5% incidence of perioperative infarction. Similarly, Wells and Kaplan reported a low incidence of ischemic complications in patients having bypass before noncardiac surgical procedures. Also, McCollum et al. saw no deaths or infarctions in 60 patients who underwent bypass grafting prior to major surgery. From these studies, many believe that the risks of perioperative MI and ischemic-related deaths are significantly lower in patients who have coronary revascularization prior to noncardiac surgery than in those with similar coronary artery disease but without previous bypass.

C. Perioperative Monitoring

   1. The ECG standard lead II provides the clinician with information on cardiac rhythm. Any number of dysrhythmias can occur under general anesthesia. Most of these remain benign and so require little, if any, treatment. However, others may serve as a forerunner of problems. An example is the development of premature ventricular contractions (PVCs) secondary to MI.

      a. When multifocal PVCs or ventricular dysrhythmias occur in runs of 8 to 10 per minute or more, treatment usually is indicated. Intravenous lidocaine will generally reduce or abolish the dysrhythmia, at least temporarily. Potential causes must then be searched for and corrected. These include hyperventilation with resultant respiratory alkalosis; hypokalemia, alone or in conjunction with metabolic alkalosis; hypoxemia; hypercarbia; and ischemia.

      b. A new onset of atrial fibrillation may or may not be benign. When it is associated with a rapid ventricular response, the reduction in ventricular filling time, as well as the loss of the atrial component of ejection, can contribute significantly to a decrease in cardiac output and, potentially, in blood pressure. Fibrillation may be secondary to ischemia, right atrial distention, hypokalemia with or without digitalis therapy, hypoxemia, or hypercarbia. Early intervention should be undertaken for hemodynamic compromise and a rapid ventricular rate, usually greater than 110 beats per minute. Patients without previous digitalis therapy respond best to cardioversion. This can be the simplest treatment, particularly in the operating room. Initially one should use the lowest energy, 20 J, and synchronize the countershock to the ECG. Progressive increases in the energy level should be utilized until the patient has been converted. The judicious use of antiarrhythmic agents such as calcium blockers can prevent return of the dysrhythmia. Procainamide, usually administered as a loading dose followed by continuous infusion, has been a mainstay.

Atrial fibrillation with a rapid ventricular response but without cardiac compromise usually can be treated pharmacologically. Calcium-blocking agents work well. Verapamil up to 5 to 10 mg given in incremental doses can slow the ventricular rate. The peripheral vasodilating action may result in some decrease in blood pressure. Beta-blockers may reduce the ventricular rate but can also diminish contractility, so generally, we do not encourage their use. Long-term control can be obtained with digitalis. Rapid digitalization requires an initial dose of 0.5 mg followed by another 0.5-mg dose in 4 hours with a final dose of either 0.5 or 0.25 mg 4 hours later. Patients already on digitalis therapy may require an increase in serum potassium levels to greater than 4.5 mEq/L. In this group, further digitalis may be administered in doses ranging from 0.125 to 0.25 mg. The response to digitalis appears independent of serum concentration of the agent.

c. Spontaneous onset of ventricular tachycardia may contribute to severe cardiovascular compromise. The situation necessitates prompt cardioversion. Prior to cardioversion, 100 mg of lidocaine may be administered intravenously. On occasion, this can correct the dysrhythmia. Ventricular tachycardia usually does not respond to calcium-blocking agents.

2. Beyond rhythm monitoring, the ECG can help detect ischemic events.

    a. Simultaneous monitoring of standard lead II and lead V5 provides information on the inferior aspect of the myocardium and lateral wall function, respectively.

    b. ST-T changes remain the best overall method available to detect ischemia. The likelihood of subendocardial or myocardial damage appears to be related not only to the severity but also to the duration of the ischemic changes.

    c. Although authorities suggest that elevations in pulmonary capillary occlusion pressure (PAOP) may herald ischemia before changes are seen in the ECG, clinically, these elevations may be extremely difficult to detect. Changes in PAOP of 3 to 4 mmHg are hard to see on the analogue trace of the pressure monitor, yet digital readouts are notoriously unreliable and do not consider variations secondary to breathing. Furthermore, changes in capillary wedge pressure can be entirely independent of any change in myocardial function or wall ischemia.

3. Invasive blood pressure monitoring

    a. Patients with significant cardiac disease require continuous monitoring of arterial pressure to detect any changes in the peripheral vascular system. Many of our interventions, including mechanical ventilation and pharmacologic agents, have direct and potentially detrimental effects on systemic blood pressure. The ability to recognize and assess these changes rapidly permits prompt intervention and correction. Moreover, anesthetic induction has a high potential for inducing cardiac depression and systemic hypotension. In order to provide the most useful information, the arterial catheter should be in place prior to the onset of anesthesia.

    b. The radial artery is the most frequently cannulated vessel. Other available sites include the ulnar, axillary, and femoral vessels. The brachial artery, with its lack of anastomotic vessels, functions as an end artery. Therefore, this site should never be used, as any obstruction can result in distal loss of the extremity.

c. The further the site of arterial cannulation is from the central aorta, the greater the discrepancy will be between measured peripheral and central blood pressure. This disparity can be exaggerated in the patient with severe arteriosclerotic disease. The lack of elasticity in the vessel walls causes perpetuation of the ejected blood pressure wave from the aortic root to the transducer system. "Overshoot" develops, and the systemic pressure appears to be considerably greater than that recorded with the blood pressure cuff. Additionally, the arterial tracing on the monitor often demonstrates extreme narrowing near the peak pressure display. This pattern correlates with absence of blood flow. Inflation of a blood pressure cuff proximal to the cannulation site will occlude the vessel. With the reduction of cuff pressure, the arterial tracing reappears on the monitor. Correlation of the first detected pressure wave with the noted cuff pressure supplies a "return to flow" reading. This value best approximates the arterial pressure when a large discrepancy exists between cuff pressures and direct readings.

4. Pulmonary artery catheterization

a. Indications for the use of the pulmonary artery catheter include congestive heart failure and ventricular dysfunction. Clinically, this generally translates into an ejection fraction of less than 40%. Patients who have significant wall motion abnormalities but in whom the ejection fraction has not been measured are also reasonable candidates for pulmonary artery catheterization. Patients with previous MI often have a significant disparity between right and left ventricular functions and may likewise benefit from preoperative placement of a pulmonary artery catheter.

b. Most attenuations in cardiac function occur

during anesthetic induction. Intuitively, then, it makes sense to place the pulmonary artery catheter prior to the induction. In the awake state, this procedure can be uncomfortable, even painful, for the patient, resulting in significant increases in systemic blood pressure and heart rate, which obviously can be detrimental because of the increased myocardial oxygen demands. Therefore, the clinician should ensure that adequate sedation and analgesia are provided prior to catheter placement. Prior discussion with the patient can reduce somewhat the need for medication to accomplish the goal. The patient generally will tolerate more pain and discomfort if aware, not only of what to expect, but also of the reasons the procedures are necessary.

c. The pulmonary artery catheter allows measurement and, ultimately, manipulation of cardiac function to maximize performance and minimize risk. Although cardiac output can be measured directly, the value alone provides little insight into cardiac function. However, the ability to separate preload or pulmonary artery occlusion pressure and calculation of system vascular resistance can provide useful information. Increases in systemic resistance generally increase left ventricular wall tension and, ultimately, ventricular afterload. Both these changes are associated with an increase in myocardial oxygen requirements. The clinician should be cautioned, however, that changes in systemic vascular resistance are indirectly related to alterations in cardiac output. Resistance is a calculated number, and one must not place too much faith in the value by itself. Rather, the entire clinical picture must be examined. If resistance is significantly elevated, the causes can include either intense vasoconstriction or diminished contractility. Most times, an elevated systemic blood pressure associated with an increase in systemic resistance signifies increased peripheral vasoconstriction. Patients in this category often respond best initially to vasodilating agents such as nitroprusside. On the other hand, a low systemic pressure coupled with a high resistance most often indicates altered contractility. Under these circumstances, an inotropic agent such as epinephrine, dopamine, or dobutamine may be the appropriate first choice. Many times, a combination of an inotrope and a vasodilator will be necessary to increase cardiac output.

    d. Cardiac output, by itself, provides little useful information. However, myocardial and systemic oxygen demands must be met. Determination of the difference between the arteriovenous oxygen content (A − VDO$_2$) provides the best clinical information as to the adequacy of cardiac output. These are global measurements and do not reflect individual organ functions such as that of the myocardium. Whenever oxygen extraction is increased, as evidenced by an A − VDO$_2$ above 5.5 ml/100 ml of blood, certain organ systems may be at risk, particularly the heart. Normally, myocardial oxygen extraction is maximal, even under the best of conditions. Therefore, when global measurements indicate an increase in oxygen extraction, myocardial failure or infarction may already be present, even if undetected by our conventional means, including ECG or wedge pressure change.

    5. Devices have recently become available that allow continuous or nearly continuous measurement of cardiac output. These include transesophageal and transthoracic Doppler devices. However, a serious drawback is the inability to make the other determinations previously discussed. The devices provide little, if any, information on filling pressures or the adequacy of cardiac output. Echocardiography still is not available on a continuous basis in the operating room. However, as this technique continues to be perfected, information will be made available continuously regarding wall function and ejection fractions.

D. Anesthetic Agents

With appropriate monitoring, the selection of the anesthetic agent is perhaps less crucial and somewhat easier.

1. Morphine appears to be the narcotic agent that most consistently causes systemic hypotension. Although it may have direct vasodilating effects, particularly if the patient is volume depleted, histamine release is a likely cause of the observed hypotension. The degree of hypotension is dose related: in doses of 1 mg/kg, hypotension should not present significant problems, but with larger doses, more profound hypotension may occur. Most authors feel that morphine has minimal direct myocardial depressant action. Because of the venodilation that develops, fluid requirements can increase. Vasodilation with reduced venous return obviously may be beneficial in patients with congestive heart failure. Morphine does not appear to be detrimental and works well in patients with coronary artery or valvular disease. Its duration of action prolongs recovery time, and this slower emergence may necessitate postoperative mechanical ventilation. On the other hand, the protracted arousal ensures a more controlled emergence from anesthesia. When coupled with maintenance of normothermia, the prolonged recovery time seems to reduce the incidence and severity of postoperative hypertension.

2. Fentanyl appears to work well in all forms of cardiovascular disease. In the usual anesthetic range of 35 to 100 µg/kg, the agent has little effect on blood pressure or cardiac contractility. In higher doses, the reduction in heart rate may be associated with a decrease in blood pressure, particularly in patients in whom cardiac output has some relation to heart rate. The more severe the cardiac disease, as evidenced by the extent of reduction of the ejection fraction, the lower the dose required to maintain anesthesia without impairing cardiovascular function.

3. Sufentanil is more potent than fentanyl but otherwise appears to have precisely the same cardiovascular actions. Some authors think that less sympathetic stimulation occurs with sufentanil than with fentanyl during surgical intervention. Because of its relatively short action, alfentanil is not efficacious for longer anesthetic procedures unless given as a constant infusion.

4. Inadequate doses of narcotic agents have often been associated with increasing blood pressure during noncardiac procedures in patients with cardiovascular disease. This is particularly so with certain painful stimuli. Anticipation of such events and pretreatment with small incremental doses of thiopental or inhalation agents can be extremely helpful.

5. Nitrous oxide seems to be declining in favor. Alone or in combination with narcotics and inhalation agents, N_2O has direct dose-related myocardial depressant effects. Because of the unpredictability of this agent and its propensity for causing myocardial depression, its use requires scrutiny in patients with myocardial or vascular disease. In addition, it appears that the agent causes significant coronary vessel vasoconstriction.

6. When inhalation agents are used in patients with cardiac disease, isoflurane is often the drug of choice. The potential benefits include its minimal myocardial depressant effects and peripheral vasodilating abilities. Also, unlike halothane, it does not seem to increase the incidence of dysrhythmias. This is true whether it is used alone or in combination with exogenous epinephrine.

In patients with coronary artery disease, debate continues over the existence of a coronary steal syndrome with isoflurane usage. Significant data exist on both sides of this issue. In our experience, this phenomenon does not seem to occur on a predictable or a regular basis.

7. Today, a popular anesthetic technique combines narcotics with small doses of inhalation agents. Usually, isoflurane is added to control increases in systemic blood pressure, with the majority of the anesthetic requirements being supplied by the narcotics. This nontraditional approach attempts to harness the benefits of both types of agents to provide the best chance of a complication-free outcome. Coupled with appropriate monitoring, as previously outlined, this method can be most effective. Induction of anesthesia in the patient with cardiovascular disease should be accomplished in a manner designed to prevent sharp changes in blood pressure, heart rate, and cardiac output. With myocardial disease, induction agents such as barbiturates or benzodiazepines can significantly affect both peripheral resistance as well as cardiac contractility. Thus, these agents must be used with care. Likewise, ketamine can cause significant increases in heart rate and blood pressure, possibly with detrimental effects. Any other agents that impact on cardiovascular function should also be avoided if other drugs are available that do not adversely affect hemodynamic stability (i.e., pancuronium *v* vecuronium).

E. Postoperative Care

1. In the postoperative period, pain and any other stimuli that will offset myocardial oxygen balance should be avoided. Increasingly, epidural narcotics for pain relief after intrathoracic and intraabdominal procedures have been utilized. These provide a constant level of analgesia without the peaks and valleys associated with the traditional intravenous or intramuscular therapies. These patients must be kept in an area where they can be monitored closely for signs of respiratory depression.

2. Patient-controlled analgesia pumps have been shown to be as efficacious as epidural narcotics. The incidence of perceived pain, as well as the overall use of narcotics, is reduced with this technique.

3. Use of intrapleural catheters with the infusion of local anesthetics may be useful in patients with upper abdominal or intrathoracic surgery in whom narcotics should be avoided.

4. Patients should remain intubated and mechanically ventilated until they demonstrate sufficient pulmonary reserve, as evidenced by an adequate vital capacity and negative inspiratory force. Obviously, patients should also be able to maintain adequate alveolar ventilation and oxygenation on modest levels of oxygen (<50%).

III. SUMMARY OF ANESTHETIC CONSIDERATIONS
Patients who have congestive heart failure or an MI within 6 months of surgery are at especially high risk for perioperative cardiac problems. High-risk patients needing anesthesia should be monitored with arterial and pulmonary artery catheters. The latter, having the ability to measure venous oxygen by oximetry, can provide continuous information on oxygen

delivery and consumption for patients needing more frequent evaluation of their hemodynamic state. ECG lead II and lead V_5 should be monitored for rhythm and signs of ischemia.

Newer devices such as transesophageal echocardiography and transthoracic Doppler instruments permit noninvasive measurement of cardiac output. The nearly continuous evaluation of cardiac output by Doppler devices allows for easier titration of anesthetic agents.

All intravenous induction agents can depress myocardial contractility and vasodilation. These agents can be safely used if titrated carefully.

Opiates, especially the synthetic derivatives, fentanyl, sufentanil, and alfentanil, are frequently used as the chief anesthetic because of minimal direct myocardial depressant action. Nitrous oxide may have direct myocardial depressant effects and may cause coronary vasculature constriction. The use of isoflurane can cause significant afterload reduction and coronary arterial shunting. However, it causes the least myocardial depression of the potent inhalation anesthetics.

In the immediate postoperative period, these patients should continue to be invasively monitored. Good postoperative analgesia should be provided to decrease sympathetic activity and oxygen consumption. Epidural opiates, patient-controlled devices, and intrapleural local anesthetics are effective alternatives to intravenous, intramuscular, or oral opiates for postoperative analgesia. Patients should remain intubated and mechanically ventilated if there is any evidence of inadequate respiratory reserve or hemodynamic instability.

Recommended Reading

Abrams J. Nitrates. Med Clin North Am 1988;72:1.

Adler DC, Bryan-Brown CW. Use of axillary artery for intravascular monitoring. Crit Care Med 1973;3:148.

Allen PD, Walman T, Concepcion M. Epidural morphine provides post operative pain relief in peripheral vascular and orthopedic surgical patients: a dose–response study. Anesth Analg 1986; 65:873.

Applefeld MM, Roffman DS. Digitalis and other positive catecholamine-like inotropic agents in the management of congestive heart failure. Am J Med 1986;80(suppl 2B):40.

Bashour TT, Andreae GE, Hanna ES, Mason DT. Reparative operations for mitral valve incompetence: an emerging treatment of choice. Am Heart J 1987;113:1199.

Baughman KL. Calcium channel blocking agents in congestive heart failure. Am J Med 1986;80(suppl 2B):46.

Belkin RN, Kisslo J. Clinical applications of echocardiography in myocardial and valvular heart disease. Prog Cardiovasc Dis 1986; 29:81.

Bonow RO: Aortic regurgitation: medical assessment and surgical intervention. Adv Intern Med 1983;28:93.

Bull A. The anesthetic evaluation and management of the surgical patient with heart disease. Surg Clin North Am 1983;63:1035.

Cannon PJ. The kidney in heart failure. N Engl J Med 1977;296:26.

Carabello B, Cohn PF, Alpert JS. Hemodynamic monitoring in patients with hypotension after myocardial infarction. Chest 1978;74:5.

CASS Principal Investigators and Associates. Myocardial infarction and mortality in the coronary artery surgery study (CASS) randomized trial. N Engl J Med 1984;310:750.

Castaner A, Betriu A, Sanz G. Natural history of severe left ventricular dysfunction after myocardial infarction. Chest 1984;85:744.

Chariker FG, Mahaffey JE. Anesthesia for patients with cardiac disease. Clin Plast Surg 1985;12:61.

Chatterjee K, Parmley WW. Vasodilator therapy for acute myocardial infarction and chronic congestive heart failure. J Am Coll Cardiol 1983;1:133.

Cheng TO. Mitral valve prolapse. Disease-a-Month 1987;33:481.

Chesebro JH, Adams PC, Fuster V. Antithrombotic therapy in patients with valvular heart disease and prosthetic heart valves. J Am Coll Cardiol 1986;8:41B.

Chung DC. Anesthetic problems associated with treatment of cardiovascular disease I: digitalis toxicity. Can Anaesth Soc J 1981;28:6.

Cohn JN. Unloading the heart in congestive heart failure. Am J Med 1984;77:67.

Cohn JN, Franciosa JA. Vasodilator therapy of cardiac failure I and II. N Engl J Med 1977;297:27 and 254.

Colucci WS. Usefulness of calcium antagonists for congestive heart failure. Am J Cardiol 1987;59:52B.

Colucci WS, Wright RF, Braunwald E. New positive inotropic agents in the treatment of congestive heart failure: mechanisms of action and recent clinical developments I and II. N Engl J Med 1986;314:290 and 349.

Coulshed N. Disorders of mitral valve function. Practitioner 1982;226:407.

Crystal GJ, Rooney HW, Salem MR. Myocardial blood flow and oxygen consumption during isovolemic hemodilution alone and in combination with adenosine-induced controlled hypotension. Anesth Analg 1988;67:539.

De Angelis J. Axillary arterial monitoring. Crit Care Med 1976;4:205.

DePace NL, Ross J, Iskandrian AS. Tricuspid regurgitation: noninvasive techniques for determining causes and severity. J Am Coll Cardiol 1984;3:1540.

Devereux RB, Perloff JK, Reichek N, Josephson ME. Mitral valve prolapse. Circulation 1976;54:3.

Dunkman WB, Leinbach RC, Buckley MJ. Clinical and hemodynamic results of intraaortic balloon pumping and surgery for cardiogenic shock. Circulation 1972;46:465.

Dzau VJ, Creager MA. Clinical response to angiotensin-converting enzyme inhibition in cardiac failure. Clin Exp Theory Prac 1987;A9(2 & 3):521.

Eisele JH, Smith NT. Cardiovascular effects of 40 percent nitrous oxide in man. Anesth Analg 1972;51:956.

Foex P. Preoperative assessment of the patient with cardiovascular disease. Br J Anaesth 1981;53:731.

Ford BM, Weich HFH, Coetzee AR. Preoperative assessment of cardiac patients for non-cardiac surgery. S Afr Med J 1984;65:237.

Francis GS. Neurohumoral mechanisms involved in congestive heart failure. Am J Cardiol 1985;55:15A.

Francis GS, Cohn JN. The autonomic nervous system in congestive heart failure. Annu Rev Med 1986;37:235.

Friedman WF, George BL. New concepts and drugs in the treatment of congestive heart failure. Pediatr Clin North Am 1984;31:1197.

Friesinger GC. The reasonable work-up before recommending medical or surgical therapy: an overall strategy. Circulation 1982;65(suppl II):21.

Frishman WH. β-Adrenergic blockers. Med Clin North Am 1988;72:37.

Fuster V, Chesebro JH. Mechanisms of unstable angina. N Engl J Med 1986;315:1023.

Goldman L, Caldera DL, Nussbaum SR et al. Multifactorial index of cardiac risk in noncardiac surgical procedures. N Engl J Med 1977;297:845.

Graves DA, Foster TS, Batenhorst RL. Patient controlled analgesia. Ann Intern Med 1983;99:360.

Harries AD, Griffiths BE. Assessment of chronic aortic valve disease in adults. Postgrad Med J 1982;58:1.

Harris P. Congestive cardiac failure: central role of the arterial blood pressure. Br Heart J 1987;58:190.

Hermanovich J. The management of the cardiac patient requiring noncardiac surgery. Surg Clin North Am 1983;63:985.

Hutton I, Hillis WS. Modern management of heart failure. Br J Hosp Med 1986;December:406.

Jeffrey CC, Kunsman J, Cullen DJ, Brewster DC. A prospective evaluation of cardiac risk index. Anesthesiology 1983;58:462.

Kaplan JA, King SB. The precordial electrocardiographic lead (V₅) in patients with coronary-artery disease. Anesthesiology 1976; 45:570.

Katz AM. Congestive heart failure: role of altered myocardial cellular control. N Engl J Med 1975;293:1184.

Kligfield P, Levy D, Devereux RB, Savage DD. Arrhythmias and sudden death in mitral valve prolapse. Am Heart J 1987;113:1298.

Kloster FE, Kremkow EL, Ritzman LW. Coronary bypass for stable angina. N Engl J Med 1979;300:149.

Knapp RB,Topkins MJ, Artusio JF. The cerebrovascular accident and coronary occlusion in anesthesia. JAMA 1962;182:332.

Knoebel SB. Chronic ischemic heart disease: from concept to fact. J Am Coll Cardiol 1983;1:20.

Kowalski SE. Mitral valve prolapse. Can Anaesth Soc J 1985;32:138.

Laragh JH. Endocrine mechanisms in congestive heart failure: renin, aldosterone and atrial natriuretic hormone. Drugs 1986; 32(suppl 5):1.

Levy D, Savage D. Prevalence and clinical features of mitral valve prolapse. Am Heart J 1987;113:1281.

Lunn JK, Stanley TH, Eisele J, Webster L, Woodward A. High dose fentanyl anesthesia for coronary artery surgery: plasma fentanyl concentrations and influence of nitrous oxide on cardiovascular responses. Anesth Analg 1979;58:390.

Mahar LJ, Steen PA, Tinker JH. Perioperative myocardial infarction in patients with coronary artery disease with and without aorto-coronary bypass grafts. J Thorac Cardiovasc Surg 1978;76:533.

Maille JG, Boulanger M, Dyrda I, Tremblay N. Anesthesia and myocardial infarction. Can Anaesth Soc J 1986;33:807.

Mancini DM, Le Jemtel TH, Factor S, Sonnenblick EH. Central and peripheral components of cardiac failure. Am J Med 1986; 80(suppl 2B):2.

McCullom CH, Garcia–Rinaldi R, Graham JM, DeBakey ME. Myocardial revascularization prior to subsequent major surgery in patients with coronary artery disease. Surgery 1977;81:302.

McIntosh HD. Aorto-coronary bypass grafting: an internist's perspective. Circulation 1982;65(suppl II):77.

Mearns AJ. Heart valve replacement. Practitioner 1982;226:443.

Moise A, Theroux P, Taeymons Y. Unstable angina and progression of coronary atherosclerosis. N Engl J Med 1983;309:686.

Morton BC. Natural history and management of chronic aortic disease. Can Med Assoc J 1982;126:477.

Newman WH. Biochemical, structural and mechanical defects of the failing myocardium. Pharmacol Ther 1983;22:215.

Nishimura RA, Schaff HV, Shub C. Papillary muscle rupture complicating acute myocardial infarction: analysis of 17 patients. Am J Cardiol 1983;51:373.

Oberman A, Jones WB, Riley CP, Reeves TJ, Sheffield LT, Turner ME. Natural history of coronary artery disease. Bull NY Acad Med 1972;49:1109.

Packer M. Mechanisms of nitrate action in patients with severe left ventricular failure: conceptual problems with the theory of venosequestration. Am Heart J 1985;110:259.

Packer M. The role of vasodilator therapy in the treatment of severe chronic heart failure. Drug 1986;32(suppl 5):13.

Passamani E, Davis KB, Gillespie MJ. A randomized trial of coronary artery bypass surgery. N Engl J Med 1985;312:1665.

Rahimtoola SH. Valvular heart disease: a perspective. J Am Coll Cardiol 1983;6:199.

Rahimtoola SH, Cheitlin MD, Hutter AM. Valvular and congenital heart disease. J Am Coll Cardiol 1987;10:60A.

Rahimtoola SH, Grunkemeier GL, Starr A. Ten year survival after coronary artery bypass surgery for angina in patients aged 65 or older. Circulation 1986;74:509.

Rao TLK, Jacobs KH, El-Etr AA. Re-infarction following anesthesia in patients with myocardial infarction. Anesthesiology 1983; 59:499.

Reeves TJ. Medical management of patient with angina pectoris: an overview of the problem. Circulation 1982;65(suppl II):3.

Remme WJ. Congestive heart failure: pathophysiology and medical treatment. J Cardiovasc Pharmacol 1986;8(suppl 1):S36.

Roberts R. Inotropic therapy for cardiac failure associated with acute myocardial infarction. Chest 1988;93(suppl):22.

Roberts R. Enzymatic diagnosis of acute myocardial infarction. Chest 1988;93(suppl):3.

Rosow C. Newer opioid analgesics and antagonists. Anesth Clin North Am 1979;6:319.

Ross J. Afterload mismatch in aortic and mitral valve disease: implications for surgical therapy. J Am Coll Cardiol 1985;5:811.

Rotmensch HH, Vlasses PH, Ferguson RK. Angiotensin-converting enzyme inhibitors. Med Clin North Am 1988;72:399.

Rubin SA, Swan HJC. Vasodilator therapy for heart failure: concepts, applications, and challenges. JAMA 1981;245:761.

Ruffolo RR, Kopia GA. Importance of receptor regulation in the pathophysiology and therapy of congestive heart failure. Am J Med 1986;80(suppl 2B):67.

Rugie N. Congestive heart failure. Med Clin North Am 1986;70:829.

Savino JA, Del Guercio LRM. Preoperative assessment of high risk surgical patients. Surg Clin North Am 1985;65:763.

Schroeder JS, Lamb I, Hu M, Stinson EB. Coronary bypass surgery for unstable angina pectoris. JAMA 1977;237:2609.

Selzer A. Changing aspects of the natural history of valvular aortic stenosis. N Engl J Med 1987;317:91.

Sheehan FH, Braunwald E, Canner P. The effect of intravenous thrombolytic therapy on left ventricular function: a report on tissue type plasminogen activator and streptokinase from the thrombolysis in myocardial infarction (TIMI Phase I) trial. Circulation 1987;75:817.

Silverman KJ, Grossman W. Angina pectoris: natural history and strategies for evaluation and management. N Engl J Med 1984;310:1712.

Stanley TH, Gray NH, Stanford W, Armstrong R. The effects of high-dose morphine on fluid and blood requirements in open heart procedures. Anesthesiology 1976;38:536.

Steen PA, Tinker JH, Tarhan S. Myocardial re-infarction after anesthesia and surgery. JAMA 1978;239:2566.

Stephenson LW, Edie RN, Harken AH, Edmunds LH. Combined aortic and mitral valve replacement in practice and prognosis. Circulation 1984;69:640.

Tarhan S, Moffitt EA, Taylor WF, Giuliani ER. Myocardial infarction after general anesthesia. JAMA 1972;220:1451.

Thompson R. Aortic regurgitation: how do we judge optimal timing for surgery? Aust NZ J Med 1984;14:514.

Thompson WL, Watton RP. The elevation in plasma histamine levels in dogs following administration of muscle relaxants, opiates and macromolecular molecules. J Pharmacol Exp Ther 1964; 143:131.

Toll MC. Direct blood pressure measurements: risks, technology evolution and some current problems. Med Biol Eng Comput 1984;22:2.

Topkins MJ, Artusio JF. Myocardial infarction and surgery. Anesth Analg 1964;43:716.

Topol EJ. Advances in thrombolytic therapy for acute myocardial infarction. J Clin Pharmacol 1987;27:735.

Waller JL, Kaplan JA. Anaesthesia for patients with coronary artery disease. Br J Anaesth 1981;53:757.

Waters J, Wilkinson C, Golmon M, Schoeppel S, Linde HW, Brunner EA. Evaluation of cardiac risk in noncardiac surgical patients [Abstr]. Anesthesiology 1981;55(3A):A343.

Weber KT, Gill SK, Janicki JS, Maskin CS, Jain MC. Newer positive inotropic agents in the treatment of chronic cardiac failure: current status and future directions. Drugs 1987;33:503.

Weber KT, Likoff MJ, Janicki JS, Andrews V. Advances in the evaluation and management of chronic cardiac failure. Chest 1984;85:253.

Wells PH, Kaplan JA. Optimal management of patients with ischemic heart disease for non-cardiac surgery by complementary anesthesiologist and cardiologist interaction. Am Heart J 1981; 102:1029.

Wiedemann HP, Matthay MA, Matthay RA. Cardiovascular–pulmonary monitoring in the intensive care unit 1. Chest 1984;85:537.

Willman VL. Management of the patient with coronary artery disease: a surgeon's perspective. Circulation 1982;65(suppl II):13.

Yusuf S. The use of beta adrenergic blocking agents, IV nitrates and calcium channel blocking agents following acute myocardial infarction. Chest 1988;93(suppl):25.

≡ Cardiac Dysrhythmias and Pacemakers

David H. Wong
Anne B. Wong
Eugene Y. Cheng

Cardiac dysrhythmias are of great concern in the perioperative period. During this time, many drugs and conditions may adversely affect existing dysrhythmias or cause new ones. Both supraventricular and ventricular dysrhythmias may compromise systemic perfusion.

Cardiac Dysrhythmias

I. ETIOLOGY
   A. Two physiologic mechanisms account for most ectopic dysrhythmias.
      1. Reentry dysrhythmias are precipitated by a variety of alterations in refractoriness, impulse formation, and conduction.
      2. Enhanced automaticity dysrhythmias result from repetitive firing from a single ectopic focus.
   B. Factors underlying dysrhythmias of either origin include hypoxia, electrolyte and acid–base abnormalities, ischemia, excess myocardial fiber stretch, altered sympa-

thetic and parasympathetic tone, and use of certain drugs.

II.   PATHOPHYSIOLOGY

Reversible causes of cardiac dysrhythmias are outlined below.

A.   Electrolytes

1.   Hyperkalemia may cause heart block or malignant ventricular dysrhythmias. Intraoperative causes of hyperkalemia include malignant hyperthermia, intravascular hemolysis, crush syndrome, and succinylcholine administration (especially to patients with burns, trauma, upper neuron disease, and intra-abdominal sepsis). Hyperkalemia, particularly if associated with myocardial ischemia and high circulating catecholamine levels, reduces the resting membrane potential (RMP), increasing the likelihood of an activation during the ventricular refractory period that will induce tachydysrhythmias.

2.   Hypokalemia also predisposes to ventricular dysrhythmias. Intraoperative hypokalemia may be secondary to respiratory alkalosis, nasogastric suction, and diuresis. Hypokalemia makes the heart more susceptible to dysrhythmias induced by catecholamines, hypoxia, hypercarbia, anticholinergics, and digitalis toxicity. Chronic hypokalemia may be more benign than acute hypokalemia. The ratio of intracellular to extracellular K^+ is probably more important than the absolute extracellular K^+ concentration in maintaining a normal gradient between RMP and the activation threshold.

3.   Hypomagnesemia and hypercalemia may provoke digitalis-induced dysrhythmias.

4.   Variations in the sodium concentration from normal produce no specific ECG changes and usually are not a cause of cardiac dysrhythmias.

B.   Myocardial Ischemia

1.   Ischemia causes a differential in the refractory periods of adjacent myocardial cells and is commonly associated with ventricular dysrhythmias.

2.   Coronary spasm (variant angina pectoris), which is characterized by pain during rest and ST segment elevation, is often associated with dysrhythmias.

3.   Enlargement of a failing left ventricle stretches myocardial cells and can enhance automaticity.

4.   Treatment of myocardial ischemia with nitrates,

beta-blockers, and calcium channel blockers may reduce or eliminate associated dysrhythmias.

C. Sympathetic and Parasympathetic Activity

    1. Increased sympathetic activity from anxiety, exercise, exogenous catecholamines, acute myocardial infarction (MI), or congestive heart failure may lead to both atrial and ventricular dysrhythmias.

    2. Vagal tone may protect against ventricular dysrhythmias in an acutely ischemic myocardium. Anticholinergic drugs, by their vagolytic action, can induce ventricular dysrhythmias.

D. Atrial bradycardia may increase the differences in the refractory periods among Purkinje fibers, enhancing the incidence of ventricular ectopy.

E. Prolonged QT Interval

    1. Prolongation of the QT interval, much like bradycardia, results in a dispersion of refractory periods among Purkinje fibers, increasing the chance of ventricular dysrhythmias.

    2. Torsade de pointes, a polymorphic ventricular tachycardia characterized by alternating electrical polarity, is typical in patients with prolonged QT intervals.

    3. Acquired causes include hypokalemia, hypomagnesemia, and certain antiarrhythmic drugs such as quinidine, procainamide, disopyramide, or amiodarone.

F. Drugs

Many drugs may affect cardiac rhythm. Dysrhythmias may occur even when drug concentrations are not in the toxic range. The following have dysrhythmogenic potential.

    1. Sympathomimetics

    2. Anticholinergics

    3. Methylxanthines

    4. Tricyclics

    5. Cholinergics

    6. Thyroid extract

    7. Phenothiazines

    8. Antiarrhythmics.

III. CARDIAC ELECTROPHYSIOLOGY

A. The RMP of the cardiac cell is determined mainly by the concentration gradient of K^+ and Na^+ across the cell membrane. The relative excess of intracellular potassium and extracellular sodium is maintained by several membrane pumps, including the Na^+ pump, which actively transports Na^+ out of cells.

B.   When an electrical stimulus is sufficient to reduce the transmembrane potential from its resting level to a critical level termed the "threshold potential," an action potential results. The RMP is approximately -95 mV. The threshold potential in cardiac fibers is about -65 mV.

C.   Five different phases of action potential are found in cardiac muscle.

    1.   Phase 0 is the initial rapid upstroke of depolarization caused by a sudden increase in cell membrane permeability to Na^+, resulting in a large influx of this ion (Fig. 1-9).

    2.   Phases 1–3 are repolarization stages.

        a.   Phase 1: Early repolarization—influx of Cl^- and efflux of K^+

        b.   Phase 2: Plateau phase of slow repolarization—release of internal Ca^{++}

        c.   Phase 3: Terminal phase of rapid repolarization—efflux of K^+.

    3.   Phase 4: Return to original RMP.

    4.   In nonpacemaker cells, phase 4 is flat. In pacemaker cells, spontaneous slow depolarization occurs in phase 4 until the threshold membrane potential is reached, and another action potential is generated.

    5.   Phase 0 produces the QRS complex, and phase 3 is responsible for producing the T wave on the electrocardiogram.

IV.   ANTIARRHYTHMIC DRUGS

A.   Antiarrhythmic drugs may be classified on the basis of their electrophysiologic properties. There are four major classes (Table 1-11).

    1.   Class I agents bind to the sodium channel and inhibit phase 0 inflow of Na^+ into the cell.

        a.   Class 1A agents (quinidine, procainamide, disopyramide): moderate phase 0 depression; slow conduction and prolong repolarization.

        b.   Class 1B agents (lidocaine, mexiletine, tocainide, phenytoin): minimal phase 0 depression; slow conduction and shorten repolarization.

        c.   Class 1C agents (lorcainide, encainide, and fle-

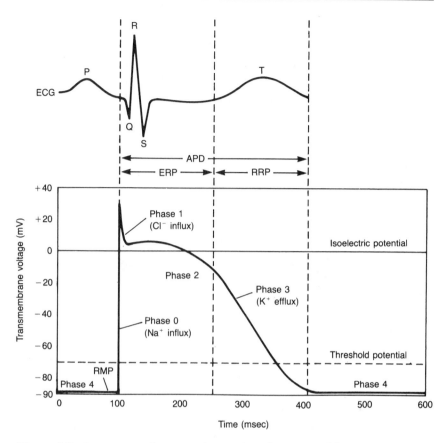

Figure 1-9 A transmembrane action potential generated by a single ventricular cell is correlated with a simultaneously recorded electrocardiogram. When excitation occurs, the massive influx of sodium ions causes depolarization (phase 0). During subsequent repolarization (phases 1, 2, and 3), the early influx of chloride ions (phase 1) and the later efflux of potassium ions (phase 3) act to restore the original resting membrane potential (RMP, phase 4). The effective refractory period (ERP) plus the relative refractory period (RRP) constitutes an action potential duration (APD). During the ERP, no impulses, regardless of intensity, can be conducted by the heart; during the RRP, only stimuli of higher than normal intensity will be propagated. The relation of these periods to the characteristic ECG waves and to the phases of depolarization and repolarization is also indicated. *(From Hutter AM. Cardiac tachyarrhythmias: Basic aspects and pharmacologic therapy. In: Rubenstein E, Federman DD (eds). Scientific American Medicine, vol. 1. New York, Scientific American, Inc., 1989.)*

Table 1–11. Electrophysiologic and Electrocardiographic Effects of Common Antiarrhythmic Drugs

Effect	Class I — Class 1A: Quinidine, Procainamide, Disopyramide	Class I — Class 1B: Lidocaine, Mexiletine, Tocainide, Phenytoin, Moricizine, Aprindine	Class I — Class 1C: Flecainide, Encainide, Lorcainide	Class II: Propranolol	Class III: Amiodarone	Class IV: Verapamil
Electrophysiologic						
Depolarization rate (phase 0)	↓	? ↓	↓ ↓	–	–	–
Conduction velocity	↓ ↑	↓	↓ ↑	↓ ←	↑ ↓	–
Effective refractory period (ERP)	↑ ↑	? ↓	↑	–	↑ ↑	→
Action potential duration (APD)	↑	? ↓	? ↑	–	↑ ↑	→
Automaticity	↓	↓	↓	↓	↓	–
ECG						
PR duration	– ↑ Procainamide; ↑ ↑ Quinidine; ↑ ↑ Disopyramide	– or ↓ Lidocaine; – or ↓ Mexiletine; – or ↓ Tocainide; ↓ Phenytoin	↑ ↓	– or ↑	↑ ↓	– or ↑
QRS duration			↑ ↑	– ↓	↑ ↑	–
QT duration					↑ ↑	–

Legend: ↑ = increase, ↓ = decrease, – = no change, ? = variable.
(SCIENTIFIC AMERICAN *Medicine*, Section 1, Subsection V. © 1988 Scientific American, Inc. All rights reserved.)

cainide): marked phase 0 depression; slow conduction with little effect on repolarization.

   2. Class II agents are beta-adrenergic receptor blockers. They slow conduction and increase the effective refractory period.
   3. Class III agents (amiodarone, bretylium) inhibit myocardial cell repolarization and increase the effective refractory period.
   4. Class IV agents are calcium channel blockers. They decrease the action potential duration.
   5. Class V: some authors consider digoxin, when used as an antiarrhythmic agent because of its cholinergic effects, a fifth class.

B. A rough estimate of the effectiveness of antiarrhythmic therapy can be made by auscultation and radial artery palpation. A preoperative 12-lead ECG should be examined for rate, rhythm, and ischemic changes. In patients with ectopy, a long rhythm strip of three ECG leads can be requested.

C. Plasma drug concentration measurement is commonly available for many antiarrhythmic agents (Table 1-12). Monitoring plasma levels helps guide drug administration.

V. CONTRIBUTING FACTORS

A. Oxygenation and ventilation abnormalities: hypoxemia, hypocarbia, especially when associated with hypokalemia, and hypercarbia.

B. Endotracheal Intubation and Suctioning
   1. Inadequate anesthesia with increased release of endogenous catecholamines
   2. Vagal stimulation (bladder and bowel distention, manipulation of the trachea and neck) may produce sinus bradycardia and permit ventricular escape mechanisms to act.

C. Anesthetic Agents
   1. Halogenated hydrocarbons such as halothane or enflurane produce dysrhythmias by a re-entrant mechanism.
   2. Halothane may sensitize the myocardium to both endogenous and exogenous catecholamines.
   3. Drugs such as cocaine and ketamine that block the reuptake of catecholamines can increase the incidence of dysrhythmias.
   4. Muscle relaxants that have vagal effects, such as

Table 1–12. Dosage and Effects of Antiarrhythmic Drugs

Drug (Trade name)	Dosage and Interval	Adverse Effects	Effective Plasma Concentrations
Quinidine (many brands)	qid PO loading: 300 mg q 3 hours PO maintenance: 324 mg q 6 hours	Diarrhea, nausea, vomiting, prolonged QT interval, thrombocytopenia, hypotension, rashes, cinchonism (vertigo, tinnitus, headache, fever, visual disturbances)	1.2–4.0 µg/ml
Procainamide (Pronestyl; others)	IV loading: 12–15 mg/kg; infusion rate not to exceed 100 mg/5 min IV maintenance: 2–4 mg/min PO loading: 14 mg/kg PO maintenance: 7 mg/kg q 4 hours	Lupus-like syndrome, confusion, diarrhea, nausea, vomiting, rash, hypotension, agranulocytosis	4–8 µg/ml
Propranolol (Inderal; others)	IV: 1–6 mg total (1 mg/2–3 min) PO: 10–80 mg q 6 hours	Heart block, hypotension, heart failure, fatigue, thrombocytopenia purpura	Not established: 50–100 ng/ml required for β-adrenergic blockade
Disopyramide (Norpace)	PO loading: 4 mg/kg PO maintenance: 150 mg q 6 hours	Anticholinergic effects, hypotension, heart failure, prolonged QT interval	2–4 µg/ml
Lidocaine (Xylocaine; others)	IV loading: 1–1.5 mg/kg over 2–3 min IV maintenance: 2–4 mg/min (30 µg/kg per min)	Confusion, seizures; cardiac depression at high concentration	1.5–6 µg/ml

Drug	Dosage	Toxicity / Side Effects	Therapeutic Level
Phenytoin	IV loading: 50 mg/5 min to a total of 1000 mg (12–15 mg/kg) IV maintenance: 200–400 mg/day PO loading: 14 mg/kg PO maintenance: 200–400 mg/day	Nystagmus, ataxia, vertigo, confusion, drowsiness, marrow depression; cardiac depression with rapid infusion	10–20 μg/ml
Bretylium	IV loading: 5 mg/kg; may repeat with 10 mg/kg IV maintenance: 1–2 mg/min	Hypotension, increased sensitivity to catecholamines, initial increase in arrhythmias	Measurement not essential
Amiodarone	PO loading: 600 mg q 12 hours for 2 weeks PO maintenance: 200–400 mg/day	Photosensitivity, corneal deposits, peripherial neuropathy, tremors, proximal muscle weakness, pulmonary alveolitis, hypothyroidism, prolonged QT interval	1.0–3.5 μg/ml
Verapamil (Calan, Isoptin)	IV loading: 5–10 mg over 2–3 min IV maintenance: 0.125–0.25 mg/min PO dose: 80–120 mg tid, qid	Heart block, hypotension, heart failure	100–300 ng/ml
Digoxin	IV loading: 1 mg over 24 hours divided into ____ doses IV maintenance: 0.125–0.25 mg/day PO loading: 1–1.5 mg over 24 hours divided into ____ doses PO maintenance: 0.125–0.25 mg/day	Nausea, vomiting, heart block; arrhythmias, especially with hypokalemia; delirium	1–1.5 ng/ml

pancuronium and succinylcholine, may cause supraventricular tachycardia and bradycardia, respectively.

D. Other Illnesses

1. Cardiac disease
   a. Existing dysrhythmias
   b. Left- or right-sided heart failure
   c. Valvular disease
   d. Myocardial ischemia
2. Illnesses and drug therapy
   a. Sympathomimetic drugs and methylxanthine derivatives used for treating bronchospasm increase the incidence of dysrhythmias associated with general anesthesia.
   b. Tricyclics, phenothiazines, and monoamine oxidase (MAO) inhibitors increase the incidence of supraventricular and ventricular dysrhythmias.
   c. Digoxin used for congestive failure can be dysrhythmogenic, especially if the patient is hypokalemic.

E. Ventricular Catheterization

Right-heart catheterization with a pulmonary artery (PA) catheter is frequently accompanied by ventricular premature contractions (VPCs). Dysrhythmias usually resolve spontaneously after the catheter tip passes into the PA. If dysrhythmias persist, intravenous lidocaine will usually control them until the catheter is repositioned or removed.

VI. MANAGEMENT

A. Perioperative monitoring for dysrhythmias should be with ECG lead II. The hemodynamic effects of dysrhythmias cannot be predicted from a single ECG. An intra-arterial catheter or a pulse oximeter can help determine the effect of supraventricular or ventricular dysrhythmias on blood pressure and peripheral perfusion.

B. Asymptomatic bradycardia with premature atrial beats does not require specific therapy.

C. Symptomatic Bradycardia

1. Stop intake of any drugs (digoxin, verapamil, β-blockers) that suppress sinoatrial or atrioventricular (AV) nodal activity.
2. Atropine (0.5–1 mg), isoproterenol (3–30 ng/kg per

min), or cardiac pacing may be needed to increase the heart rate and blood pressure.

D. Patients with suspected sick sinus syndrome should be investigated before any elective surgery and a decision made as to whether temporary or permanent cardiac pacing is necessary. In the presence of supraventricular dysrhythmias in patients suspected of having sick sinus syndrome, a temporary pacemaker should be placed before use of digoxin, verapamil, or β-blockers.

E. Supraventricular Tachydysrhythmias
  1. In the absence of heart failure, sinus tachycardia may be treated with small amounts of a β-blocker.
  2. Patients with atrial fibrillation, atrial flutter, and paroxysmal atrial tachycardia should have ventricular rates well controlled (<100 beats/min) with oral digoxin, verapamil, or β-blockers before surgery.
  3. Acute onset of supraventricular dysrhythmia with a rapid ventricular rate should be treated with intravenous verapamil, digoxin, or a β-blocker (Table 1-13). If there is life-threatening hypotension or failure to respond to drugs, synchronized DC conversion or overdrive pacing should be used.

F. Ventricular Dysrhythmias
  1. Ventricular premature contractions
     a. Chronic VPCs, if previously asymptomatic and untreated, do not require medical therapy in the perioperative period.
     b. Acute perioperative onset of VPCs may be associated with conditions that can be corrected readily, such as hypoxemia, hypercarbia, hypokalemia, ischemia, stress, or bradycardia. If VPCs are frequent (>5/min) or cause symptoms of hypoperfusion, a lidocaine bolus and infusion should be used to suppress the dysrhythmia for essential surgery (Table 1-13). In cases of ventricular dysrhythmias that are resistant to lidocaine, procainamide or bretylium may be alternatives.
  2. Ventricular tachycardia and fibrillation
     a. Ventricular tachycardia
        Initially, drug therapy may be tried if perfusion pressure is being maintained. In the presence

Table 1–13. *Treatment of Common Dysrhythmias*

Dysrhythmia	Treatment of Choice	Alternatives
Atrial fibrillation	Digoxin	Verapamil or propranolol to control ventricular rate Quinidine, disopyramide, or procainamide may be used for long-term suppression Cardioversion
Atrial fibrillation (associated with Wolf–Parkinson–White syndrome)	Procainamide	Phenytoin to control ventricular rate Cardioversion
Atrial flutter	Digoxin	Same as atrial fibrillation
Supraventricular tachycardia	Verapamil	Digoxin Propanolol Phenylephrine Edrophonium Cardioversion
Ventricular premature complexes (VPC)	Lidocaine	Procainamide Quinidine Tocainide Mexiletine Flecainide Encainide
Ventricular tachycardia	Cardioversion	Lidocaine Procainamide Bretylium
Digitalis-induced tachyarrhythmias	Lidocaine KCl	Phenytoin Procainamide Propranolol

of ineffective cardiac contractility, defibrillation is the treatment of choice followed by a lidocaine infusion. Surgery should be postponed if at all possible until the etiology of the dysrhythmia is found.

b. Ventricular fibrillation
Immediate asynchronous DC cardioversion with postponement of surgery for evaluation of potential causes of dysrhythmia is indicated.

VII. SUMMARY OF ANESTHETIC CONSIDERATIONS
Before surgery, reversible causes of dysrhythmias, such as electrolyte abnormalities, myocardial ischemia, and drug toxicity, should be corrected.

Antiarrhythmic medications should be taken preoperatively. Intravenous lidocaine or other antiarrhythmics that the patient is known to have responded to should be readily available. Anesthetic induction and maintenance should minimize the sympathetic response to stressful stimuli. Drugs such as halothane, ketamine, cocaine, and pancuronium can increase the incidence of intraoperative dysrhythmias, and their use should be avoided. Elective surgery should be delayed if there is new onset of supraventricular or ventricular dysrhythmias until the etiology is determined and effective therapy initiated.

Cardiac Pacemakers

Cardiac pacing has evolved greatly since its beginnings 25 years ago. Complete AV block, once one of the primary indications for pacing, now accounts for only one of many. Today, cardiac pacing is used to treat symptoms of organ hypoperfusion from bradydysrhythmias and for prophylaxis in patients with a high-degree AV block, especially in the setting of acute MI.

I. TEMPORARY PACING
  A. Indications
    1. Bradydysrhythmias and heart block
      a. First-degree heart block is usually asymptomatic and is not an indication for pacing.
      b. Second-degree heart block may be a harbinger of worsening conduction abnormalities. There are two types of second-degree block: the Mobitz Type I or Wenckebach and the Mobitz Type II. Mobitz Type I is often transient and seldom, if ever, necessitates pacing. Mobitz Type II block usually indicates destruction of the conduction system at the level of or below the bundle of His. Temporary pacing is generally indicated for acute management of Mobitz Type II block, with subsequent permanent pacemaker placement in the majority of patients.
      c. Acute development of third-degree heart block or complete AV block generally require immediate temporary pacing to maintain blood pressure and prevent ventricular escape beats.
      d. Severe sinus bradycardia after MI, during instances of profuse vagotonia, or during over-

doses of drugs that affect the conduction system, such as cholinergic agents, calcium channel antagonists, beta-blockers, and digoxin, may necessitate temporary pacing.

e. Other bradydysrhythmias, including atrial fibrillation with slow ventricular response, asystole, and bradydysrhythmias after cardioversion, and patients who are pacemaker dependent with pacemaker dysfunction are indications for temporary pacing.

2. Tachydysrhythmias

a. When tachydysrhythmias are refractory to drugs in circumstances when cardioversion is relatively contraindicated, such as digoxin therapy, anticipated prolonged asystole, or symptomatic bradycardia after cardioversion, or in the presence of pulmonary hypertension, temporary cardiac pacing can provide rapid effective treatment.

b. Temporary pacing is the therapy of first choice in managing patients with bradycardia-dependent ventricular tachycardia. Paroxysmal atrial tachycardia also responds well to temporary pacing. These two dysrhythmias are usually re-entrant rhythms with unidirectional block and slow conduction.

c. Overdrive pacing at rates 130% to 150% of spontaneous rates is recommended for interruption of the tachydysrhythmia. Once the abnormal rhythm is stopped, the pacemaker rate can be decreased to a more normal heart rate, used temporarily until antiarrhythmic therapy is established, or be stopped abruptly and reinstituted if necessary.

3. Prophylactic pacing

a. The prime prophylactic indication is acute MI complicated by various combinations of intraventricular, fascicular, and AV blocks. The most common situation is left anterior fascicular block and right bundle branch block, together with PR prolongation in the acute phase of anterior MI.

b. Other combinations include right bundle branch block and left posterior fascicular block, complete left bundle branch block, complete left bundle branch block with or without first-degree AV block, or Mobitz Type II second-degree AV block.

    c. Prophylactic pacing is rarely necessary in acute inferior-wall MI.

  4. Perioperative pacing

    a. Indications for inserting a temporary electrode preoperatively are based on the factors mentioned previously.

    b. Regional techniques and intravenous and general anesthesia have all been successful in patients with temporary cardiac pacemakers.

    c. There is no evidence that any of these anesthetic techniques will alter pacemaker thresholds or sensing capabilities.

B. Patient Evaluation

  1. Temporary cardiac pacing is usually considered for the patient with symptoms such as syncope, congestive heart failure, or angina secondary to a bradydysrhythmia or tachydysrhythmia. However, certain ECG changes in an asymptomatic patient with acute MI would indicate the need for prophylactic pacing, as previously mentioned, although further investigation may reveal a central nervous system, autonomic nervous system, or metabolic disorder.

  2. A variety of drugs may also cause ECG changes and symptoms (i.e., digoxin, propranolol, calcium channel blockers) in which careful observation or "reversal" drugs would be adequate therapy. In these cases, temporary pacing may not be necessary and may even be detrimental.

  3. Initial diagnostic tests should always include an ECG, chest radiograph, and measurement of hemoglobin and serum electrolytes. A pacing threshold and sensing potential should be established daily once a temporary pacemaker has been placed.

C. Pacemaker Identification

The type of pacing is best described by the International Classification of Heart Diseases (ICHD). The first letter of the code signifies the chamber(s) paced, the second letter the chamber(s) sensed, and the third letter the mode of response to a sensed P or R wave. Additional letters and

Table 1–14. Intersociety Commission for Heart Disease Code for Cardiac Pacemakers

I Chamber(s) Paced	II Chamber(s) Sensed	III Mode of Response(s)	IV Program- mable Functions	V Special Tachydys- rhythmia Function

V Ventricle
A Atrium
D Double
	V Ventricle
	A Atrium
	D Double
	0 None
		T Triggered
		I Inhibited
		D Double
		R Reverse
			P Program-
			  mable
			M Multipro-
			  grammable
			C Commun-
			  icating
			0 None
				B Bursts
				N Normal
				  rate
				  competition
				S Scanning
				E External

positions are intended primarily for permanent pacemakers (Table 1-14).

D. Transvenous Pacemakers

   1. Pacing modes

    a. The asynchronous pacemaker was the first and simplest. This pacemaker will emit impulses no matter what the patient's heart rate. The asynchronous pacemaker is wasteful of energy and has a remote chance of causing ventricular fibrillation if the pacemaker impulse occurs while the myocardium is repolarizing. In the ICHD system, ventricular and atrial asynchronous pacemakers are coded VOO and AOO, respectively.

    b. The synchronous pacemaker has replaced the asynchronous type. This pacemaker is capable of detecting P or R waves. If the pacemaker detects a wave and immediately emits an impulse into the refractory myocardium, then it is a triggered pacemaker. When the patient's heart rate is less than the pacemaker rate, the generator paces the ventricle. However, if the patient's heart rate is greater than the pacemaker rate, competition does not occur because the pacemaker impulses will be triggered to discharge into the QRS complex. If the pacemaker detects a wave and the generator impulse is stopped, the pacemaker is an inhibited (demand) type. This type of pacemaker eliminates competition and is practical in terms of energy conservation.

c. The most common pacing mode is VVI, or R-wave inhibited, where pacing and sensing occur via a single lead in the ventricle, and the pacemaker's output is inhibited when an R wave is sensed during the pacemaker's escape interval. Similarly, the AAI mode is P-wave-inhibited pacing.

d. Dual-chamber pacing is ideal because the atrial contribution to ventricular stroke volume is preserved. Dual-chamber pacing requires electrodes in the atrium and ventricle. The most common temporary dual-chamber pacing is the AV sequential (DVI) mode. The AV sequential mode paces the atrium and the ventricle. R-wave detection above the set pacemaker rate will inhibit atrial and ventricular pacing. This pacemaker is "blind" to atrial activity, and atrial pacing may compete with the patient's own intrinsic atrial rhythm. A temporary fully automatic AV universal (DDD) pacemaker is available but rarely used. The DDD pacemakers sense and pace in both chambers; they will inhibit when a spontaneous QRS is sensed in the ventricle, and a native P wave will trigger a ventricular output stimulus after a set electronic AV interval. Thus, the DDD ECG may show atrial pacing, AV sequential pacing, or P-wave-triggered ventricular pacing.

e. Selection of the most suitable temporary pacing mode is based on four considerations: therapeutic objectives; electrophysiologic findings, i.e., rhythm and conduction; hemodynamic needs; and technical factors.

1) If the object of temporary pacing is to provide prophylactic rate support, then single-chamber ventricular pacing usually will suffice. If the goal is to optimize cardiac function, one should select the most physiologic approach.

2)   Single-chamber atrial pacing (AAI) may be adequate for individuals with slow sinus rates and intact AV conduction. Atrial pacing is contraindicated in the presence of AV block, and it is ineffective in the presence of atrial fibrillation.

3)   Sequential AV pacing in patients with AV block or atrial pacing maintains AV synchrony and preserves the normal sequence of ventricular depolarization. Compared with ventricular pacing, atrial and AV sequential pacing increase stroke volume 10% to 20% by augmenting preload. Also, mean atrial pressures are reduced by eliminating AV dissociation.

4)   The DDD offers the same hemodynamic advantages as atrial or AV sequential pacing but also provides rate responsiveness. The DDD pacemaker will vary its pacing rate on the basis of sinus node activity that usually will increase with an increase in the need for blood flow.

E.   Leads and Insertion Techniques

1.   Any of the temporary transvenous pacing electrodes may be introduced into the central circulation through a large-bore catheter placed by the Seldinger technique (needle and guidewire). In most cases, the subclavian or internal jugular approach is used to provide both better lead stability and greater patient freedom. The brachial and femoral veins have also been utilized.

2.   Temporary pacing electrodes or catheters are available for single- and dual-chamber pacing. The flow-directed (balloon-tipped) catheters have largely replaced the stiff woven Dacron catheters because the latter require fluoroscopy for placement. Moreover, the stiff catheters are more likely to perforate a vessel or to become displaced than are the more flexible flow-directed catheters.

3.   The simple balloon-tipped ventricular catheter is easily placed but unstable. Newer catheters have flared tips, which may help prevent lead movement. Two pacing Swan-Ganz catheters are available. One has external electrodes for atrial and ventricular

pacing. These electrodes are placed so that they should be in reasonable position to pace the atrium and ventricle after the catheter has been correctly positioned in the PA. The other type has a separate lumen to insert a pacing electrode into the right ventricle.

F. Pacemaker Evaluation

    1. Pacing threshold

        a. Good lead performance is present when the threshold of stimulation is low and the intracardiac signal (R or P wave) has sufficient amplitude for sensing. Pacing thresholds of less than 1 mA would be optimal for atrial or ventricular leads.

        b. Testing the pacing threshold is accomplished by slowly lowering the milliamperage until the paced QRS (or P wave) complex disappears, leaving only the pacemaker spikes and ECG signs of the patient's spontaneous heart activity. Then the milliamperage is slowly raised to the pacing threshold where the pacing spike is coupled to the QRS complex.

        c. The threshold of stimulation rises after lead insertion because of an inflammatory response or necrosis at the electrode–tissue interface. The magnitude of the threshold rise may be as much as threefold to fourfold. To compensate for the potential increase in pacing threshold, the pacemaker is set at two to three times the electrical threshold.

        d. Ordinarily, a newly implanted catheter electrode should pace at 3 mA or less. If pacing threshold is greater than 6 mA, the catheter should be repositioned.

    2. Sensing potential

        a. With the use of a demand pacemaker, the sensing of the catheter electrode must also be tested to determine if the catheter tip is able to detect electrical stimuli (R or P wave) from the endocardium, which allows the generator to be inhibited or act in a "demand" mode.

        b. A QRS-inhibited (VVI) pacemaker usually has a sensing threshold of approximately 2 to 3 mV. Therefore, the amplitude of the QRS complex of a bipolar lead from the right ventricular cavity should be at least 1 to 2 mV greater than the sensing threshold to make certain it is strong enough to trigger the pacemaker. In the case of the VVI pacemaker, this means inhibition of the electrical pacing signal.

c.   When a bipolar catheter electrode is used, the signal from the electrode at the catheter tip and the signal from the electrode proximal to the tip should be checked individually by taking a unipolar lead ECG from each of these locations. With an intracardiac ECG, 1 mV causes a 1-cm deflection. Turning the standardization to one-fourth will usually allow the entire endocardial deflection to be seen. The sensitivity of the sensing threshold may be changed from a small QRS complex (demand setting) preventing triggering of the pacemaker to a setting where the largest QRS complex will not inhibit the pacemaker (asynchronous mode). If the QRS complex has a small endocardial amplitude of less than 2 mV, the electrode tip should be repositioned. In most circumstances, setting the electrical sensing dial on the generator on demand or up to 3 to 4 mV is adequate for pacing needs without testing for sensitivity threshold.

G.   Conditions Affecting Transvenous Pacemakers

1.   Pacing failure
Failure to obtain an adequate threshold or intracardiac signal may be attributable to poor contact between the electrode and endocardium, local endocardial necrosis or fibrosis, hypoxia or acidosis, hypokalemia, or drug effects, particularly with type I antiarrhythmics. Specific causes of pacing failure intraoperatively are the use of electrocautery and the myopotentials from muscle fasciculations caused by succinylcholine or shivering.

2.   Complications

a.   The principal complications of temporary cardiac pacing are related to placement, presence of a foreign body, and improper functioning. Catheter placement may be complicated by refractory dysrhythmias, pneumothorax, hemothorax, cardiac perforation and tamponade, and arterial puncture and bleeding. Infection may occur at any point in the pacemaker system, with resultant sepsis. As with most invasive catheters, the skin site is the usual source of bacteria. Thrombosis and thrombophlebitis are not uncommon at the site of insertion, which will increase the risk of infection.

b. After the initial placement of the electrode lead, complications such as lead displacement, extracardiac muscle stimulation, lead fracture, induction of dysrhythmias, and cardiac perforation may occur.

c. Sometimes, it is necessary to remove the temporary pacing electrode because of malfunction. The majority can be pulled out by gentle traction. Complications of forceful prolonged traction include ventricular tachycardia, ventricular fibrillation, shock from invagination of the right ventricular wall to the tricuspid valve, intracardiac lead rupture, and tear of the right side of the heart.

H. Perioperative Considerations

1. Potassium

a. Preoperative correction of serum potassium is especially important in patients with pacemakers. The normal intracellular-to-extracellular potassium ratio maintains a resting membrane potential of -90 mV. Acutely increasing the extracellular potassium by rapid potassium administration, tissue ischemia, muscular fasciculation, or hypoventilation will lower the usual 30:1 ratio, creating a less negative resting membrane potential. The preoperative pacemaker output setting then can more easily stimulate the myocardium to contract, increasing the potential for ventricular tachycardia or fibrillation. The opposite occurs when the potassium ratio rises acutely.

b. Hyperventilation or intraoperative diuresis producing an extracellular potassium decrease, making the resting membrane potential more negative, could cause a loss of pacing capture.

2. Electrical interference

   a. Electrocautery

     1) The use of electrocautery is a significant cause of pacemaker failure. With temporary pacemakers, the external generators can simply be adjusted to the asynchronous mode when the electrocautery is being used frequently.

     2) Implanted VOO or AOO nonprogrammable generators are not affected by electrocautery.

     3) The newer ventricular-inhibited nonprogrammable pacemakers (VVI) revert to asynchronous activity after they have turned off for one impulse because of electromagnetic interference. Once the interference is removed, the pacemaker will revert to the VVI mode. The older VVI generators were completely inhibited by electromagnetic interference. A magnet over the pacer generator was necessary to convert the pacemaker from the demand mode to an asynchronous mode.

     4) Multiprogrammable pacemakers should be programmed to asynchronous activity preoperatively, or one should have a programmer device on hand that can immediately reprogram the pacemaker to a VVI or VOO mode. The danger with programmable pacemakers is the potential for random reprogramming with electrocautery, especially if a magnet is used.

     5) To help decrease the interference from electrocautery, recommendations are to use electrocautery in short bursts, use bipolar electrocautery, locate the ground plate as far as possible from the pacer generator (never have the generator between the ground pad and the pacing electrode), and set the electrocautery current at the lowest functional level.

6) Less likely complications are inhibition of generators by myopotentials from muscle fasciculations caused by succinylcholine and postoperative shivering. This problem can be circumvented by reprogramming the generator to the asynchronous mode or to decreased R-wave sensitivity.

3. Patients with congestive heart failure and a cardiac pacemaker may be anticoagulated. Therefore, caution must be used when using regional anesthesia techniques. There is the potential for dislodging the pacing electrode with central venous catheters; however, if a central venous pressure line or PA catheter is needed, its use should not be prohibited.

I. Alternatives to Temporary Transvenous Cardiac Pacing

1. External transcutaneous pacing

The external transcutaneous pacemaker (ETCP), originally described by Zoll in 1952, has been reintroduced in the form of an improved device that operates in the demand mode (VVI). The ETCP is easy to use and noninvasive, making it ideal for use in the field or while preparing a patient for transvenous pacing.

a. Large external electrode pads of high impedance are placed on the precordium and on the back at the cardiac level between the left scapula and the spine, and the monitor leads are attached to the generator. The pacing rate is set above the patient's intrinsic rate. The pacemaker output is lowered to 0, and the power is turned on. The pacemaker amplitude is increased until a stimulated QRS response follows the pacing artifact. The pacing current is kept just above the electrical threshold, and the pacing rate is adjusted to the rate desired.

b. Ventricular pacing thresholds are usually between 40 and 70 mA. At the lower end of the range, the pacing sensation is tolerable, with a mild thumping feeling and pectoral twitching. Higher pacing currents may cause a severe thumping sensation, an intense burning or stinging, and intolerable muscle twitching.

2. Transesophageal pacing

Transesophageal pacing is another noninvasive

technique that may be used by individuals not trained in transvenous pacing electrode placement or when pacing needs to be established rapidly prior to correction of coagulopathies or in the presence of venous abnormalities. Ventricular pacing by the transesophageal route works well in the infant and small child.

    a.   In the adult, atrial pacing is easily achieved with pacing currents between 20 and 30 mA. Because of the distance of the ventricle from the esophagus, ventricular pacing is difficult to achieve, and the pacing threshold is high, making pacing in an awake patient extremely uncomfortable.

    b.   The generator is usually the AAI or VVI type.

    c.   Because of the simplicity, ease of application, and more dependable ventricular pacing, transcutaneous pacing has relegated transesophageal pacing to a rarely used temporary modality.

3.   Transthoracic pacing

In the past, the transthoracic approach has been successful in emergency circumstances. However, with the introduction of an effective transcutaneous cardiac pacemaker, the transthoracic approach is rarely warranted, generally being used only if no other form of pacing is available.

    a.   This method of temporary pacing has significant complications, which include pneumothorax, coronary artery perforation, mediastinal bleeding, and cardiac tamponade.

    b.   The transthoracic entry site is just to the left of the sternum in the fourth intercostal space with the needle and stylet being directed perpendicular to the chest wall. Another approach has the needle enter just to the left of the xiphoid process, aiming down at a 45° angle toward the left nipple. Connecting the stylet and needle to the V lead of a standard ECG yields an "injury current" upon penetration of the right ventricular wall, providing that there is not complete ventricular asystole. Subsequent removal of the stylet and aspiration of blood allows the pacing electrode to be passed through the needle into the right side of the heart. The electrode is then connected to a standard external transvenous pacemaker generator.

II. PERMANENT PACING

A. Preoperative Evaluation

    1. History

During the preoperative visit, a detailed history of cardiac pacemaker performance is obtained. Signs of pacemaker malfunction should be sought: symptoms of decreased cerebral perfusion; inappropriate pacing of pectoral muscle or diaphragm twitching (likely attributable to faulty lead insulation), skipped beats (secondary to myopotential oversensing); and weakness, orthostatic hypotension, or decreased exercise tolerance (pacemaker syndrome). Pain over the pulse generator pocket may be the result of infection or tissue erosion.

    2. Diagnostic tests

        a. Chest radiograph should be checked for lead position or fracture.

        b. Electrocardiogram

            1) The 12-lead ECG is examined for pacemaker rate, pacemaker QRS morphology, and the relation of the pacemaker spikes to the spontaneous and paced QRS. The morphology of the paced QRS complex indicates the paced site: the paced QRS has a left bundle branch block (**LBBB**) pattern if the paced site is in the right ventricle (**RV**) and a right bundle branch block (**RBBB**) pattern if the paced site is the left ventricle (**LV**), distal coronary sinus, or right ventricular septum. If the RV is supposed to be the pacing site and the ECG shows an RBBB pattern, the lead may be pacing the right ventricular septum, or it may have perforated the septum.

            2) Attenuated pacemaker spikes suggest battery failure, electrical short circuit, or lead fracture. If the pacemaker spike is not followed by a QRS pattern, the pacemaker is not capturing. Failure to capture may be attributable to lead dislodgment, subthreshold stimulus secondary to a low battery or inappropriately low programmed energy output, lead fracture, or perielectrode fibrosis, which may occur 1 to 8 weeks after pacemaker insertion. Failure to capture may also be the result of decreased thyroid function, decreased serum potassium, type I antiarrhythmic drugs, or excessive digoxin levels.

3) Unipolar lead systems show greater amplitude in the pacemaker spike because of the larger distance between the cathode (intracardiac) and the anode (the generator). The amplitude does not necessarily reflect the voltage output. These pacemakers are more susceptible to oversensing of pectoralis muscle myopotentials and extraneous radio signals (electrocautery).

3. Evaluation of capabilities of a demand pacemaker

a. One way to test the pacemaker is to slow the patient's intrinsic heart rate below the preset demand rate by a Valsalva maneuver or small doses (2–10 mg IV) of edrophonium. Carotid sinus massage is not recommended because of the risk of arteriosclerotic plaque embolizing to the brain.

b. As a general rule, sensing capabilities are lost before pacing. If the generator is less than 2 years old, the chest radiograph shows no breaks in the lead, and no inappropriate pacing impulses appear on the ECG, then the pacing portion of the generator probably is working correctly. Present-day pulse generators last 7 to 10 years on a lithium battery.

c. When a magnet is applied over the pacemaker generator, it closes a reed switch, eliminates the sensing circuit, and converts the demand pacemaker to an asynchronous mode, pacing at a preset rate. If magnet application does not produce pacemaker spikes, then the power source is depleted, a component has failed, or an incomplete circuit exists secondary to lead fracture or a loose connection between the lead and the generator. Pacemaker units with non-adjustable rates should not differ by more than 2 beats/min from the programmed rate. If the magnet rate is decreased by 6 beats/min or 10% from the set rate, the pacemaker battery needs replacement. It is important to know the end-of-life indicators for specific pacemakers (provided by the manufacturer) because some pacemakers indicate end of life by an increase in rate.

    d. Dysrhythmias caused by magnet application are rare. However, magnets should not be used with programmable units, because this may permit random reprogramming by the electrocautery. The magnet turns on a receiver that enables the pacemaker to receive rate programming instructions. Random radio signals sent by electrocautery, particularly spark-gap type unipolar electrocautery, may then reprogram the pacemaker.

4. Evaluation of sensing function

    a. Undersensing is the failure of the pacemaker to sense atrial or ventricular depolarizations that fall outside the programmed refractory period. This can be the result of an inadequate intracardiac signal, battery failure, lead fracture, perielectrode fibrosis, inappropriately low sensing settings, high serum potassium, or high serum levels of class I antiarrhythmic agents.

    b. Oversensing may lead to pauses in the paced rhythm and may be secondary to false signals caused by lead fracture or contact of two electrodes in the same cardiac chamber, pectoralis muscle myopotentials, and electromagnetic interference (EMI). Persistent EMI may lead to asynchronous pacing when the preset interference rate is reached.

B. Perioperative Problems with Permanent Pacemakers

    1. If a demand pacemaker is not programmable, it can be converted to an asynchronous mode when necessary by applying an external magnet. With multi-programmable units, the pacemakers should be programmed preoperatively to either the ventricular asynchronous or the ventricular demand mode.

2. To prevent pacemaker problems with EMI, the EMI ground pad is placed as close to the operative site as possible. The ground plate should be located so that the current path from the electrocautery tip is as far as possible from the pulse generator and lead. If the current path and pacemaker electrode intersect, current induction in the electrode will be minimized if the intersection is perpendicular. Electrocautery is limited to brief bursts. Most present-day pacemakers will revert automatically to an asynchronous mode in the presence of EMI. Contact between the electrocautery probe and the pacemaker generator must be avoided, as this may overheat and destroy the pacemaker circuitry.

3. Unipolar pacemakers can be inhibited by myopotentials generated by voluntary or involuntary muscle movements (e.g., seizures, succinylcholine-induced fasciculations, myoclonic movements). This is especially true with passively fixed (temporary) endocardial electrodes or recently implanted actively fixed (screw-in) endocardial electrodes. After a period of 4 to 6 weeks of electrode stabilization, this should not be a problem with actively fixed endocardial electrodes.

4. Intraoperative hyperventilation, hypokalemia, and class I antiarrhythmics may necessitate increased energy output for capture and pacing.

5. Automatic implanted cardiac defibrillators (AICD) can be discharged accidently with electrocautery or other electrical signals generated by surgical equipment. Therefore, AICDs should be turned off preoperatively and turned back on in the postanesthetic care unit.

III. SUMMARY OF ANESTHETIC CONSIDERATIONS

The principal indications for cardiac pacing are symptomatic bradydysrhythmias and heart block, tachydysrhythmias, and prophylaxis in acute anterior myocardial infarctions with high-degree heart block. After placement of transvenous cardiac pacemakers, sensing and pacing capabilities should be established. If excess energy levels are required for pacing, then the pacing electrodes should be repositioned before surgery. Inhalational anesthetics will not affect the pacing threshold. Regional anesthesia can be used without interfering with pacemaker function unless large doses of local anesthetic are given with significant systemic absorption. Changes in serum potassium concentration, shivering, muscle fasciculation from administration of succinylcholine, and electrocautery can interfere with pacemaker function. Changing cardiac pacemakers to the asynchronous mode with either an external magnet or a pacemaker reprogrammer will prevent electrical interference from inhibiting pacemaker function. Patients with AICD should have the unit switched off preoperatively, because electrical activity from the surgical field can cause accidental discharge. Alternatives to transvenous pacing include external transcutaneous, transesophageal, and transthoracic cardiac pacing.

Recommended Reading

Atlee JL III. Perioperative cardiac dysrhythmias: mechanisms, recognition, management. Chicago: Year Book Medical Publishers, 1985.

Atlee JL III. Pacemakers and cardioversion. In: Kaplan J, ed. Cardiac anesthesia. 2nd ed. New York: Grune and Stratton, 1987:855.

Backofen JE, Schauble JF, Rogers MC. Transesophageal pacing for bradycardia. Anesthesiology 1984;61:777.

Bhatia S, Goldschlager N. Office evaluation of the pacemaker patient: detection of normal and abnormal pacemaker function. JAMA 1985;254:1346.

Chung EK. What's new in cardiac pacing in myocardial infarction. Hosp Cardiol 1979;12:22.

Dreifus LS, Michelson EL, Kaplinski E. Bradyarrhythmias: clinical significance and management. J Am Coll Cardiol 1983;1:327.

Gallagher JJ, Smith WM, Kerr CR, et al. Esophageal pacing: a diagnostic and therapeutic tool. Circulation 1982;65:336.

Goldberger E. Treatment of cardiac emergencies. 4th ed. St Louis: CV Mosby, 1985:243.

Hauser RG, Vicari RM. Temporary pacing: indications, modes, and techniques. Med Clin North Am 1986;70:813.

Higgins JR. Temporary cardiac pacemakers. In: Civetta JM, Taylor RW, Kirby RR, eds. Critical care. New York: JB Lippincott, 1988:227.

Okumura K, Henthorn RW, Epstein AE, Plumb VJ, Waldo AL. Further observations on transient entrainment: importance of pacing site and properties of the components of the re-entry circuit. Circulation 1985;72:1293.

Perry RS, Illsley SS. Basic cardiac electrophysiology and mechanisms of antiarrhythmic agents. Am J Hosp Pharm 1986;43:957.

Pillar LW, Lennelly BM. Myopotential inhibition of demand pacemakers. Chest 1977;66:418.

Schrager BR, Cully J, Chahine RA. Temporary cardiac pacing. In: Sprung CL, Grenvik A, eds. Invasive procedures in critical care. New York: Churchill Livingstone, 1985:167.

Serwer GA, Eckerd JM, Kelly EE, et al. Emergency ventricular pacing from the esophagous in infancy. Am J Cardiol 1986;58:1105.

Shively B, Goldschlager N. Progress in cardiac pacing. Arch Intern Med 1985;145:2103.

Simon AB. Perioperative management of pacemaker patient. Anesthesiology 1977;46:127.

Singh BN, Opie LH, Harrison DC, et al. Antiarrhythmic agents. In: Opie LH, ed. Drugs for the heart. New York: Grune and Stratton, 1983.

Waldo AL, Wells JL, Cooper TB, Maclean WAH. Temporary cardiac pacing: applications and techniques in the treatment of cardiac arrhythmias. Progr Cardiovasc Dis 1981;23:451.

Weng JT, Smith DE, Moulder PV. Antiarrhythmic drugs: electrophysiological basis of their clinical usage. Ann Thorac Surg 1986;41:106.

Zaidan JR. Pacemakers. Anesthesiology 1984;60:319.

Zaidan JR, Curling PE, Craver JM. Effect of enflurane, isoflurane and halothane on pacing stimulation thresholds in men. PACE 1985;8:32.

Zaidan JR. Pacemakers and programmable defibrillators. ASA Annual Refresher Course Lectures 1988;114:1.

Zoll PM, Zoll RH, Falk RH, et al. External noninvasive temporary cardiac pacing: clinical trials. Circulation 1985;71:937.

≡ Pericardial Disease and Cardiomyopathies

Peter J. Papadakos

Cardiac Tamponade

I.   DEFINITION

Cardiac tamponade is compromise of the heart muscle by an external influence sufficient to cause hemodynamic effects. Usually caused by the accumulation of fluid, blood, or air within the pericardial sac, it may also be caused by the extra-pericardial compression by fluid-filled, overdistended, non-compliant lungs.

II. ETIOLOGY

The causes of cardiac tamponade can be grouped into three categories.

A. Trauma, Blunt and Sharp

In trauma cases, tamponade may be lifesaving, in that it prevents exsanguination from the wounds to the heart or great vessels. This group may also include intrapericardial rupture from retrograde dissection of an aortic aneurysm.

B. After Open Heart Surgery

The classic signs of cardiac tamponade may be absent in patients in whom surgery has opened the pericardial sac and released uniform pressure. In this form of compression, only one chamber may be affected. A high degree of suspicion should be held in any patient with increasing intracardiac pressures after cardiac surgery.

C. Enlarging Pericardial Effusions

Etiologies include bacterial or viral infection, which are the most common cause, malignancy, uremia, radiation, connective tissue diseases, and bleeding secondary to anticoagulants. These effusions usually accumulate slowly and may attain large volumes before causing symptoms and hemodynamic effects.

III. PATHOPHYSIOLOGY

Normal intrapericardial pressure (IPP) is subatmospheric and is equal to intrapleural pressure. The determinants of IPP include intrapericardial volume and pericardial compliance. In the normal state, IPP has negligible effects on venous return and right-sided filling pressures. During tamponade, IPP increases so that the increased pressure in the pericardial sac becomes the principal factor influencing ventricular filling. The rate of fluid accumulation and the prior condition of the pericardium determine the effect of increasing IPP. If the accumulation is slow or the pericardium loose, a large amount of material may collect before hemodynamic changes occur. Conversely, the rapid accumulation of as little as 100 ml of material may result in marked hemodynamic instability.

A. Hemodynamic Effects of Pericardial Effusion

1. Stroke volume decreases.

2. Ventricular end-diastolic volume falls.

3. Ventricular filling pressures increase in relation to the rise in IPP so that eventually, with cardiac tamponade, diastolic pressure across the heart is equal:

$$IPP = RAP = RVEDP = PAOP = LVEDP$$

B. Increasing adrenergic discharge compensates for falling stroke volume producing the following compensatory mechanisms.
  1. Increasing heart rate is the most important compensatory mechanism in tamponade. Cardiac output and blood pressure become critically dependent on heart rate, because the stroke volume falls and eventually is fixed in response to external pressure.
  2. Peripheral resistance is increased by arteriolar constriction in order to maintain the systemic blood pressure.
  3. Venoconstriction facilitates preload.
  4. Increased contractility may increase ejection fraction and maintain stroke volume.

IV. CLINICAL FEATURES
  A. Signs and Symptoms
    1. The classic clinical features are tachycardia, tachypnea, orthopnea, dyspnea, and diaphoresis.
    2. Another common finding is pulsus paradoxus, which is an exaggeration (>10 mmHg) of the decrease in systolic blood pressure that normally occurs with inspiration.
    3. The combination of elevated central venous pressure, systemic hypotension with a decreased pulse pressure, and distant muffled heart sounds with an indeterminant apical impulse is known as Beck's triad. It is common in cardiac tamponade associated with trauma.
  B. Diagnostic Tests
    1. Chest radiography usually shows a nonspecific enlargement of the cardiac silhouette.
    2. Electrocardiogram changes are likewise nonspecific. There may be low voltage across all leads or electrical alternans of either the P wave or the QRS complex.
    3. The diagnostic gold standard is the echocardiogram, which will demonstrate echo-free spaces between the heart and pericardium representing pericardial fluid.

V. ANESTHETIC MANAGEMENT
  A. Cardiac tamponade or significant pericardial effusion should be drained preoperatively. With adequate fluid removal, signs and symptoms of tamponade should resolve.
  B. With resolution of pericardial compression, cardiac function should normalize, in which case special anesthetic preparation is not necessary.
  C. In the case of underlying myocardial dysfunction or the possibility of rapid reaccumulation of pericardial fluid, invasive monitoring with arterial and pulmonary artery (PA) catheterization is indicated.

Constrictive Pericarditis

I. DEFINITION
Constrictive pericarditis, like cardiac tamponade, causes hemodynamic changes by restricting ventricular filling. This restriction is caused by a stiff, fibrosed, unyielding pericardium rather than by accumulation of fluid.

II. ETIOLOGY
  A. Bacterial or Viral Infection
  B. Malignancy
  C. Radiation
  D. Uremia
  E. Connective Tissue Disease
  F. Idiopathic.

III. PATHOPHYSIOLOGY
The greatest inhibition of ventricular filling in constrictive pericarditis occurs in the last two-thirds of diastole, whereas in tamponade, it occurs throughout diastole. The stroke volume is usually maintained in constrictive pericarditis because left ventricular end-diastolic volume is preserved by the rapid filling in early diastole. The degree of elevation of ventricular filling pressures is dictated by the severity and duration of the constriction and intravascular blood volume. Equalization of right and left ventricular pressures and passive elevation of PA pressure indicates severe constrictive disease.

IV. CLINICAL FEATURES
  A. Symptoms include gradually increasing fatigue and dyspnea.
  B. Signs of increasing venous pressure are engorged neck veins, ascites, and peripheral edema.

    C. Pulsus paradoxus does not occur because the rigid pericardial sac is unable to transmit respiratory changes in the pleural pressure.

V. DIAGNOSTIC TESTS

    A. Chest radiography may show a normal or enlarged cardiac silhouette. Pulmonary congestion usually is absent.

    B. The ECG may be normal. Low voltage, left atrial hypertrophy, atrial fibrillation, or atrial flutter may be present.

    C. The echocardiogram is nonspecific. There may be an inspiratory increase in right ventricular diameter, an inspiratory decrease in left ventricular diameter, and respiratory changes in the motion of the aortic or mitral valve leaflets.

    D. Cardiac catheterization is the best method to differentiate constrictive pericarditis from other cardiac pathology. There should be equalization of diastolic pressures and between right and left ventricular filling pressures. Cardiac output is normal or reduced at rest and fails to increase appropriately with exercise.

VI. ANESTHETIC PLAN FOR PERICARDIECTOMY

    A. Preoperative medication must be given cautiously. Hypotension or a decrease in preload is poorly tolerated.

    B. Invasive monitors are necessary to help optimize preload and for titration of vasoactive drugs.

        1. Arterial catheterization should be accomplished preoperatively to have beat-to-beat blood pressure monitoring during induction.

        2. A Swan-Ganz catheter would be more beneficial than a central venous catheter. With the PA catheter, both right- and left-sided filling pressures can be measured, and it is possible to determine cardiac output.

    C. Intraoperative Anesthesia

        1. Anesthetic agents, such as potent inhalational agents, which cause myocardial depression should be avoided. Histamine-releasing drugs (morphine, *d*-tubocurarine) should not be used because of the possibility of decreasing preload.

        2. Drugs that preserve heart rate, such as pancuronium or ketamine, are useful.

        3. Positive measures, such as volume expansion, infusion of inotropes, oxygen supplementation, and afterload reduction, may improve intraoperative oxygen delivery and hemodynamics.

4. Antiarrhythmic agents and extracorporeal circulation may be needed during pericardiectomy when the surgical manipulation of the heart leads to dysrhythmias and failing cardiac output.

D. Postoperative Care

The patient's hemodynamic condition usually improves after surgical release of the constrictive process, and patients usually can be weaned rapidly from inotropic agents. Routine postoperative care in an ICU should include hemodynamic support and observation for postoperative dysrhythmias. A sudden decrease in mediastinal chest tube output and poor response to fluid challenges and inotropic agents may indicate reaccumulation of pericardial fluid and possible cardiac tamponade.

Hypertrophic Cardiomyopathy

I. PATHOPHYSIOLOGY

A. Hypertrophic cardiomyopathy (idiopathic hypertrophic subaortic stenosis, IHSS) is characterized by obstruction to left ventricular outflow secondary to asymmetrical hypertrophy of the intraventricular septum. It is a primary disease of the myocardium.

1. The subvalvular obstruction shows a beat-to-beat variability, unlike the obstruction of a fixed valvular stenosis. The mechanism of this process is an early to mid-systolic apposition of the anterior leaflet of the mitral valve and the intraventricular septum, which worsens with increased contractility. A pressure gradient develops between the left ventricular cavity and the aortic outflow tract.

2. The associated left ventricular hypertrophy is an attempt to overcome the obstruction to flow. The hypertrophy may reduce the volume of the left ventricular chamber.

B. Left ventricular systolic function is usually supernormal. This hyperfunction of the chamber often results in a cavitary obliteration during systole. Ejection fractions of 80% and greater are common. Heart failure is rare. If it does occur, it is in the late phase of the disease, usually related to a myocardial infarction or the progression of mitral regurgitation.

    C. Diastolic relaxation is markedly impaired in IHSS because isovolumic relaxation is prolonged and the fall in diastolic pressure extends to the middle of diastole, thereby shortening filling time. Diastolic compliance is also reduced, causing a rise in end-diastolic pressure that further impedes left ventricular filling and coronary perfusion.

II. CLINICAL FEATURES

    A. Symptoms of IHSS include chest pain, dyspnea, "graying-out" spells, and exercise-induced syncope.

    B. Signs of IHSS are presystolic apical thrust, pulsus biferiens, and a variable systolic murmur.

III. DIAGNOSTIC TESTS

    A. The ECG may demonstrate left ventricular hypertrophy with or without strain patterns. A Q wave may be present in leads 2, 3, or aVF or leads V_4–V_6. The common dysrhythmias are atrial and ventricular ectopic beats and also ventricular or supraventricular tachycardias with or without fibrillation.

    B. Echocardiography may make the diagnosis, as can cardiac catheterization.

IV. ANESTHETIC PLAN

    A. The key goal during anesthesia for patients with IHSS is to decrease the pressure gradient across the left ventricular outflow tract. This can be done by decreasing myocardial contractility, increasing ventricular volume, or increasing afterload.

    B. Anesthetic Drugs

        1. An ideal induction agent is thiopental. It is readily available and has a mild myocardial and sympathetic depressant effect.

        2. Nitrous oxide plus halothane is excellent for the maintenance of anesthesia in that it causes a mild myocardial depression without a marked decrease in systemic vascular resistance and blood pressure.

        3. Narcotic anesthesia is not as good as inhalational anesthesia, because narcotics do not have a significant myocardial depressant effect and they also decrease systemic vascular resistance.

        4. A cardiovascularly stable muscle relaxant should be used (vecuronium, atracurium). Those such as pancuronium that increase heart rate and myocardial contractility should not be used.

    C. Perioperative Complications

        1. Intraoperative and postoperative hypotension is

best treated with fluid loading, an alpha-1-receptor agonist, or both. Positive inotropic agents should not be used.

   2. Sinus rhythm should be preserved. Beta-blockers may be used for junctional, atrial, and ventricular tachycardia. Verapamil is an effective alternative to beta-blockers for slowing atrial tachycardias. Both agents must be titrated carefully because either can cause significant myocardial depression and hypotension that will worsen outflow obstruction.

V. MONITORING

   A. Arterial catheterization should be used to provide continuous monitoring of blood pressure.

   B. Central venous pressure and PA catheters are not helpful because of the wide variability in intraventricular pressure from changes in the obstructive process.

   C. Intraoperative echocardiography may be useful in determining the effectiveness of anesthetic management.

Congestive Cardiomyopathy

I. DEFINITION AND ETIOLOGY

Dilated cardiomyopathies are acute or chronic disorders that affect the myocardium diffusely or in a multifocal fashion and decrease contractility. The progressive nature of the process leads to the signs and symptoms of congestive heart failure. Etiology ranges from idiopathic to collagen vascular disease, infections, nutritional deficiencies, or drug toxicity.

II. PATHOPHYSIOLOGY

As myocardial contractility fails, the heart maintains its output by increasing left ventricular end-diastolic volume, causing the heart to dilate (Frank-Starling principle). As the heart dilates, the ejection fraction will also decrease, usually to about 40% or less. Ultimately, as the heart fails, the entire left ventricle becomes hypokinetic. Compensatory mechanisms include tachycardia and increased systemic vascular resistance, which will eventually worsen cardiac failure.

III. CLINICAL FEATURES

   A. Patients usually present with chronic fatigue, diminished exercise tolerance, dyspnea, and chest pain.

   B. Signs of significant heart failure include jugular venous distention, peripheral edema, ascites, hepatomegaly, and an S3 gallop.

IV. DIAGNOSTIC TESTS

    A. The chest radiograph usually demonstrates pulmonary congestion and cardiomegaly.

    B. The ECG may show left bundle branch block, left ventricular hypertrophy, poor R-wave progression, or variable ST segment changes. Dysrhythmias are common, with atrial fibrillation occurring in 20% of cases. Ventricular ectopics and bursts of ventricular tachycardia are also common.

V. ANESTHETIC PLAN

    A. The main goal is to maintain myocardial performance. Myocardial depressive inhalational agents should be avoided.

    B. A narcotic–oxygen technique is ideal in that it maintains a good depth of analgesia with minimal myocardial depression.

    C. Preoperative optimization of myocardial function with intravenous inotropic agents often helps with intraoperative hemodynamic stability. Afterload reduction with nitroprusside if blood pressure is stable also will augment cardiac output. If pharmacologic treatment fails, insertion of an intra-aortic balloon should be considered.

    D. Postoperative intravenous inotropic agents are often helpful until patients can be returned to their preoperative medication for congestive failure.

VI. INTRAOPERATIVE MONITORING

Appropriate monitoring depends on the severity of the heart failure.

    A. In general, invasive arterial blood pressure monitoring is necessary, especially because many patients may become hemodynamically unstable with administration of anesthetic drugs.

    B. PA catheterization is usually necessary for evaluation of left ventricular filling pressure. Biventricular failure and increased pulmonary artery pressure from chronic failure make central venous pressures an inaccurate reflection of left ventricular filling pressures.

Summary of Anesthetic Considerations

Patients with large pericardial effusions or cardiac tamponade usually have tachycardia, tachypnea, orthopnea, dyspnea, and diaphoresis. Combinations of jugular venous distention, hypotension, decreased pulse pressure, pulsus paradoxus, and muffled heart sounds are often found. Preoperative evaluation with chest radiography and ECG will show nonspecific changes. Echocardiography is best for evaluating the amount of pericardial fluid. If this fluid compromises hemodynamic stability, it should be drained preoperatively. With the resolution of pericardial compression, cardiac function usually normalizes, and no special anesthetic preparation is necessary. In the case of underlying myocardial dysfunction or a possibility of rapid accumulation of pericardial fluid, invasive monitoring with a PA catheter is indicated.

Patients with symptomatic constrictive pericarditis will present much as do those with large pericardial effusions. In these patients, pericardiectomy should precede other noncardiac procedures. Cardiac catheterization is the best method of differentiating constrictive pericarditis from other cardiac pathology. Any perioperative hypotension or decreased preload is poorly tolerated. Invasive monitoring is necessary intraoperatively. However, postoperatively, with the constrictive process removed, hemodynamic status usually normalizes, and invasive hemodynamic monitors and inotropic agents are rarely needed.

Hypertrophic cardiomyopathy (IHSS) is best diagnosed with an echocardiogram or cardiac catheterization. Symptoms include chest pain, dyspnea, and exercise-induced syncope. These symptoms are worsened by conditions that increase myocardial contractility. The key goal during anesthesia for these patients is to decrease the pressure gradient across the left ventricular outflow tract. This can be done by decreasing myocardial contractility, increasing ventricular volume, or increasing afterload.

The clinical presentation of congestive cardiomyopathy and its work-up are similar to those in patients with congestive heart failure from coronary artery disease. The main goal is to maintain myocardial performance by avoiding myocardial depressive inhalational agents or using inotropic agents. Invasive intraoperative monitoring should be considered for patients in failure or with minimal cardiac reserve as indicated by a low ejection fraction.

Recommended Reading

Adair JH, Gold JA, Thomas SJ. Less common cardiac diseases. In: Thomas SJ, ed. New York: Churchill Livingston, 1984.

Canedo MI, Frank MJ, Abdulla AM. Rhythm disturbances in hypertrophic cardiopathy: prevalence, relation to symptoms and management. Am J Cardiol 1980;45:848.

Fowler NO. Constrictive pericarditis: new aspects. J Am Coll Cardiol 1982;50:1014.

Johnson RA, Palacios I. Dilated cardiomyopathies of the adult I. N Engl J Med 1982;307:1051.

Moller CT, Schoonbee CG, Rosendorff C. Hemodynamics of cardiac tamponade during various modes of ventilation. Br J Anesth 1979;51:409.

Shabetai R, Fowler NO, Guntheroth WG. The hemodynamics of cardiac tamponade and constrictive pericarditis. Am J Cardiol 1970;26:480.

Spodick DH. The normal and diseased pericardium: current concepts of pericardial physiology, diagnosis and treatment. J Am Coll Cardiol 1983;1:240.

≡ Right-sided Heart Failure and Pulmonary Hypertension

Richard Prielipp

Recent appreciation of the role of right ventricular function in overall myocardial performance has led to earlier diagnosis of and intervention in states of deteriorating right ventricular performance. Pulmonary hypertension, defined as a mean pulmonary artery pressure (PAP) exceeding 20 mmHg, is the underlying pathophysiologic process that links the many diverse etiologies for right-sided heart failure (cor pulmonale). Cor pulmonale defines a condition involving pulmonary hypertension-induced disruption of right ventricular structure (dilation and hypertrophy) and function.

This chapter will review the etiology and pathophysiology of pulmonary hypertension and cor pulmonale, the modalities of therapy available and the rationale for their utilization in pulmonary hypertension, and the pertinent anesthetic issues and recommendations for patients with pulmonary hypertension undergoing surgery.

I.   ETIOLOGY OF COR PULMONALE

    A.   Right ventricular failure is most commonly associated with left ventricular failure, but it is important to determine when intrinsic pulmonary hypertension represents the precipitating cause for right ventricular dysfunction.

    B.   Before making the diagnosis of cor pulmonale, one must eliminate left ventricular failure and congenital heart disease (e.g., left-to-right shunts such as atrial or ven-

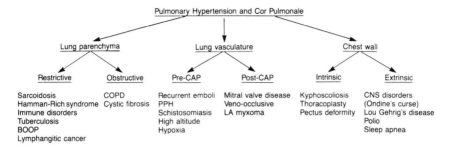

Figure 1-10 Classification of cor pulmonale by primary pathologic process. *BOOP* = bronchiolitis obliterans with organizing pneumonia; *COPD* = chronic obstructive pulmonary disease; *PPH* = primary pulmonary hypertension; *LA* myxoma = left atrial myxoma.

tricular septal defects) as contributory. Anatomic classification is useful based on the site of primary pathology: lung parenchyma, pulmonary vasculature, or chest wall (Figure 1-10).

II. PATHOPHYSIOLOGY OF PULMONARY HYPERTENSION

    A. Normal Pulmonary Circulation

        1. The normal pulmonary circulation accommodates nearly the whole flow of the systemic circulation (approximately 5 L/min at rest; up to 25 L/min during heavy exercise) while operating at one-sixth of the systemic pressure. The quantity of blood within the pulmonary circulation is approximately 0.5 to 1.0 L, whereas only 80 ml (approximately one cardiac stroke volume) is exposed to the gas-exchanging surface of the capillary network at any specific moment.

        2. Pulmonary vascular resistance is linearly distributed, with 50% to 60% of the resistance in the precapillary vessels and 40% to 50% within the postcapillary vasculature. Resistance normally decreases as cardiac output increases via the mechanisms of recruitment and distention within the pulmonary vasculature. Distention probably plays a prominent role in dependent (zone 3) segments of the lung, whereas recruitment is the primary compensating mechanism acting in nondependent lung (zone 1). Both of these compensatory mechanisms may diminish significantly or disappear in diseased lungs.

B. Pulmonary Hypertension
At least a 50% reduction in the effective cross-sectional area of the pulmonary vascular bed must occur for resting PAP to rise. Either active vasoconstriction or anatomic obliteration or obstruction of the vessels may elicit pulmonary hypertension.

1.   Vasoconstriction
Hypoxia is a potent vasoconstrictor and may be significantly potentiated by acidosis. High altitude, obesity, hypoventilation, and severe chronic obstructive lung disease can elevate PAP via a hypoxic mechanism. Direct pharmacologic vasoconstrictors such as alpha-receptor agonists, serotonin (in carcinoids), and thromboxane-A_2 (in septic shock) also increase pulmonary vasomotor tone.

2.   Anatomic disorders
Pulmonary vessels may be distorted by severe compression in scoliosis, progressively eliminated as in destructive emphysema, or physically obstructed by recurrent thromboemboli. Diseases such as primary pulmonary hypertension combine elements of reactive vascular constriction and occlusion. Once established, pulmonary hypertension may be modified by factors such as cardiac output, erythrocytosis, and blood volume.

3.   Right ventricular response to pulmonary hypertension
The right ventricle functions at a much greater compliance than the left ventricle, and acute pressure loads on the right side of the heart may induce rapid deterioration. High PAP may precipitate right ventricular distention, thereby increasing wall tension to a failure threshold (law of Laplace, $T = r \times p$, where T is wall tension, r is ventricular chamber radius, and p is intraventricular pressure). On the other hand, slow, chronic changes in pulmonary artery pressures allow time for right ventricular hypertrophy to compensate for the increased ventricular wall stress. The right side of the heart has an intrinsically greater capacity to hypertrophy in infancy and early childhood. Congenital heart lesions such as ventricular septal defects or pulmonic stenosis may lead to striking muscular hypertrophy with long-term compensation of pressures ap-

proaching those of the systemic circulation. However, this maximally compensated right ventricular mechanism may fail when subjected to stress such as hypoxemia, acidosis, or fluid overload.

III. DIAGNOSIS
  A. Clinical Features
   1. The initial clinical signs of cor pulmonale may not appear as striking as the symptoms of left ventricular failure and may easily be confused with signs of a respiratory disorder. Right ventricular failure may be preceded by a period of clinically silent pulmonary arterial hypertension. In a few cases, subclinical pulmonary hypertension can be detected noninvasively by echocardiography; however, right heart catheterization is usually required for diagnosis.
   2. The symptoms are retrosternal pain, cough, dyspnea on exertion, weakness, fatigue, and early exhaustion. Occasionally, hoarseness secondary to left recurrent laryngeal nerve compression by the enlarged pulmonary artery (PA) is present.
   3. Physical signs
     a. Prominent "a" wave of jugular venous pulse.
     b. Cardiac heave or thrust along the left sternal border.
     c. Presence of a fourth heart sound secondary to significant right ventricular hypertrophy.
     d. Loud second component of the second heart sound (increased P_2).
     e. Possible murmur of pulmonic and tricuspid insufficiency.
     f. Cyanosis, clubbing, peripheral dependent edema, and ascites are late signs. Increased intravascular and extravascular volume is secondary to the release of renin, aldosterone, and antidiuretic hormone.
  B. Roentgenographic Changes in Pulmonary Hypertension
   1. Dilation of the main pulmonary artery and central branches.
   2. Narrowing of the peripheral pulmonary arteries, resulting in a marked falloff in size from the central to the peripheral arteries ("pruning") and producing relatively clear lung fields.
   3. Possible calcification of the main pulmonary artery.
   4. Right ventricular hypertrophy and dilation, appre-

ciated on the lateral chest radiograph view as a reduced size of the retrosternal space between the upper cardiac border and the sternum.

    5.   Subtle changes are usually appreciated only when analyzed over time by viewing a sequence of chest films.

C. ECG Changes

    1.   "P pulmonale" in leads II, III, and aVF, associated with a p-wave axis of $+70$ to $+90$ degrees.

    2.   Rightward shift of the QRS axis.

    3.   Clockwise rotation of the main cardiac vector.

    4.   Right ventricular hypertrophy (tall R waves in V_1 to V_3 and deep S wave in V_6).

    5.   Compensatory T wave inversions may be seen in V_1-V_6.

    6.   Partial or complete right bundle branch block.

    7.   Low voltage of QRS complex in all leads may be prominent feature of underlying chronic obstructive lung disease.

D. Pulmonary Function Tests

Bedside or formal pulmonary function testing results may reflect derangements of the primary pulmonary disorder; e.g., restrictive lung volumes of severe kyphoscoliosis or decreased expiratory flow rates of severe obstructive lung disease.

E. Right Heart Catheterization

    1.   Right heart catheterization helps to differentiate cor pulmonale secondary to left-sided heart failure from pulmonary hypertension without left-sided dysfunction.

        a.   Left-sided heart failure or early mitral stenosis will demonstrate a normal pulmonary artery diastolic (PAD)-to-pulmonary artery occlusion pressure (PAOP) gradient; i.e., a normal calculated pulmonary vascular resistance (Appendix A).

        b.   Pulmonary hypertension-induced cor pulmonale will demonstrate a widening in the PAD–PAOP pressure gradient to >8 mmHg.

    2.   Mean pulmonary artery pressure (PAP) is usually highest in obliterative vascular diseases such as primary pulmonary hypertension, recurrent thromboembolic disease, and Eisenmenger's syndrome.

IV. THERAPY

Optimal preoperative preparation, crucial to successful anesthetic induction and recovery, has five key components.

A. Oxygen

Significant evidence substantiates the efficacy of oxygen therapy in chronic obstructive lung disease (COLD) in improving symptoms and possibly in decreasing PAOP and PAP. Therefore, one should utilize supplemental oxygen to avoid acute hypoxic episodes and to prevent cardiac decompensation.

B. Infection Control

Sputum is examined preoperatively for color, viscosity, quantity, and odor. The patient is questioned regarding recent changes in baseline sputum characteristics, noting any significant changes. A low threshold for instituting antibiotic therapy should be utilized. Nontoxic patients may be given a 10- to 14-day course of oral broad-spectrum antibiotics. Toxic patients (fever, elevated leukocyte count, infiltrates on chest radiography) should have intravenous therapy initially with broad-spectrum antibiotics until sputum cultures can be used to direct more specific antibiotic coverage.

C. Bronchodilation

Bronchodilator responsiveness is assessed by pulmonary function tests (Appendix C), the results being used to titrate optimal bronchodilator therapy. Inhaled β_2-agonists such as albuterol should yield maximum benefit while minimizing arrhythmias or other systemic toxic effects. Anticholinergics such as ipratropium bromide may be added for synergistic action with sympathomimetic bronchodilators, especially in patients with COLD. Aminophylline, if given, must be carefully maintained in a therapeutic nontoxic range (8–15 µg/ml).

D. Fluid Control

Patients with right-sided heart failure require optimized preload, for fluid underload or overload may result in poor right ventricular function. Therefore, invasive monitoring often proves necessary to assess left and right ventricular filling individually. Fluid management must be cautious: excessive crystalloid may increase lung lymph flow and compromise marginal ventilatory reserve, whereas dehydration will limit cardiac output and oxygen delivery and will compromise microcirculatory perfusion by increasing blood viscosity. All insensible, deficit, and third-space fluid losses should be considered in fluid replacement.

   E. Cardiac Glycosides in Cor Pulmonale

Patients with chronic respiratory disease and cor pulmonale sometimes have increased susceptibility to digoxin toxicity. Whereas digoxin may optimally control certain supraventricular arrhythmias, it may worsen others (i.e., multifocal atrial tachycardia) even in low doses. The therapeutic index of digoxin preparations is considerably narrowed in this patient population, necessitating careful titration.

     1. Advantages of digoxin

        a. Decreases right ventricular end-diastolic pressure.

        b. Improves right ventricular contractility.

        c. Especially beneficial to patients with coexisting left-sided heart failure.

     2. Drawbacks of digoxin

        a. After digitalization, systolic pulmonary artery pressures tend to rise because of increased cardiac output and a small but consistent rise in pulmonary vascular resistance.

        b. Patients with cor pulmonale sometimes experience significant hypoxemia after digitalization.

        c. The neuroexcitatory and catecholamine effects of digitalis on the myocardium may increase the incidence of arrhythmias.

   F. Preoperative Optimization of the Hematocrit

     1. The adverse effects of high viscosity secondary to severe erythrocytosis (hematocrit >60%) outweigh the potential benefits of increased oxygen-carrying capacity.

     2. Euvolemic erythrapheresis or phlebotomy to a hematocrit of 50% to 55% appears to have immediate favorable hemodynamic effects.

        a. Significant reduction in the blood viscosity shear rate.

        b. Small (2–3 mmHg) but significant decrease in PAP.

        c. Small (0.3 L/min per m^2) but significant increase in the cardiac index.

        d. Significant increase (18%) in effective renal plasma flow.

    3. Cautions

        a. Phlebotomies are most safely carried out in small quantities (300 ml) every 1 to 2 days, with a recovery interval of 48 hours prior to elective surgery.

        b. No further favorable shifts are documented by decreasing the hematocrit to less than 50%.

        c. Oxygen delivery is decreased after erythrapheresis despite the small favorable increase in cardiac output.

V. ANESTHESIA

  A. Premedication

    1. Because sedative effects are potentiated in these debilitated patients, "routine" doses for premedication must be significantly reduced or the drug eliminated. Opiates may dangerously depress the carbon dioxide response curve and generally should be avoided. Sedation is most safely titrated in the operating room by the anesthesiologist.

    2. The use of anticholinergics should be limited because of the undesirable side effects of increasing the physiologic dead space and increasing the heart rate during the anesthetic induction.

    3. Safe transport to the operating room should include supplemental oxygen to avoid hypoxemia.

  B. Monitoring

Extensive monitoring, which is required in these patients, should be established prior to anesthetic induction. Local infiltrative anesthesia with carefully titrated intravenous sedation will provide a stress-free preinduction period.

    1. ECG, with lead II and V_5, which combine to detect most arrhythmias and left ventricular ischemia. The V_4R lead can be used for detection of right ventricular ischemia.

    2. Pulse oximetry

    3. Temperature

    4. Urine output via Foley catheter

    5. Peripheral nerve stimulator

    6. Continuous arterial pressure monitoring

7. End-tidal CO_2 (may markedly underestimate arterial CO_2 tension)

8. Pulmonary artery catheterization, because the majority of these patients will require invasive hemodynamic monitoring to record right and left ventricular performance accurately and to optimize fluid replacement. Mixed venous oxygen saturation catheters allow closer examination of right ventricular performance and oxygen delivery. The role of transesophageal echocardiography monitoring for right ventricular dysfunction has yet to be determined.

9. Potent inhalation agent monitoring.

C. Induction and Maintenance of Anesthesia

1. Regional anesthetic techniques

Conduction anesthesia may decrease undesirable respiratory alterations induced by general anesthesia (e.g., loss of functional residual capacity, decrease in ciliary activity, increased ventilation–perfusion mismatching) and may prove advantageous for extremity or lower abdominal procedures. Also, when it is combined with general anesthesia, a lower concentration of inhalational agent is needed. Epidural (v intrathecal) administration has the advantages of titration to a selected spinal level in a slower, more controlled fashion; ability to extend the duration as long as necessary; and optimization of postoperative analgesia via epidural narcotics.

2. General Anesthesia

No single agent has documented superiority in patients with pulmonary hypertension and associated right-sided heart dysfunction. A smooth, controlled induction and emergence should limit the stress response and corresponding catecholamine-induced increases in PAP. During all stages of anesthesia, manipulations that increase PAP must be avoided. Five key principles are: keep the patient well oxygenated; avoid acidosis; avoid exogenous/endogenous vasoconstrictors; avoid stimuli that increase sympathetic tone; and avoid hypothermia.

a. Induction

A smooth induction must avoid hypoxia, hypercarbia, catecholamine response to laryngoscopy, and drug-induced histamine release. Preoxygenation should be utilized whenever possible. Muscle relaxants such as metocurine, *d*-tubocurarine, and atracurium that have a tendency to release histamine should be avoided. Lidocaine (1.5 mg/kg) may be administered intravenously 3 minutes prior to laryngoscopy to further obtund the sympathetic response to intubation.

b. Maintenance

A deep plane of anesthesia should be maintained to blunt responses to surgical stimuli. Nitrous oxide may increase pulmonary hypertension. Therefore, if nitrous oxide is necessary, one must proceed cautiously and monitor its effect on pulmonary hemodynamics closely. No evidence clearly favors any one potent agent in this patient population. All inspired gases must be appropriately warmed and humidified prior to delivery.

c. Vasodilator therapy

Pulmonary vasodilators may prove necessary in select cases refractory to conventional treatment (Table 1-15). Invasive hemodynamic monitoring is a prerequisite to initiation of vasodilator therapy. The hemodynamic goal is to decrease right ventricular wall tension by decreasing PAP and to increase the right ventricular ejection fraction, thereby improving cardiac output and perfusion. One must approach these objectives by observing several precautions, because systemic hypotension, right ventricular ischemic failure, exacerbation of pulmonary hypertension, and increased pulmonary shunting are potential complications. A drug with preferential pulmonary vasodilator effects would minimize the risk of systemic complications while effectively lowering pulmonary resistance. Available drugs have systemic vasodilator potencies as great as or greater than their pulmonary vasodilator potencies. Prostaglandin E_1 (PGE_1), nitroglycerin, and isoproterenol exhibit relatively greater selectivity for the pulmonary vascula-

Table 1–15. Vasodilator Drugs for Pulmonary Hypertension*

Drug	Trade Name	Dose Range
Hydralazine	Apresoline	0.05–0.1 mg/kg bolus
Sodium nitroprusside	Nipride	0.3–5.0 µg/kg per min
Nitroglycerin	Nitrostat	0.25–1.5 µg/kg per min
Nifedipine	Procardia	5–10 mg po or subling
Isoproterenol	Isuprel	0.02–0.08 µg/kg per min
Prostaglandin E_1	Alprostadil Prostin VR	0.03–0.10 µg/kg per min

*Represents author's opinion; significant variation in drug response is to be expected in this patient population.

ture in select cases, and limited clinical experience has documented some favorable results. Careful monitoring must accompany pulmonary vasodilator administration in this setting.

   d. Emergence

A stress-free emergence is the goal. Prior to extubation, complete muscle reversal is documented with a peripheral nerve stimulator, and sufficient narcotic analgesia is ensured before elimination of anesthetic vapor. Not all patients may be extubated immediately postoperatively because of underlying pulmonary dysfunction. Oxygen supplementation should be provided for all patients. Adequate arterial oxygenation should be confirmed with blood gas analysis or pulse oximetry.

VI. POSTOPERATIVE MONITORING AND CARE

The same level of care and monitoring that supported the patient through the operative phase must continue into the postoperative and intensive care settings. Invasive monitoring is used until the patient is stable and extubated, no further significant fluid shifts are anticipated, and all hemodynamic vasodilator or vasopressor infusions are discontinued.

VII. SUMMARY OF ANESTHETIC CONSIDERATIONS

Patients with right-sided heart failure have nonspecific complaints of retrosternal pain, cough, dyspnea on exertion, weakness, and early fatigue. Physical signs consistent with right-

Heart Rate	Cardiac Output	PAP	Predominant Vasodilator Effects
+1	+1	0/−1	Systemic >>> pulmonary
0/+1	0	−1/−2	Systemic > pulmonary
0/+1	0	−2	Systemic > pulmonary
0/+1	0/+1	−1	Systemic >> pulmonary
+3	+2/+3	0/−1	Systemic = pulmonary
0/+1	+1/+2	−3	Systemic = pulmonary

sided failure are a prominent "a" wave of the jugular venous pulse, S_4, loud second component of the second heart sound, and peripheral edema. Right heart catheterization is needed to determine the extent of heart failure and pulmonary hypertension and to help differentiate cor pulmonale secondary to left-sided heart failure from pulmonary hypertension without left-sided failure.

Preoperative oxygen therapy, pulmonary infection control, bronchodilator therapy, and fluid control will help reduce pulmonary hypertension and right-sided failure. The use of digoxin is most beneficial for right-sided heart failure if there is coexisting left-sided heart failure.

Premedication in patients with cor pulmonale should be kept to a minimum. Any sedative agent could cause CO_2 retention and worsen pulmonary hypertension and right-sided failure. Anticholinergic agents may increase physiologic dead space and increase the heart rate. Supplemental oxygen should be provided for these patients throughout the perioperative period.

Regional anesthesia is acceptable for patients with cor pulmonale. Any reduction in preload should be corrected immediately. No single inhalational agent has been documented to be superior in patients with pulmonary hypertension. Whether the patient is to receive regional or general anesthesia, the important principles to remember are: keep the patient well oxygenated, avoid acidosis, avoid the administration of vasoconstrictors, avoid stimuli that will increase sympathetic tone, and avoid hypothermia.

Perioperative monitoring for cor pulmonale should always include arterial and pulmonary artery catheterization. Occasionally, patients with severe cor pulmonale who are refractory to conventional perioperative therapy will need pulmonary vasodilators to decrease pulmonary hypertension and increase cardiac output.

Recommended Reading

Ashutosh K, Dunsky M. Noninvasive tests for responsiveness of pulmonary hypertension to oxygen. Chest 1987;92:393.

Bergofsky EH. Tissue oxygen delivery and cor pulmonale in chronic obstructive pulmonary disease. N Engl J Med 1983;308:1092.

Green LH, Smith TW. The use of digitalis in patients with pulmonary disease. Ann Intern Med 1977;87:459.

Hilgenberg JC, McCammon RL, Stoelting RK. Pulmonary and systemic vascular responses to nitrous oxide in patients with mitral stenosis and pulmonary hypertension. Anesth Analg 1980; 59:323.

Hines RL. Monitoring for right ventricular ischemia: is it necessary? [editorial]. J Cardiothorac Anesth 1987;1:95.

Janicki JS, Weber KT, Likoff MJ, et al. The pressure–flow response of the pulmonary circulation in patients with heart failure and pulmonary vascular disease. Circulation 1985;72:1270.

Juhl J, Crummy A. Paul and Juhl's essentials of radiological imaging. 5th ed. Philadelphia: JB Lippincott, 1987:864.

Klein HO, Tordjman T, Ninio R, et al. The early recognition of right ventricular infarction: diagnostic accuracy of the electrocardiographic V4R lead. Circulation 1983;67:558.

Lakshminarayan S. Ipratropium bromide in chronic bronchitis/emphysema. Am J Med 1986;81(suppl 5A):76.

Lynch CL. Perioperative right ventricular ischemia. J Cardiothorac Anesth 1987;1:126.

McCammon RL, Hilgenberg JC, Stoelting RK. Hemodynamic effects of diazepam and diazepam–nitrous oxide in patients with coronary artery disease. Anesth Analg 1980;59:438.

Morrison DA. Pulmonary hypertension in chronic obstructive pulmonary hypertension: the right ventricular hypothesis. Chest 1987;92:387.

Packer M. Vasodilator therapy for primary pulmonary hypertension. Ann Intern Med 1985;103:258.

Rich S, Levy PS. Characteristics of surviving and nonsurviving patients with primary pulmonary hypertension. Am J Med 1984;76:573.

Schulte–Sasse U, Hess W, Tarnow J. Pulmonary vascular responses to nitrous oxide in patients with normal and high pulmonary vascular resistance. Anesthesiology 1982;57:9.

Smith DE, Bissett JK, Phillips JR, et al. Improved right ventricular systolic time intervals after digitalis in patients with cor pulmonale and chronic obstructive pulmonary disease. Am J Cardiol 1978;41:1299.

Trager MA, Feinberg BL, Kaplan JA. Right ventricular ischemia diagnosed by an esophageal electrocardiogram and right atrial pressure tracing. J Cardiothorac Anesth 1987;1:123.

Wallis PJW, Cunningham J, Few JD, et al. Effects of packed cell volume reduction on renal haemodynamics and the renin–angiotensin–aldosterone system in patients with secondary polycythaemia hypoxic cor pulmonale. Clin Sci 1986;70:81.

Weisse AB, Moschos CB, Frank MJ, et al. Hemodynamic effects of staged hematocrit reduction in patients with stable cor pulmonale and severely elevated hematocrit levels. Am J Med 1975;58:92.

≡ Aortic Aneurysms and Peripheral Vascular Disease

Eugene Y. Cheng

I. DEVELOPMENT OF AORTIC DISEASE AND LARGE ARTERY DISEASE

   A. Pathogenesis

      1. Atherosclerosis

Atherosclerosis, the formation of atheromatous plaques in large and medium-sized arteries, is the most common form of arteriosclerosis. In the early stages of plaque formation, the lesions may be reversible with diet and medication, but later, the plaques become necrotic, fibrotic, and calcified and probably are permanent.

      2. Atherogenesis

Atherogenesis probably begins by proliferation of smooth muscle in the intima. Cholesterol and other lipids then accumulate within the muscle cells, forming simple plaques. Platelet aggregation and thrombosis in response to nonspecific arterial wall injury and increased plasma epinephrine and lipid levels may contribute to the primary process.

B. Risk Factors
1. Hyperlipoproteinemia
Increased atherosclerosis is related to total cholesterol levels greater than 180 mg/dl and to elevation of low-density lipoprotein (LDL) in particular. Elevation of high-density lipoprotein (HDL) has a protective effect, possibly by transporting cholesterol from smooth muscle to the liver for metabolism. The ratio of total cholesterol to HDL is a better predictor of coronary artery disease than is the level of either fraction alone. The normal HDL fraction is 20% to 25% of the total cholesterol. A favorable ratio in adults of total cholesterol to HDL is 4.5:1 or lower.
2. Hypertension
Increased physical stress on the arterial wall and the change in flow patterns contribute to accelerated atherosclerosis.
3. Smoking
Cigarette smoking is a causative risk factor in coronary artery disease (CAD). The primary process probably is related to coronary thrombosis and not secondary to enhanced atherosclerosis. Nicotine and hypoxemia from carbon monoxide inhalation enhance platelet aggregation and vasoconstriction.
4. Lifestyle
Two popular beliefs are that a Type A personality and lack of exercise predispose people to atherosclerosis and CAD. However, scientific data do not consistently support the positive relation between Type A behavior and CAD. Exercise may increase plasma HDL, but actual increases in coronary collateral vessels and regression of atheromatous changes are not well documented.
5. Diabetes mellitus
6. Obesity
Obesity is not itself an independent risk factor. However, it frequently is associated with other risk factors such as hypertension, diabetes mellitus, and hyperlipoproteinemia.

II. AORTIC DISEASE
A. Thoracic Aneurysms
1. Incidence
Thoracic aortic aneurysms become more common with age, reaching a peak in the fifth, sixth, and

seventh decades. Medial degeneration from atherosclerosis, cystic medial necrosis, and trauma are common causes.

2. Prognosis

The 5-year survival rate of untreated symptomatic patients is less than 10%, with most patients dying from rupture. Progressive enlargement carries a particularly poor prognosis. Rupture has almost a 100% mortality rate. Asymptomatic aneurysms discovered radiologically in normotensive patients are compatible with longer survival.

3. Clinical features

a. Pain: compression of adjacent nerves; erosion of ribs, sternum, and vertebrae.

b. Superior vena caval syndrome: obstruction of the superior vena cava or innominate vein.

c. Cough and dyspnea: tracheobronchial obstruction.

d. Angina and heart failure: dilatation of the aortic root, separating valve leaflets with resultant regurgitation, heart failure, and ischemia; tamponade.

e. Unconsciousness and death: antegrade dissection or rupture into the pleural space, esophagus, or tracheobronchial tree.

4. Diagnostic studies

a. Diagnosis is suggested by mediastinal widening on the chest radiograph.

b. Screening for thoracic aneurysm can be done with computed tomography (CT) and contrast digital subtraction angiography.

c. Definitive diagnosis is accomplished with aortography of the arch and descending aorta.

5. Treatment

Surgical treatment of aneurysms is the only effective method. The operative mortality rate is 10% in the older patient with other medical illnesses, but the risk falls strikingly in younger patients and those without complicating illnesses.

B. Abdominal Aortic Aneurysm

1. Incidence

Aneurysms are much more common in the abdominal than the thoracic aorta. More than 95% are secondary to atherosclerosis. Rarely, trauma, syphilis, mycotic infection, or Marfan's syndrome are responsible. The highest occurrence is in the sixth and seventh decades.

2. Prognosis

Patients with untreated asymptomatic and symptomatic aneurysms have five-year survival rates of 20% and less than 10%, respectively. The smallest detectable aneurysms are approximately 4 cm. The risk of rupture increases with size: a 5-cm aneurysm has a 10% chance of rupture per year compared with 40% in a 7-cm aneurysm. Ruptured aneurysms have a mortality rate of greater than 40%.

3. Clinical features

   a. The majority of abdominal aortic aneurysms are asymptomatic and usually are found at the time of routine abdominal examination.

   b. Abdominal symptoms range from vague discomfort to severe pain. Pain in the flank or back suggests leakage or rupture.

   c. Physical examination usually can detect aneurysms 4 cm or larger. The pulsating mass may be tender.

4. Diagnostic studies

   a. Plain films of the abdomen, especially the lateral view, may show calcification in the wall of the aneurysm.

   b. Abdominal ultrasonography and CT usually provide accurate noninvasive assessment of aneurysm size and location.

   c. Arteriography provides the most accurate evaluation of the aneurysm. If surgery is being considered seriously, this procedure is necessary to evaluate the circulation of the aortic branches.

5. Treatment

   a. Patients with asymptomatic aneurysms less than 7 cm may be treated medically, especially if they have other illnesses. Onset of symptoms or enlargement of the aneurysm mandates surgery.

   b. Elective aneurysmectomy is associated with a 2% to 5% mortality rate.

   c. Emergency surgery to repair a leaking or ruptured aneurysm entails an operative mortality risk of 25% to 50%. Elderly patients with aneurysms and severe associated medical problems have an operative mortality rate of 20% to 60%.

C. Dissecting Aneurysms of the Aorta

A dissecting aortic aneurysm is distinct from an aortic aneurysm. It arises from a tear in the intima, resulting in extravasation of blood into a false channel within the media. The hematoma may dissect for variable distances causing no trouble, or it may occlude side branches or rupture through the adventitia, causing end-organ failure.

1. Classification and incidence
   a. DeBakey classification
      1) Type I: Starts at the ascending aorta and involves the entire length of the aorta
      2) Type II: Limited to the ascending aorta
      3) Type III: Starts distal to the left subclavian artery and spreads distally.
   b. Modified classification
      1) Type A: Ascending dissection
      2) Type B: Descending dissection
      3) Type C: Fatal and inoperable dissection.
   c. Types A and B account for 50% to 60% and 40% of aortic dissections, respectively. Dissections are three times more common in men and occur most frequently between the ages of 50 and 70 years.
2. Clinical features
   a. Pain is the most frequent symptom. It has been described as a sudden onset of a tearing, throbbing, or ripping sensation. The pain may initially be confined to the abdomen, back, or chest area but may radiate to the lower and upper extremities.
   b. Dyspnea
   c. Nausea and vomiting
   d. Physical examination may show hypotension, differences in the blood pressures of the two upper extremities, or neurologic deficits, depending on the arch vessels involved.
3. Diagnostic studies
   a. Electrocardiography may show left axis deviation, left ventricular hypertrophy, ischemic

              changes, or concurrent myocardial infarction, conduction defects, and dysrhythmias.

    b. The chest radiograph is usually abnormal, with a dilated aorta, widened mediastinum, cardiomegaly, and pulmonary edema.

    c. An aortogram is required to confirm the diagnosis. This study will reveal splitting and distortion of the contrast column and aortic insufficiency.

  4. Treatment

    a. Indications for surgical therapy

      1) Ascending aortic dissection

      2) Rupture or progression of descending aortic dissection

      3) Inability to control pain or arterial pressure in those with descending aortic dissection.

    b. Indication for medical therapy: uncomplicated dissections (no end-organ damage) of the descending aorta.

    c. Untreated ascending aortic dissections have almost a 0% 1-year survival rate. Surgical mortality rates in acute ascending dissections are between 10% and 20%, with long-term survival approaching 60%. In patients with descending aortic dissections, the mortality rate for surgical or medical treatment is approximately 10% to 20% in the first year. With optimal medical or surgical therapy, long-term survival rate also approaches 60%.

III. ILIOFEMORAL ARTERIAL DISEASE

  A. Causes of Acute Arterial Occlusion

    1. Embolism from mural thrombus in the left ventricle

    2. Embolism from atheromatous lesions in the abdominal aorta or iliofemoral artery

    3. Thrombosis, usually involving an existing atheromatous lesion.

  B. Causes of Chronic Arterial Occlusion

    1. Nearly always atherosclerotic

      a. Peripheral atherosclerosis most frequently involves the common femoral or superficial femoral arteries.

      b. Atherosclerosis of the distal abdominal aorta or the iliac arteries most frequently occurs in men younger than 60 years.

        c. Elderly or diabetic persons are at higher risk for distal atherosclerosis.

    2. May be the result of thromboangiitis obliterans (Buerger's disease), an inflammatory disease primarily of young male smokers.

C. Clinical Features

    1. Claudication distal to the site of occlusion

    2. Loss of pulse at the site of and distal to the occlusion

    3. Decreased skin temperature and cyanosis, especially in more distal obstructions with poor collateral circulation.

D. Diagnostic Studies

    1. In most cases, the history and physical examination is adequate for diagnosis.

    2. Doppler ultrasound is useful for assessing the pulsatile blood flow profile in arteries distal to the obstructing lesions.

    3. Arteriography is necessary to assess the extent of obstructive disease and the feasibility of reconstructive surgery.

E. Treatment

    1. Vasodilators usually are not effective with fixed atherosclerotic disease.

    2. Hemorrheologic agents (pentoxifylline) reduce blood viscosity and increase red cell flexibility, which can increase blood flow distal to obstructive lesion.

    3. Transluminal angioplasty and laser photodynamic therapy are effective for localized stenoses.

    4. Reconstructive arterial surgery is effective for symptomatic aortoiliac disease.

    5. Surgery for femoropopliteal disease should be reserved for patients with severe claudication because of the high failure rate of bypass grafts.

IV. PREANESTHETIC EVALUATION

A. Atherosclerotic Heart Disease

    1. Incidence in surgical candidates

Of patients undergoing major vascular surgery, 50% to 70% have atherosclerotic heart disease. Of those patients with CAD, approximately 35% will have no previous cardiac history (myocardial infarction, angina pectoris, or ECG changes suggestive of CAD). Myocardial infarction accounts for 40% to 70% of deaths after vascular surgery. Because these patients tend to be sedentary and exercise tolerance is hard to determine by history or exercise testing, other modalities may be necessary to evaluate the extent of CAD.

2. Diagnostic tests
    a. Echocardiography localizes areas of nonfunctioning or poorly functioning myocardium and permits gross estimation of left ventricular ejection fraction and valvular function.
    b. Radionuclide imaging (MUGA scan) localizes wall motion abnormalities and provides a better estimate of left ventricular ejection fraction than does echocardiography.
    c. Dipyridamole–thallium ^{201} perfusion scan is able to differentiate fixed ischemic and infarcted areas from reversible ischemic areas without the necessity of exercise testing.
    d. Coronary arteriography evaluates coronary anatomy, ejection fraction, wall motion, and valvular function.
    e. Prior to any major vascular surgery, evaluation of the left ventricular wall motion and ejection fraction should be done with either echocardiography or a MUGA scan. To determine the presence of any reversible ischemic areas, a dipyridamole–thallium perfusion scan should be used. If any significant reversible ischemic areas are found, coronary arteriography is necessary to determine the suitability of the patient for myocardial revascularization prior to any elective major vascular surgery.

B. Renal Disease
    1. Many patients with vascular insufficiency have the potential for renal disease. Diabetes mellitus, hypertension, nephrosclerosis, and renal vascular disease are common coexisting medical diseases that may affect renal function. Additional renal insults are likely with aortic crossclamping or intraoperative hypotension. Assessing renal function preoperatively provides a baseline for postoperative comparison and a predictor of postoperative function.
    2. Preoperative urinalysis and serum urea nitrogen and creatinine should be routine. A 12- or 24-hour creatinine clearance test will quantitate the renal insufficiency associated with an increased serum creatinine.

C. Cerebral Vascular Disease

    1. The likelihood of atherosclerotic disease in the carotid vasculature is high if the patient has hypertension, diabetes mellitus, and evidence of vascular narrowing elsewhere in the systemic circulation.

    2. Prior to elective aortic aneurysm or peripheral vasculature surgery, carotid endarterectomies may be indicated for patients with transient ischemic attacks or mild strokes who have retained good neurologic function.

    3. Asymptomatic carotid bruits are not an indication for delaying surgery, as there is no evidence that these patients are at increased risk for stroke, although they are at higher risk for perioperative cardiac morbidity. The necessity of a work-up of asymptomatic carotid bruits is controversial.

D. Pulmonary Disease

    1. Smokers and patients with other pulmonary disease are at increased risk for postoperative pulmonary complications, especially after upper abdominal or thoracic surgery.

    2. To help delineate the extent of pulmonary disease, baseline chest radiography, pulmonary function tests, and arterial blood gas measurements are helpful.

    3. Preoperative maneuvers to decrease the extent of postoperative pulmonary complications would include proper deep breathing and coughing and incentive spirometry techniques, clearing retained secretions with pulmonary clapping and drainage, antibiotics if indicated, and initiating or optimizing bronchodilator therapy.

V. PREMEDICATION

    A. Sedative and anxiolytic agents are useful in patients with vascular disease. The majority of these patients have hypertension, and decreasing their fear and anxiety with a preoperative visit and sedative/anxiolytic medication will diminish the rises in blood pressure.

    B. The elderly and patients with pulmonary, cardiovascular, or multisystem disease will be very sensitive to the usual amounts of preoperative medication. Therefore, the doses of all sedatives and anxiolytic and opiate agents should be reduced, especially when drugs are used in combinations.

    C. All antihypertensive medications should be continued to the day of surgery. The only exceptions are monoamine oxidase inhibitors, which should be discontinued several weeks prior to surgery.

    D. Platelet-inhibiting drugs such as salicylates need to be discontinued 10 days prior to major vascular surgery.

    E. Preoperative hydration should be considered for patients on diuretics, those who have received bowel-cleansing preparations, and those who will have a major regional block.

VI. MONITORING

    A. All the usual anesthetic monitors are indicated: ECG lead V_5 and lead II, esophageal stethoscope, temperature probe, pulse oximeter, blood pressure cuff, and capnography or mass spectroscopy.

    B. Invasive arterial monitoring is required in all aortic and most peripheral vascular surgery cases. Clamping and unclamping the aorta causes large changes in blood pressure, and the existence of significant end-organ damage necessitates close observation of blood pressure and access for arterial blood sampling.

    C. A pulmonary artery catheter for estimation of left ventricular preload and cardiac output is essential for the optimal care of any patient having aortic surgery. With aortic crossclamping, systemic vascular resistance can be acutely elevated 40% to 50% with an associated decrease in cardiac output. Increasing pulmonary artery occlusion pressure (PAOP) may be one of the early indications of myocardial ischemia. Measurement of mixed oxygen tension with oximetric pulmonary artery catheters provides a continuous and sensitive index of the adequacy of tissue perfusion. The PAOP helps guide fluid replacement, especially during periods of rapid fluid shifts.

    In general, central venous pressures (CVP) is not a reliable reflection of left ventricular end diastolic volume. The CVP catheter is useful in providing a secure access to the central circulation and may indicate volume status in nonaortic vascular surgery in patients without significant cardiac or pulmonary problems.

    D. Esophageal two-dimensional echocardiography can supplement information from the pulmonary artery catheter about left ventricular end-diastolic volume and function. Changes in left ventricular wall movement are an early indicator of myocardial ischemia.

E. Urine output from a Foley catheter is a useful indicator of renal perfusion.

F. Somatosensory evoked potential (SSEP) monitoring should be considered during aortic surgery that may compromise spinal blood flow. All anesthetics will affect the SSEP to some degree. This monitor thus will require a technician knowledgeable about the effects of anesthetics to differentiate changes caused by perfusion defects and those attributable to anesthetics.

G. Electroencephogram (EEG) monitoring may be useful in surgery involving the aortic arch. However, interpretation of the EEG is complicated by the effects of anesthetics and hypothermia.

VII. INDUCTION

A. A smooth controlled induction is ideal. Laryngoscopy and intubation with inadequate suppression of the sympathetic system may result in hypertension and tachycardia. Excess suppression of the sympathetic nervous system by induction drugs can cause circulatory arrest. Fasciculations induced by succinylcholine can increase intra-abdominal pressure and cause aneurysmal rupture.

B. Drugs other than the ultra-short-acting barbiturates, benzodiazepines, and opiates can be used during induction to blunt the sympathetic response to intubation.

    1. Lidocaine: 1–1.5 mg/kg IV 1 minute before intubation

    2. Labetalol: 0.25–0.5 mg/kg IV infused over 5 to 10 minutes prior to intubation

    3. Esmolol: 40–80 mg IV infused over 10 minutes prior to intubation.

C. Treatment of Hypotension Produced During Induction

    1. Fluid boluses can readily reverse hypotension.

    2. In the presence of good left ventricular function and adequate intravascular volume, a pure alpha-receptor agonist (phenylephrine, 50–200 μg IV bolus, repeated as necessary [may be contraindicated with bradycardia]) can be used.

    3. Left ventricular dysfunction or an ischemic myocardium may necessitate use of an agent with inotropic as well as vasoconstrictive activity.

        a. Ephedrine: 5–25 mg IV as a bolus, repeated as necessary

        b. Dopamine: 1–10 μg/kg per min as a continuous infusion

      c. Epinephrine: 20–50 μg IV bolus, repeated as necessary, or continuous infusion at 0.03–0.3 μg/kg per min.

VIII. MAINTENANCE

    A. Inhalational agents may be used for most vascular cases. For patients with significant congestive heart failure, the direct myocardial depressant effects of enflurane and halothane may overshadow the benefits of decreased afterload and oxygen consumption. Isoflurane does not have as much myocardial depressant effect as enflurane and halothane, but in patients with CAD, there is the potential for cardiac failure secondary to coronary steal.

    B. Opiate-based anesthesia may be more appropriate for patients with severe myocardial dysfunction. This technique has minimal cardiac depressant effects and will also permit use of a high concentration of oxygen if needed. Usually, extremely high doses of opiates are required to produce amnesia. To help ensure amnesia, a long-acting benzodiazepine such as diazepam or lorazepam can be given preoperatively or during induction. Opiate-based anesthesia will not cause as marked a depression of the sympathetic nervous system. Occasionally, despite high doses, tachycardia and hypertension occur that will not be responsive to additional boluses of opioids. With isolated hypertension, a vasodilator such as nitroprusside, nitroglycerin, trimethaphan, or hydralazine can be used. If both tachycardia and hypertension occur, a careful titration of a β-blocking agent may be needed.

    C. Regional anesthesia by continuous or bolus local anesthetic is useful for many major vascular procedures either alone or in conjunction with general anesthesia. The safety of epidural catheters during surgical cases in which anticoagulation is started after catheter placement has been fairly well established. In cases with preexisting anticoagulation, where high levels of anticoagulation are needed, or in the presence of thrombocytopenia or bleeding disorders, regional anesthesia should be avoided. Sensory and sympathetic blockade by epidural anesthesia will decrease the general anesthetic requirement and attenuate the reflex mesenteric and renal cortical vasoconstriction. Higher blood flow through vascular grafts may occur with improved distal perfusion. Additional benefits are the ability to provide postoperative analgesia with epidural opioids and the reduction of postoperative deep vein thrombosis by increasing intraoperative venous flow and early postoperative ambulation.

IX. SPECIAL INTRAOPERATIVE CONSIDERATIONS

A. Aortic Clamping and Unclamping

Clamping the aorta will acutely increase the systemic vascular resistance (SVR), arterial blood pressure, and PAOP and decrease cardiac output. Intravenous nitroprusside or nitroglycerin given immediately prior to the clamping of the aorta will counteract excessive increases in SVR, blood pressure and PAOP. If normalizing SVR, blood pressure, and PAOP does not improve cardiac output, dobutamine or dopamine should be used.

Unclamping the aorta is usually associated with hypotension. The etiologies may include the systemic effects of acidosis and metabolites released on unclamping, a decrease in distal vasomotor tone, and reactive hyperemia distal to the clamp site. Discontinuation of any vasodilators (including inhalational agents), optimizing preload, and close communication with the surgeon during unclamping will help diminish episodes of hypotension.

B. Renal Flow

Infrarenal aortic crossclamping is associated with approximately a 40% decrease in renal blood flow. Suprarenal aortic crossclamping will result in an 85% to 95% reduction in renal blood flow. Kidneys with extremely low or no blood flow can develop acute tubular necrosis within 30 minutes. The incidence of renal failure after elective abdominal aortic aneurysm repair is approximately 5%. Prior to interrupting aortic flow, intravenous administration of mannitol, 0.5 mg/kg, optimizing intravascular volume, and infusing dopamine at dopaminergic doses (≤ 3 μg/kg per min) will increase urine output and may provide some renal protection. Ideally, urine output should be maintained at 1 to 2 ml/kg per hour.

C. Ventilation

For most aortic surgery, the patient is supine, and both lungs are ventilated. With descending thoracic aortic aneurysms, the right lateral decubitus position is frequently used and one-lung ventilation utilized to improve the visibility of the surgical field. Proper tube position for one-lung ventilation can easily be established with a fiberoptic bronchoscope. One-lung ventilation may result in unacceptably low PaO_2. Placing PEEP on the dependent lung or continuous positive airway pressure on the nondependent lung frequently improves oxygenation without compromising the surgical field.

X.   POSTOPERATIVE CONSIDERATIONS

    A. Cardiovascular

After extensive intra-abdominal surgery, hemodynamic status can change rapidly because of continued third spacing of fluid into the peritoneal cavity, accumulation of interstitial edema, bleeding, or changes in myocardial contractility and vascular tone. Significant shifts in intravascular volume may occur as late as 48 hours after major surgery. The pulmonary artery catheter is helpful in determining the requirements for fluid, inotropic support, vasopressors, or afterload-reducing agents.

    B. Pulmonary

Postoperative extubation as soon as a patient is awake and has adequate respiratory muscle strength may result in pulmonary complications. Large volumes of fluid and blood products are given during aortic surgery. Postoperatively, the extra fluid that accumulated in the interstitial and third space will return to the intravascular space. In the case of renal failure or myocardial dysfunction where urine output is decreased, pulmonary edema may develop, necessitating reintubation. Prior to extubation, in addition to having adequate arterial blood gases (PaO_2 >80 mmHg, $PaCO_2$ <45 on an FIO_2 <0.5) and spontaneous respiratory measures (negative inspiratory force >-25; forced vital capacity >15 ml/kg), the patient should have a stable cardiovascular system, no evidence of significant bleeding, and a reasonable urine output without need for fluid challenges or large amounts of inotropic drugs.

XI.   SUMMARY OF ANESTHETIC CONSIDERATIONS

Patients requiring surgery for aortic aneurysms or peripheral vascular disease should be evaluated preoperatively for CAD and myocardial dysfunction. If any significant reversible ischemic areas are found, coronary arteriography is necessary to determine the suitability of the patient for myocardial revascularization prior to elective major vascular surgery. Renal and cerebral vascular disease are likely in patients with aortic aneurysms and peripheral vascular disease, and the existence of these problems should be identified preoperatively. Moderate to heavy preoperative sedation is useful to decrease stress and anxiety and diminish increases in blood pressure. It is very important to administer all antihypertensive medications until the time of surgery, especially in patients with aortic aneurysms. Any large changes in blood pressure and pulse rate could cause myocardial ischemia, decreased peripheral perfusion, and aneurysm rupture.

Extensive hemodynamic monitoring is required in these patients, because clamping and unclamping of the aorta and other major arterial vasculature can cause marked changes in SVR, mean arterial pressure, cardiac output, and regional metabolic balance.

General anesthesia is utilized for most vascular cases, but regional anesthesia is reasonable for many vascular procedures either alone or in conjunction with general anesthesia. Important goals are to minimize the sympathetic response to noxious stimuli and to treat immediately any hypotension or hypertension. Significant shifts in intravascular volume can occur postoperatively. The invasive hemodynamic monitor should be left in postoperatively until fluid challenges and inotropic support are no longer needed. Patients also should be left intubated until fully awake and without signs of cardiovascular instability.

Recommended Reading

Botta GC, Contini S, Adorni A. Abdominal aortic aneurysms: Some controversial points. J Cardiovasc Surg 1983;24:481.

Boucher CA, Brewster DC, Darling C, et al. Determination of cardiac risk by dipyridamole–thallium imaging before peripheral vascular surgery. N Engl J Med 1985;312:389.

Casthely PA, Fyman PN, Abrams LM, et al. Anesthesia for aortic arch aneurysm repair: experience with 17 patients. Can Anaesth Soc J 1985;32:73.

Chambers BR, Norris JW. The case against surgery for asymptomatic carotid stenosis. Stroke 1984;15:964.

Cheitlin MD. Finding the high-risk patient with coronary artery disease. JAMA 1988;259:2271.

Cooley DA, Carmichael MJ. Abdominal aortic aneurysm. Circulation 1984;70(suppl I):5.

DeSanctis RW, Doroghazi RM, Austen WG, et al. Aortic dissection. N Engl J Med 1987;317:1060.

Diehl JT, Cali RF, Hertzer NR, et al. Complications of abdominal aortic reconstruction: an analysis of perioperative risk factors in 557 patients. Ann Surg 1983;197:49.

Gamulin Z, Forster A, Morel D, et al. Effects of infrarenal aortic cross-clamping on renal hemodynamics in humans. Anesthesiology 1984;61:394.

Goldman L, Caldera DL, Nussbaum SR, et al. Multifactorial index of cardiac risk in noncardiac surgical procedures. N Engl J Med 1977;297:845.

Grotta, JC. Current medical and surgical therapy for cerebrovascular disease. N Engl J Med 317:1505.

Hertzer NR, Beven EG, Young JR, et al. Coronary artery disease in peripheral vascular patients: a classification of 1000 coronary angiograms and results of surgical management. Ann Surg 1984;199:223.

O'Donnell TF, Callow AD, Willet C, et al. The impact of coronary artery disease on carotid endarterectomy. Ann Surg 1983;198:705.

Odoom JA, Sih IL. Epidural analgesia and anticoagulant therapy: experience with one thousand cases of continuous epidurals. Anaesthesia 1983;38:254.

Rao TLK, El-Etr AA. Anticoagulation following placement of epidural and subarachnoid catheters: an evaluation of neurologic sequelae. Anesthesiology 1981;55:618.

Silverstein PR, Caldera DL, Cullen DJ, et al. Avoiding the hemodynamic consequences of aortic cross-clamping and unclamping. Anesthesiology 1979;50:462.

Tomatis LA, Fierens EE, Verbrugge GP. Evaluation of surgical risk in peripheral vascular disease by coronary arteriography: a series of 100 cases. Surgery 1972;71(3):429.

Youngberg J. Anesthesia for aortic and peripheral vascular surgery. ASA Annual Refresher Course Lectures 1984;235:1.

≡ Hypertension

Eugene Y. Cheng

High blood pressure is the most significant risk factor for cardiovascular disease and an important cause of renal failure and stroke. There are a wide variety of types and causes of hypertension, of which essential or primary hypertension is the most common. Pathologic conditions such as renovascular disease, pheochromocytoma, Cushing's syndrome, primary aldosteronism, renal parenchymal disease, acute increased intracranial pressure, and coarctation of the aorta are causes of secondary hypertension (Table 1-16). This chapter will be limited to the perioperative evaluation and care of the patient with primary hypertension.

Primary hypertension affects well over 90% of hypertensive patients. The etiology of the disorder is poorly understood, and the condition is generally asymptomatic until complications develop. Estimates are that 15% to 25% of the adult population in the United States is hypertensive. The World Health Organization defines hypertension as a systolic blood pressure (SBP) >160 mmHg and a diastolic blood pressure >95 mmHg. However, with chronic hypertension, the associated morbidity and mortality may start with SBP >130 and DBP >95 mmHg.

I. PATHOGENESIS

Blood pressure is normally regulated by a series of feedback mechanisms. Changes are sensed by aortic and carotid baroreceptors, which after information processing in the central nervous system, modulate changes in autonomic output. Derangements in the neuroendocrine and autonomic systems may be the etiology of primary hypertension.

A. Renin–Angiotensin–Aldosterone System

Renin is a proteolytic enzyme produced by modified af-

Table 1–16. Causes of Secondary Hypertension

Cardiovascular

Severe aortic atherosclerosis
Coartation of the aorta
Aortic valve insufficiency
Patent ductus arteriosus

Endocrine

Hyperthyroidism
Cushing's disease
Primary hyperaldosteronism
Congenital adrenogenital
  syndromes
Pheochromocytoma
Acromegaly
Hyperparathyroidism

Neurogenic

Increased intracranial pressure
Psychogenic
Polyneuritis
Spinal cord section

Renal

Pyelonephritis
Glomerulonephritis
Polycystic renal disease
Renovascular stenosis
Arterial nephrosclerosis
Renal vasculitis
Diabetic nephropathy
Renin-secreting tumors
Obstructive uropathy

Drugs

Oral contraceptives
Amphetamines
Steroids
Thyroxine

ferent arteriolar smooth-muscle cells in the juxtaglomerular apparatus. Renin acts on renin substrate synthesized in the liver to release angiotensin I. This decapeptide is then cleaved by a membrane-bound converting enzyme in the lung to angiotensin II, a potent vasoconstrictor, regulator of renal tubular reabsorption, and stimulus for adrenocortical production of aldosterone. The exact role of this system in primary hypertension is uncertain, but the effectiveness of angiotensin-converting enzyme (ACE) inhibitors in lowering blood pressure suggests a significant contribution.

B. Kallikrein–Kinin System

Kallikrein is a renal enzyme that acts on kininogen, a plasma substrate, to release bradykinin. Bradykinin has vasodilator properties. Studies are ongoing to determine if decreases in renal kallikrein excretion are a pathogenetic factor.

C. Vasopressin

Vasopressin, or antidiuretic hormone, is a potent vasoconstrictor that usually acts only in acute hypovolemic hypotension before other autonomic reflexes and the renin system become maximally activated. Vasopressin may also play a role in certain volume-dependent forms of hypertension.

D. Natriuretic Factor

Natriuretic hormone has oaubain-like properties. The hormone may be secreted by the hypothalamus in volume-expanded animals and certain hypertensive patients. The inhibition of Na^+, K^+-ATPase, with a resultant increase in intracellular calcium, increases vasoconstriction. Secretion of natriuretic factor and a genetic abnormality in Na^+, K^+, and Cl^- cotransport have been suggested as the underlying etiology of primary hypertension.

E. Atrial Natriuretic Factor

This peptide isolated from atrial extracts promotes natriuresis by increasing glomerular filtration rate and inhibiting aldosterone production and renin secretion. The role of this hormone in hypertension has not been determined.

II. PREOPERATIVE HISTORY

Initially, individuals with primary hypertension are asymptomatic and without end-organ changes for 5 to 10 years. In the following 10 years, reversible damage occurs in target organs such as the heart, brain, and kidneys. Finally, after 20 to 30 years of uncontrolled hypertension, permanent organ damage is seen.

A. Cardiovascular Status

    1. One of the leading causes of death in the untreated hypertensive patient is cardiac failure. Accelerated atherosclerosis and left ventricular hypertrophy increase the risk of myocardial ischemia and dysfunction.

    2. Patients often complain of angina, fatigue, shortness of breath on exertion, nocturnal dyspnea, and nocturia.

    3. Claudication may be present secondary to peripheral vascular disease.

    4. The elderly and patients with disabling peripheral vascular disease may have asymptomatic coronary artery disease (CAD).

B. Cerebrovascular Status

    1. Hypertension is the principal risk factor for both thrombotic and hemorrhagic strokes. The risk of stroke is related to the degree of elevation of the blood pressure, especially the systolic pressure. The precise relation between the extent of hypertension and morbidity is unclear.

    2. Headache, transient ischemic attacks, visual changes, and encephalopathy are associated with increased blood pressure.

C. Renovascular Disease

Signs and symptoms of renal involvement are uncommon until significant renal failure develops and fluid retention occurs.

III. PHYSICAL EXAMINATION

A. Hypertension should not be diagnosed from a single measurement. Initially elevated readings should be confirmed on at least two subsequent visits. Pressures from both arms should be measured and the higher pressure recorded.

B. Cardiac examination may reveal increased rate, increased size, precordial heave, clicks, murmurs, dysrhythmias, and S_3 or S_4 heart sounds.

C. The funduscopic examination will show little evidence of damage early in mild hypertension. Worsening hypertensive injury will be manifested in arteriolar narrowing, arteriovenous compression, hemorrhages, exudates, and papilledema.

D. The neck may reveal carotid bruits, decreased arterial pulsation, or distended veins.

E. The abdomen should be examined for bruits, enlarged kidneys, and dilatation of the aorta.

F. Extremities may have diminished or absent peripheral arterial pulsations, bruits, edema, and cyanosis.

IV. DIAGNOSTIC TESTS

Specialized studies may be needed for the diagnosis of secondary hypertension such as renal vein renin level, intravenous urogram, renal artery angiogram, thyroid function tests, and plasma levels of catecholamines and aldosterone. In general, these tests are not appropriate for preoperative evaluation and should be performed well before any planned operative procedure. Only a few relatively simple tests need be performed before surgery, looking specifically for target-organ damage.

A. Electrocardiogram: left ventricular hypertrophy, ischemic changes, myocardial infarction, conduction defects, and drug effects.

B. Chest radiograph: cardiac enlargement, infiltrates, mediastinal widening, pulmonary congestion, and rib notching.

C. Urinalysis: proteinuria and hematuria.

D. Blood tests: hemoglobin and hematocrit, sodium, potassium, chloride, bicarbonate, urea nitrogen, creatinine, and glucose.

E. Cardiac stress test: useful objective test if history, physical examination, and other diagnostic tests suggest CAD.

V. DRUG THERAPY

The goal of treating patients with hypertension is to prevent target-organ changes that increase morbidity and mortality. The objective with either nonmedical or medical therapy is to maintain the arterial blood pressure below 140/90 mmHg.

Antihypertensive drug therapy is usually aimed at diminishing sympathetic activity. With the number of available drugs and the possible drug interactions, the anesthesiologist should have a thorough knowledge of the pharmacology of the drugs used to treat hypertension. Patients whose DBPs fall between 90 and 94 mmHg who have no other significant cardiovascular risk factors are usually treated with nonpharmacologic approaches (exercise, diet). Initial recommended therapy for refractory mild hypertension or higher diastolic and elevated systolic pressures is frequently with thiazide-type diuretics or β-blockers. Recently, ACE inhibitors and calcium antagonists have proved useful as single agents.

A. Antihypertensive Drugs (Table 1-17)

    1. Diuretics

        a. Thiazides (hydrochlorothiazide, chlorthalidone) act by decreasing the renal tubular reabsorption of Na^+ and relaxing vascular smooth muscle. Their side effects are orthostatic hypotension, hypokalemia, hyponatremia, hypomagnesia, hyperglycemia, and metabolic alkalosis.

        b. Loop diuretics (furosemide, bumetanide) act by inhibiting Na^+ and Cl^- reabsorption, primarily in the distal tubules and the loop of Henle. Their side effects are hypovolemia, hypokalemia, hyponatremia, hypocalcemia, hypomagnesesia, tinnitus and reversible hearing impairment, and metabolic alkalosis.

        c. Potassium-sparing agents (spironolactone, triamterene, amiloride) act as an aldosterone antagonist (spironolactone) or inhibitors of tubular electrogenic sodium transport (triamterine, amiloride). They may cause hyponatremia and hyperkalemia.

    2. Beta-blockers (nonselective: propranolol, nadolol, timolol, pindolol; selective $β_1$: atenolol, metoprolol, acebutolol)

        a. Mechanism of action

            1) Nonselective and selective $β_1$ blockers inhibit the β-receptor agonist effects of norepinephrine and epinephrine.

            2) Nonselective β-blockers will also lower blood pressure by decreasing renin secretion.

        b. Side effects are congestive heart failure, heart block, masking of signs of hypoglycemia, bronchospasm, and peripheral arterial insufficiency.

    3. The $α_1$-adrenergic blocker (prazosin hydrochloride) acts through blockade of postsynaptic α-receptors stimulated by endogenous catecholamines. Its side effects are "first-dose" syncope, orthostatic hypotension, and palpitations.

    4. Centrally acting adrenergic inhibitors (clonidine,

Table 1–17. Antihypertensive Drugs and their Use

Type of Drug	Trade Names	Usual Dose (mg)	Dosing Interval	Usual Maximum mg/day
Diuretics				
Thiazides				
Hydrochlorothiazide	Esidrex, Hydrodiuril	25	qd	100
Chlorthalidone	Hygroton	25–100	qd	200
Loop Diuretics				
Furosemide	Lasix	20–80	bid	320
Bumetanide	Bumex	0.5	bid	5
Indapamide	Lozol	2.5–5.0	qd	5
Potassium-sparing agents				
Spironolactone	Aldactone	25–50	tid	100
Triamterene	Dyazide, Maxzide	50–100	bid	300
Amiloride	Moduretic	5	qd	10
Beta-Blockers				
Nonselective				
Propranolol	Inderal	20–80	bid–qid	480
Nadolol	Corgard	20–40	qd	320
Timolol	Blocadren	10–20	bid	80
Pindolol	Visken	10–20	bid	60
Selective β_1				
Atenolol	Tenormin	25–50	qd	150
Metoprolol	Lopressor	50–100	bid	200
Acebutolol	Sectral	400–800	qd	1600
Alpha-1 Adrenergic Blocker				
Prazosin	Minipress	2–4	bid–tid	20
Centrally Active Adrenergic Inhibitors				
Clonidine	Catapres	0.1–0.4	bid	2.4
Guanabenz	Wytensin	4–8	bid	32
Guanfacine	Tenex	1	bid	3
Methyldopa	Aldomet	250	qd–tid	2000
Peripherally Acting Adrenergic Inhibitors				
Guanadrel	Hylorel	10–25	bid	100
Guanethidine	Esimil, Ismelin	10	qd	150
Reserpine	Hydropres	0.1	qd	0.25

Table 1–17. Antihypertensive Drugs and their Use (*continued*)

Type of Drug	Trade Names	Usual Dose (mg)	Dosing Interval	Usual Maximum mg/day
Combined Alpha–Beta Adrenergic Blocker				
Labetalol	Normodyne, Trandate	200–300	bid	1200
Direct Vasodilators				
Hydralazine	Apresoline	50	bid–qid	300
Minoxidil	Lonitin	2.5–5	bid	80
ACE Inhibitors				
Captopril	Capoten	12.5–25	bid–tid	150
Enalapril	Vasotec	2.5–5	qd	40
Lisinopril	Zestiril	10–20	qd	40
Calcium Channel Blocker				
Verapamil	Calan, Isoptin	80–120	tid–qid	480
Diltiazem	Cardizem	30–60	tid–qid	360
Nifedipine	Adalat, Procardia	10–20	tid–qid	180

guanabenz, guanfacine hydrochloride, methyldopa) stimulate central α-adrenergic receptors, inhibiting sympathetic outflow. Their side effects are sedation, fatigue, and sexual dysfunction.

5. Peripherally acting adrenergic inhibitors (guanadrel, guanethidine, reserpine) prevent release of neurotransmitters from peripheral adrenergic neurons (guanadrel sulfate, guanethidine monosulfate) or deplete stores of catecholamines in presynaptic nerve endings, the adrenal medulla, and brain (reserpine). Their side effects are diarrhea, sexual dysfunction, and orthostatic hypotension (guanadrel sulfate, guanethidine monosulfate) and lethargy, nasal congestion, and depression (reserpine).

6. The only combined α–β adrenergic blocker is labetalol. Its nonselective β-adrenergic receptor-blocking activity is greater than its α_1 adrenergic blocking activity. (The usual receptor blocking ratio is $7:1$ [$\beta:\alpha$].) Its side effects are bronchospasm and orthostatic hypotension.

7. Direct vasodilators (hydralazine, minoxidil) act by direct vascular smooth-muscle relaxation (arterioles more than veins). The side effects are headache, tachycardia, fluid retention, positive antinuclear antibody test (hydralazine), and hypertrichosis (minoxidil).

8. ACE inhibitors (captopril, enalapril, lisinopril) prevent the conversion of inactive angiotensin I to the active angiotensin II. Their side effects are "first-dose" hypotension, reversible renal failure in patients with renal artery stenosis, angioneurotic edema, hyperkalemia, and dysgeusia.

9. Calcium antagonists (verapamil, diltiazem, nifedipine) act by blockade of calcium channels and inhibition of renin release. Side effects are heart block (greatest with verapamil), edema, and tachycardia (greatest with nifedipine).

B. Drugs for Hypertensive Crises

Accelerated (malignant) hypertension is a state in which end-organ damage from hypertension occurs in a brief period of time. Diastolic blood pressure usually exceeds 120 mmHg, and symptoms such as restlessness, confusion, somnolence, blurred vision, headache, nausea, and vomiting occur. The syndrome of hypertensive encephalopathy is characterized by visual disturbances, focal neurologic deficit, and seizures. Stupor or coma may develop. If left ventricular failure develops, pulmonary edema or acute myocardial infarction can occur. Renal damage usually manifests itself early as proteinuria, hematuria, and azotemia. Oliguria may also be seen. If therapy is delayed, permanent end-organ damage is possible. Initial treatment should be given parenterally in an intensive care unit (Table 1-18). Oral therapy is possible but can be harder to titrate (Table 1-19).

1. Nitroprusside acts by direct vasodilatation. Its side effects are hypotension, thiocyanate toxicity (weakness, hyperreflexia, confusion, delirium, tachyphylaxis, coma), cyanide toxicity (metabolic acidosis), decreased platelet adhesiveness, and methemoglobinemia.

2. Trimethaphan camsylate acts by ganglionic blockade. Its side effects are hypotension, rapid development of tachyphylaxis, and sympathetic blockade (urinary retention, constipation, ileus, pupillary dilation).

Table 1–18. Parenteral Drugs for Treatment of Hypertensive Emergencies

Drug	Trade Name	Dose	Onset Time (min)	Duration of Action
Vasodilators				
Sodium nitroprusside	Nipride, Nitropress	0.1–8 μg/kg per min IV infusion	<0.5	3–5 min
Nitroglycerin	Nitrostat, Nitrol	0.1–10 μg/kg per min IV infusion	1–3	3–5 min
Hydralazine	Apresoline	5–20 mg IV bolus 0.5–2.0 μg/kg per min IV infusion	10	2–6 hours
Diazoxide	Hyperstat	50–150 mg IV bolus	1–3	6–12 hours
Adrenergic Inhibitors				
Labetalol	Normodyne, Trandate	5–50 mg IV bolus 2 mg/min IV infusion	2–5	1–6 hours
Trimethaphan	Arfonad	5–30 μg/kg per min IV infusion	1–2	10–15 min
Esmolol	Brevibloc	500 μg/kg (1-min) bolus 25–200 μg/kg per min IV infusion	1	10–15 min
Phentolamine	Regitine	5–15 mg IV bolus	1–2	10–15 min
Methyldopa	Aldomet	250–500 mg IV infusion	30–60	6–10 hours

3. Labetalol (see previous section)
4. Esmolol is a selective β_1-blocker. Its side effects are hypotension and bradycardia.
5. Nifedipine (see previous section)
6. Nitroglycerin is a direct vasodilator (venous more than arterial at low doses). Its side effects are hypotension, headache, nausea and vomiting, methe-

Table 1–19. Oral Drugs for Treatment of Hypertensive Emergencies

Drug	Trade Name	Recommended Dose (mg)	Frequency (Hours)
Captopril	Capoten	12.5–25	1–2
Clonidine	Catapres	0.1–0.2	1–2
Labetol	Normodyne, Trandate	200–400	3–4
Minoxidil	Lonitin	2.5–5	2–3
Nifedipine	Adalat, Procardia	10–20	0.5–1

moglobinemia, tachyphylaxis, and platelet dysfunction.

7. Diazoxide is also a direct vasodilator. Its side effects are hypotension and aggravation of angina pectoris.

8. Hydralazine (see previous section)

VI. ANESTHETIC CARE

    A. General Considerations

        1. In the early days of antihypertensive drug therapy, many reports described severe hypotension and bradydysrhythmias leading to an increase in perioperative morbidity and mortality rates. Recommendations then were to discontinue drug therapy for at least 2 weeks prior to any planned anesthetic. Anesthetic drugs and techniques have improved, and current recommendations are to continue all antihypertensive drugs up to the day of surgery except for monoamine oxidase (MAO) inhibitors, which should be stopped 2 weeks prior to the date of surgery. (Note: MAO inhibitors are no longer recommended for the treatment of hypertensive patients).

        2. Untreated or poorly controlled hypertensives tend to have a greater hypotensive response to vasodepressive intravenous and inhaled anesthetics. Conversely, an exaggerated sympathetic response may manifest itself as hypertensive episodes under light anesthesia. Most hypertensive patients may undergo elective surgery despite poorly controlled blood pressure without an increased risk; the excep-

tion is those with DBP >120 mmHg with end-organ damage.

3. Patients at highest risk of perioperative cardiac complications are those who experience an intraoperative blood pressure decrease of 50% from their preoperative values or a 33% decrease for more than 10 minutes. Autoregulation of brain blood flow is shifted to the right with persistent hypertension. Most hypertensive patients are tolerant of drops in blood pressure of approximately 20% without compromising cerebral perfusion. Renal blood flow autoregulation is also shifted to the right, and any decrease from the usual preoperative blood pressure will decrease glomerular filtration rate.

B. Recommendations

1. Preoperative evaluation

   a. Unexpected abnormalities on preoperative history, physical examination, or tests, especially concerning the cardiovascular, central nervous system, and renal systems, should be documented and carefully evaluated.

   b. Elective surgery should be postponed if DBP exceeds 120 mmHg or in the presence of extreme lability in blood pressure.

2. All antihypertensive medications (except MAO inhibitors) should be continued until the time of surgery.

3. Monitoring

   a. Continuous ECG monitoring using a V_5 lead to detect the earliest indications of cardiac ischemia.

   b. Invasive arterial pressure monitoring is indicated if significant blood pressure changes are anticipated, in the presence of significant target-organ damage, to monitor use of parenteral antihypertensive medications, and for long procedures.

   c. Urinary output, especially in long procedures, to provide some indication of renal function.

   d. Monitoring with pulmonary artery catheterization is advised in patients with significant left ventricular dysfunction and if large fluid shifts are anticipated in the presence of significant end-organ damage.

    e.   Transesophageal echocardiography provides noninvasive identification of cardiac dysfunction by regional wall motion abnormalities.

    f.   Electroencephalogram (EEG) monitoring for assessing cerebral perfusion during anesthesia has not become a standard of practice. Common problems are slow response time, difficulty in interpretation, and interference from electrocautery.

4. Induction of anesthesia

    a.   Most intravenous induction agents inhibit the sympathetic nervous system. Many hypertensive patients will have a decreased plasma volume from poorly controlled hypertension or the use of diuretics. Hypotension frequently results from the combination of decreased plasma volume and large doses of induction agents. Fluid challenges will usually correct decreases in blood pressure brought on by induction. Preinduction hydration should be considered in patients on diuretics.

    b.   An exaggerated sympathetic response to intubation or other painful stimuli will cause hypertension in patients who are inadequately anesthetized. This response may be attenuated by intravenous lidocaine (1.5 mg/kg) 1 minute prior to induction or intravenous administration of a sympatholytic agent prior to induction (esmolol 40–80 mg over 4–5 min).

5. Maintenance of anesthesia

    a.   General anesthesia is well tolerated by most hypertensive patients. The most important consideration is the maintenance of intraoperative blood pressure so as not to vary more than 30% from preoperative values.

    b.   Regional anesthesia may be advantageous in patients with high systemic resistance, as the sympathetic block will help control blood pressure without the use of other pharmacologic agents. Preinduction hydration should be considered in patients having epidural and spinal blocks. Hypotension may occur with rapid onset of sympathetic block. Fluid challenge will readily resolve this problem. In situations such as congestive heart failure, in which additional volume may worsen an underlying medical condition, a sympathomimetic agent given as intermittent intravenous bolus (ephedrine, phenylephrine) or infusion (dopamine) may be used.

6. Postoperative care

    a. The postoperative period can be the most difficult in which to maintain a stable blood pressure because of surgical pain and resolving anesthesia. Hypoxia, hypercarbia, and a distended bladder also exacerbate underlying essential hypertension. During this time, close monitoring of target-organ function is as important as it is intraoperatively. Invasive arterial monitoring may be required because of wide oscillations of the pressure from excessive sympathetic stimuli and drugs given to control blood pressure.

    b. The intravenous route should be utilized for antihypertensive agents in the postanesthetic care unit for rapid control. Peripheral circulation may be compromised, and drug absorption from intramuscular injection sites and cutaneous patches may be erratic. Ileus from the surgery or anesthetic prevents reliable drug uptake from the enteral route.

C. Hypertensive emergencies

    1. Severe hypertension (DBP >120 mmHg with signs or symptoms of end-organ injury) is an emergency.

    2. Preoperatively, all elective surgery should be postponed until blood pressure is controlled to avoid these problems.

    3. Severe intraoperative and postoperative hypertension may cause cerebral edema, seizures, hemorrhagic stroke, left ventricular failure, myocardial infarction, renal failure, and increased surgical bleeding.

    4. Common causes of severe hypertension that can easily be treated postoperatively are pain, hypoxia, hypercarbia, full bladder, or hypervolemia. Less common causes are acute cerebrovascular accident, hypoglycemia, thyroid storm, malignant hyperthermia, and pheochromocytoma.

5. Initially, hypertensive emergencies should be treated with intravenous antihypertensive agents aided by invasive arterial monitoring.

6. Overly aggressive treatment of hypertension may also impair perfusion. Attempts should be made to keep blood pressure within 70% of the preoperative baseline values.

7. Oral preoperative antihypertensive drugs should be started as soon as possible postoperatively to help control hypertension. Rebound hypertension occurs especially after discontinuation of β-blockers or clonidine.

VII. SUMMARY OF ANESTHETIC CONSIDERATIONS

In most instances, patients with primary hypertension may undergo surgery without an increase in perioperative complications. Evidence of any target-organ damage or diastolic pressures >120 mmHg will increase anesthetic risks, so surgery should be postponed. Blood pressure should be stabilized and end-organ damage assessed.

All hypertensive drugs except MAO inhibitors should be continued to the day of surgery. Blood pressure should be carefully monitored throughout the induction, intraoperative, and postanesthetic periods to avoid changes of greater than 30% from preoperative values.

Hypotension caused by decreased sympathetic tone from intravenous or inhaled anesthetic agents responds well to fluids. Sympathomimetic agents should be given if fluid challenges do not normalize blood pressure.

Severe perioperative hypertension should be treated with short-acting intravenous agents to assure uptake and to provide a method of responding rapidly to changes in pressure.

Recommended Reading

Brown BR Jr. Anesthesia for the patient with essential hypertension. Semin Anesth 1987;6:79.

Burris JF, Freis ED. Hypertensive emergencies. Cardiovasc Clin 1986;16:163.

Fremes SE, Weisel RD, Baird RJ, et al. Effects of postoperative hypertension and its treatment. J Thorac Cardiovasc Surg 1983;86:47.

Frohlich ED. Hemodynamic considerations in clinical hypertension. Med Clin North Am 1987;71:803.

Goldman L, Caldera DL. Risks of general anesthesia and elective operation in the hypertensive patient. Anesthesiology 1979;50:285.

Goodloe SL. Essential hypertension. In: Stoelting RK, Dierdorf SF, eds. Anesthesia and co-existing disease. New York: Churchill Livingstone, 1983:99.

Haber E, Slater EE. High blood pressure. In: Rubenstein E, Federman DD, eds. Medicine. New York: Scientific American, 1988:1.

Hancock WE. Coronary artery disease—epidemiology and prevention. In: Rubenstein E, Federman DD, eds. Medicine. New York: Scientific American, 1988:1.

Joint National Committee. The 1988 report of the Joint National Committee on Detection, Evaluation, and Treatment of High Blood Pressure. Arch Intern Med 1988;148:1023.

McRae RP Jr, Liebson PR. Hypertensive crisis. Med Clin North Am 1986;70:749.

Miller ED Jr. Anesthesia and the hypertensive patient. International Anesthesia Research Society Review Course Lectures 1987;6.

Moser M. Implications of the recent clinical trials in hypertension. NY State J Med 1987;87:5.

Prys—Roberts C, Meloche R, Foex P. Studies of anesthesia in relation to hypertension I: cardiovascular responses of treated and untreated patients. Brit J Anaesth 1971;43:122.

Rodriguez PR, Mangano DT. Anesthesia and hypertension. Semin Anesth 1982;1:226.

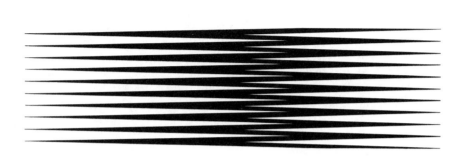

Pulmonary Disorders

Douglas B. Coursin
Steven Croy
Susan L. Goelzer

Pulmonary diseases encompass a wide range of problems and are one of the most frequent acute or chronic illnesses that anesthesiologists must deal with in the perioperative period. The lung has three major functions; gas exchange, metabolism, and host defense. Any of these functions may be altered in the preoperative period, intraoperatively, or postoperatively (predictably or randomly). Diminution or loss of these vital functions may be transient intraoperatively or may persist into the postoperative period, depending on the underlying physical and psychological status of the patient; the type, location, and duration of surgery; and the method of anesthesia and postoperative analgesia. Postoperative respiratory complications may be simply an accentuation of these physiological alterations or may be more severe if there is significant underlying pathology, poor patient education and motivation, or lack of a coordinated perioperative plan.

This chapter will deal with the perioperative management of asthma, chronic lung disease, pulmonary oxygen toxicity, aspiration pneumonitis, pulmonary embolism, chest trauma, and adult respiratory distress syndrome (ARDS).

Asthma

I.   CLINICAL FEATURES
- **A.** Incidence
  Asthma is a common disease that can significantly increase morbidity and mortality rates in the perioperative period. It affects 2% to 5% of adults and 7% to 10% of children, roughly 10 to 20 million persons in the US.
- **B.** Pathogenesis
  1. Asthma is a condition of reversible airway hyperresponsiveness and inflammation caused by chemical, pharmacologic, psychological, or physical stimulation.
  2. Asthmatic episodes of bronchoconstriction and inflammation appear to be neurally and humorally mediated.
  3. Possible inciting extrinsic and intrinsic factors include dusts, fumes, upper respiratory infections, exercise, cold, aspirin, nonsteroidal anti-inflammatory agents, dyes, and stress.
  4. In addition to the physical and emotional stress of surgery, intubation and direct physical irritation of the airway during anesthesia may precipitate bronchospasm.

II. PREOPERATIVE EVALUATION
  A. History
    1. The frequency and severity of asthmatic attacks and the need for emergency room visits and hospitalizations suggest the severity of the disease process in a particular patient.
    2. Patients in whom emotional stress and direct physical stimulation frequently incite asthmatic attacks that necessitate hospitalization should be presumed to be at risk for severe bronchospasm in response to intubation and anesthesia.
    3. The efficacy of the bronchodilator drugs used routinely or on an emergency basis should be known.
    4. Patients should be questioned about steroid use within the last year.
  B. Diagnostic Tests
    1. Pulmonary function tests are an inexpensive, noninvasive means of determining the presence of airway diseases and the degree of reactivity and reversibility (Table 2-1).
      a. During an acute attack, forced expiratory volume in 1 second (FEV_1), mid-forced expiratory flow rate (FEF 25–75%), and forced vital capacity (FVC) will be markedly diminished.
      b. Clear response to bronchodilator therapy usually will increase flow and measured volumes by 20%.
      c. Residual volume (RV) and functional residual volume (FRC) are usually increased (measured by helium dilution, nitrogen washout, or plethysmography).
    2. Arterial blood gas analysis (normal values: Appendix D)
      a. At the onset of an acute asthmatic attack, mild hypoxemia and hypocarbia is found.
      b. As the episode worsens, hypoxemia worsens, and normocarbia or hypercarbia develops.
    3. Chest radiograph
      a. The film may be normal or show hyperinflation of the lung.
      b. Pneumonia, pneumothorax, pulmonary edema, and pulmonary hypertension may be the cause or complication of asthma.

Table 2–1. Interpretation of Spirometry Results

Functional Class	Description
Class 0	Breathlessness appropriate to activity
Class I (minimal)	Dyspnea on rapidly climbing stairs and hills and while running
Class II (moderate)	Dyspnea with routinely climbing stairs and hills, especially during pulmonary infections
Class III (severe)	Dyspnea during walking; dyspnea at rest only with respiratory infections
Class IV (very severe)	Dyspnea at rest or with minimal activity—talking, dressing

    4.   Electrocardiogram (ECG)

During acute attacks, the ECG may be normal or show premature ventricular beats, right bundle branch block, and evidence of right atrial or ventricular strain or enlargement.

III. MEDICATIONS

    A. β-Adrenergic Receptor Agonists (Table 2-2)

        1. Commonly used drugs: metaproterenol, terbutaline, albuterol.

        2. Mechanism of action: activate adenylate cyclase to increase intracellular cAMP, which dilates bronchi and inhibits the release of bronchoconstricting mediators.

        3. Routes of administration: inhalation, oral, parenteral.

    B. Methylxanthine Derivatives

        1. Commonly used drugs

            a. Theophylline is offered in several oral dosage forms: tablets and capsules (designed for timed release), elixirs, syrups, and suspensions.

            b. Aminophylline is the most commonly used soluble theophylline salt. It contains 85% anhydrous theophylline and is used primarily for intravenous and intramuscular injection.

Obstructive*				Restrictive			
MVV	*VC*	*RV*	*FEV₁*	*MVV*	*VC*	*RV*	*FEV₁*
% of predicted			*% VC*	*% of predicted*			*% VC*
>80	>80	80–120	>75	>80	>80	80–120	>75
65–80	>80	<150	60–75	>80	60–80	80–120	>75
45–65	>80	150–175	40–60	>80	50–60	80±	>75
30–45	↓	>200	<40	60–80	35–50	<80	>75
<30	↓ ↓	>200	<40	<60	<35	<80	>75

*Obstructed patients should be tested with a properly administered dose of bronchodilators. A positive response to bronchodilators is usually stated to have occurred if FEV_1 or flow rates increase by more than 20%.

    2. Mechanism of action

The exact mechanism is not known. Postulated mechanisms are inhibition of phosphodiesterase, prostaglandin antagonism, stimulation of endogenous catecholamine release, β-receptor agonist activity, and adenosine receptor antagonism.

    3. Routes of administration: oral, parenteral.

C. Parasympatholytics (Table 2-3)

    1. Commonly used drugs: atropine, glycopyrrolate, ipratropium.

    2. Mechanism of action: decrease acetylcholine output by the vagus nerve, thereby decreasing bronchial constriction mediated by cGMP.

    3. Routes of administration: inhalation, parenteral.

D. Corticosteroids

    1. Commonly used drugs: hydrocortisone, methylprednisone, prednisone (see Appendix E for steroid potency table), beclomethasone (inhaled).

    2. Mechanism of action: influence at the level of DNA the synthesis of proteins that regulate cellular synthesis and release of bronchoconstricting mediators.

    3. Routes of administration: oral, parenteral, inhalation.

Table 2–2. Inhaled Beta-Agonist Bronchodilators

Drug (Trade Name)	Effectiveness	Onset (min)	Peak (min)
Isoproterenol (Mistometer, Medihaler-Iso, Norisodrine)	+ + +	2–5	5
Isoetharine (Bronkosol, Bronkometer)	+	10–25	25
Albuterol (Proventil, Ventolin)	+	5–10	15
Metaproterenol (Alupent, Metaprel, MDI)	+	10–20	15
Terbutaline (Brethaire)	+ +	5–15	25

    E. Mast Cell Inhibitor
       1. Commonly used drug: cromolyn sodium.
       2. Mechanism of action: decreases mediator (histamine, leukotrienes) release from pulmonary mast cells by non-cAMP-related mechanism.
       3. Route of administration: inhalation.
    F. Calcium Channel Blockers
       1. Commonly used drugs: verapamil, nifedipine.
       2. Mechanism of action: decrease mediator release from mast cells that have a calcium-dependent process.
       3. Routes of administration: oral, parenteral.
IV. PERIOPERATIVE MEDICATION
    A. Bronchodilator therapy should be optimized by monitoring the clinical response, pulmonary function tests, and, if possible, serum levels (therapeutic theophylline level: 10–15 μg/ml).
    B. All oral bronchodilators should be given on the day of surgery. The use of an aerosol inhaler preoperatively is particularly advantageous, as it delivers medications directly to their site of action.
    C. Steroid supplementation should be supplied for any patient on suppressive doses of steroids (greater than prednisone 5 mg or other steroid of equivalent amount for longer than 2 to 3 weeks) within the previous year. A total of 150 to 300 mg of hydrocortisone over the initial 24 hours perioperatively is more than sufficient. Patients

Duration (hrs)	Dose (μg/puff)	Dysrhythmia/ Tachycardia	Side Effects
1–4	125	+ + + +	Tachyphylaxis, cardiac, ventricular fibrillation
1–2	340		Tachyphylaxis
4–6	90	+	Muscle tremors
3	65	+ +	
3–4	200	+ +	Muscle tremors

using inhaled steroids usually do not need supplemental coverage. If there is a question of adrenal reserve, then preoperative testing wth synthetic ACTH stimulation can be performed.

V. ANESTHETIC MANAGEMENT
    A. Preoperative Medication
        1. Current baseline and supplemental asthma medications are given as outlined above.
        2. Narcotic medications should be used with care, especially avoiding agents that stimulate histamine release (meperidine, morphine).

Table 2–3. *Anticholinergic Bronchodilators*

Drug	Dose	Route of Administration	Onset (min)	Peak (min)	Duration (hrs)
Atropine sulfate	0.025–0.075 mg/kg	Inhalation	15–30	30–170	3–5
	0.4–1 mg	Oral	NA	NA	NA
Atropine methonitrate	1–1.5 mg	Inhalation	15–30	40–60	4–6
Glycopyrrolate	0.0044 mg/kg	Inhalation	15–30	30–45	2–8
		Intramuscular	15–30	30–45	2–7
Ipratropium	20–40 μg	Inhalation	3–30	90–120	3–8

NA = Not available.

3. The amount of sedative/anxiolytic agents, such as midazolam or diazepam, should be tailored to the individual need. Caution should be used in administering intravenous benzodiazepines, because rapid administration of sedative doses can cause apnea.

B. Regional Anesthesia

1. Regional anesthetic techniques avoid to some extent the possibility of bronchospasm caused by intubation or airway manipulation.

2. Schnider and Papper showed a 1.9% incidence of wheezing during regional anesthesia in 159 asthmatic patients compared with a 1.6% incidence in nonintubated patients during general anesthesia and a 6.4% incidence in intubated patients undergoing general anesthesia.

C. Induction

1. Thiopental itself does not induce bronchospasm. Relatively large doses (4–7 mg/kg) of thiopental should be administered, depending on age, hemodynamic stability, and concurrent sedative/narcotics, to ensure an adequate depth of anesthesia prior to airway manipulation.

2. Lidocaine intravenously, but not intratracheally, prior to intubation blunts airway reactivity.

3. Ketamine can be used as an alternative induction agent. It has bronchodilatory effects secondary to release of endogenous catecholamines. Corssen et al. studied ketamine in 40 asthmatic patients. Wheezing subsided after induction in 17 cases. This improvement lasted from 6 to 8 minutes. However, in patients with an upper respiratory tract infection, ketamine has caused paroxysmal coughing. To prevent excess salivation in patients receiving ketamine, pretreatment with atropine or glycopyrrolate is recommended.

4. Halothane is felt to be the agent of choice for inhalational induction, because it does not produce upper airway irritation such as may occur with isoflurane or enflurane.

5. If a rapid-sequence induction is required, such as in the patient with a full stomach or the pregnant patient, ketamine is probably the agent of choice because of its bronchodilator effects.

      6.   Regardless of the technique of induction, intubation should be performed only after the patient is deeply anesthetized.

      7.   The muscle relaxants of choice are succinylcholine, vecuronium, and pancuronium. Atracurium and *d*-tubocurarine should be avoided because of their potential to release histamine.

D. Intraoperative Management

      1.   Routine monitoring should include inspired O_2 analysis, pulse oximetry, and end-tidal CO_2 (may have poor correlation with $PaCO_2$ in severe asthma) measurements.

      2.   Patients should be hydrated and receive adequately warmed and humidified gases to avoid drying and inspissation of secretions.

      3.   Devices are commercially available to allow in-line administration of metered doses of inhaled bronchodilators as needed.

      4.   For maintenance of anesthesia, equipotent concentrations of halothane, isoflurane, and enflurane are probably equally effective in preventing and reversing bronchoconstriction. In the presence of therapeutic theophylline levels and beta agonists, serious ventricular dysrhythmias have been noted in those patients receiving halothane. These dysrhythmias are much less likely with isoflurane or enflurane.

      5.   Intravenous aminophylline can be used for bronchospasm unresponsive to inhaled bronchodilators or increasing inhaled anesthetic concentration, but toxic levels can be easily reached if patients have a significant serum level preoperatively.

E. Management of Intraoperative Bronchospasm

      1.   Bronchospasm during anesthesia is detected by continuous ausculation via an esophageal or precordial stethoscope and by monitoring of airway pressures and ease of ventilation.

      2.   All that wheezes intraoperatively is not asthma: the differential diagnosis includes laryngospasm, severe atelectasis, pneumothorax, light anesthesia, congestive heart failure, cuff herniation, ball valve effect of secretions in the endotracheal tube, foreign body in the airway, secretions, and bronchospasm from exacerbation of chronic obstructive lung disease or anaphylaxis.

3. Overall evaluation of the patient, airway, endotracheal tube, anesthesia machine, and arterial blood gases should be performed as necessary.

F. Emergence

1. Reversal with neostigmine or other cholinesterase inhibitors can precipitate bronchospasm secondary to cholinergic stimulation, but this reaction is readily prevented by concurrent administration of an anticholinergic such as atropine or glycopyrrolate.

2. Deep extubation is favored unless the patient is at high risk for aspiration. This is performed to avoid the potential for bronchospasm on emergence from general anesthesia with an endotracheal tube still in place.

3. Patients at high risk for postoperative aspiration should be made comfortable with opioids after the anesthetic is discontinued. Patients may be extubated when fully awake and with good muscle tone.

VI. STATUS ASTHMATICUS

All three major volatile agents have been successful in treating status asthmaticus after aggressive conventional therapy has failed. Particular attention must be given to the mode of ventilation, airway pressure, drug interactions, and the hemodynamic effects of the volatile agents. With newer ventilators such as the Siemens Servo 900-C, a vaporizer can be placed in-line and inhalational anesthesia administered in the ICU setting. Appropriate scavenging of waste anesthetic gases is imperative in this setting.

VII. SUMMARY OF ANESTHETIC CONSIDERATIONS

Asthmatic patients with frequent attacks secondary to emotional or physical stimulation are at increased risk during the perianesthetic period, especially during intubation and emergence. Preoperatively, bronchodilator therapy should be optimized. If the patient is steroid dependent, steroid supplementation can be given orally or intravenously.

Whenever possible, regional anesthesia should be utilized to avoid manipulation of the airway. When initiating general anesthesia, the patient should be under deep anesthesia prior to intubation. All medications that can cause histamine release should be avoided. For maintenance of general anesthesia, equipotent concentrations of halothane, enflurane, and isoflurane are equally effective in preventing and reversing bronchospasms. Intraoperative bronchospasm can be treated by increasing the concentration of inhaled anesthesia, delivery of inhaled bronchodilators, or intravenous bronchodilators. Postoperatively, deep extubation is favored unless the patient is at high risk for aspiration.

Chronic Obstructive Lung Disease

I.   GENERAL CHARACTERISTICS
  A.   Chronic Obstructive Lung Disease
      Chronic obstructive lung disease (COLD) commonly includes chronic bronchitis and pulmonary emphysema. Many patients have elements of several processes and not a pure form of any one disorder. COLD is most prevalent in men after the fourth decade of life. The principal predisposing factor is tobacco abuse. This disease process is important to anesthesiologists because of its prevalence and its high perioperative morbidity and mortality rates. Postoperative death in these patients is four times as likely as is death from all other causes in the general surgical population.
  B.   Emphysema
      Pulmonary emphysema is characterized by the destruction of the alveolar walls, resulting in irreversible enlargement of the alveoli. The lung loses its elastic recoil, with resultant airway collapse on expiration and increased airway resistance. This collapse with obstruction to air flow also creates a potential for the formation of bullae. These patients have an increased work of breathing secondary to the loss of the elastic recoil. Therefore, patients may present with severe dyspnea. Although the principal predisposing factor is cigarette smoking, in some patients ($<15\%$), there is an inherited deficiency of alpha-1-antitrypsin that results in chronic lung injury.
  C.   Chronic Bronchitis
      Chronic bronchitis is characterized by the chronic secretion of excessive mucus into the bronchi, resulting in decreased airway diameter and resistance. Recurrent infections with the pneumococcus, *Haemophilus influenzae*, viruses, and *Mycoplasma* are common. Arterial hypoxemia and CO_2 retention tend to occur earlier in the course of this disease than in pulmonary emphysema.

D. Restrictive Lung Disease

Restrictive lung disease, although not included in the definition of COLD, is often a component in patients with COLD. The hallmark of this disease is a decrease in total lung capacity (TLC). The inherent disease process may alter the elastic property of the lung or affect the chest wall, respiratory muscles, or parapulmonary structures (pleura, abdomen), limiting lung expansion. In general, there is little effective therapy.

II. PREOPERATIVE ASSESSMENT

A. The preoperative evaluation and the anesthetic management are essentially the same for patients with pulmonary emphysema and chronic bronchitis. The preoperative evaluation should determine the extent of the disease and elucidate any reversible components such as bronchospasm or infection. Preoperative recognition and treatment of COLD will lessen the incidence of postoperative pulmonary complications.

B. History

  1. The history should provide information concerning the type, frequency, and duration of symptoms. Functional impairment can be addressed by assessing the degree of exertion that brings on typical symptoms such as wheezing, fatigue, dyspnea, coughing, or dizziness and whether any of these symptoms occur at rest.

  2. Recent exacerbations, inciting events, duration, and recent change in treatment provide an idea of the dynamic nature of the disease and may indicate whether any further medical management should precede elective surgery.

  3. Current and previous drug therapy may provide an idea of disease progression.

  4. Changes in sputum quality and quantity may reflect respiratory tract infection.

C. Physical Examination

  1. An obstructive pattern is often characterized by the use of accessory muscles of breathing and by maneuvers to prolong the expiratory phase such as pursed lips. The inspiration : expiration (I : E) ratio decreases from 1 : 2 to 1 : 3 or less. The time required to exhale from TLC to RV will be longer than 4 seconds. Pursed-lip breathing may be utilized as a mechanism of "respiratory hold."

2. The patient with a restrictive disease often breathes with smaller lung volumes at a more rapid rate.

3. The chest is examined for its shape and the amount of expansion from RV to total lung capacity. A normal chest circumference should expand 3.5 to 5 cm at the level of the nipples. The diaphragm can be percussed at RV to identify overinflation and the amount of diaphragmatic movement (normal = 2–4 cm). Patients with severe COLD have minimal chest wall and diaphragm movement.

4. Auscultation may reveal adventitious sounds such as wheezes or rhonchi that indicate airflow obstruction. A right ventricular heave or palpable P_2 may be found in patients with pulmonary vascular disease.

D. Diagnostic Studies

1. Chest radiography

In the preoperative chest radiograph, the trachea and major bronchi are evaluated for patency and position and the presence of any abnormal masses. A globular or boot-shaped heart may be associated with right ventricular hypertrophy. The proximal pulmonary artery (PA) may be dilated and the distal vessels "pruned" in patients with pulmonary vascular disease. A low, flat diaphragm is commonly seen in emphysematous or bronchitic patients secondary to air trapping with resultant hyperinflation. Finally, the lung fields themselves are reviewed. Infiltrates, masses, and bullae are noted for their size and location. Any evidence of pneumothorax should be sought. In addition, the location of the endotracheal tube and any vascular catheters or chest tubes are noted.

2. Pulmonary function tests (PFT)

a. Testing will provide some information about preoperative lung volumes and airflow and will aid in categorizing the type and amount of functional impairment. Routine spirometry is a simple and helpful test. The FVC is the entire volume exhaled, whereas the FEV_1 is the volume exhaled in 1 second. The peak or maximal expiratory flow rate (PEFR or MEFR) represents the maximum forced flow the patient is able to generate. The slope between 25% and 75% of the FVC is called the FEF_{25-75}. The ratio of FEV_1/FVC and FEF_{25-75} provides an indication of airflow obstruction.

b. An FEV_1/FVC ratio of less than 75% indicates moderate obstructive disease, whereas a ratio less than 50% indicates severe disease. A diminished FEF_{25-75} also indicates airflow obstruction and is said to be an early indicator of small-airways disease when other pulmonary function tests are still within normal limits. In addition, the FEF_{25-75} is much less effort dependent. Numerous other tests are available that measure closing capacity, diffusing capacity, TLC, maximal ventilatory volume (MVV), and compliance, among others. The MVV is often used in assessing patients with chronic lung disease. It requires the patient to inhale and exhale as hard as possible for 12 seconds. This test is highly effort dependent and so requires a cooperative patient to obtain useful data.

c. A decrease in the absolute value of the FEV_1 and FVC with a normal FEV_1/FVC is indicative of restrictive pulmonary disease. Restrictive disease is found in patients with intrinsic pulmonary pathology such as asbestosis, silicosis, interstitial lung disease, and others, as well as in those with thoracic cage deformities such as kyphoscoliosis or after trauma, or those with muscle or neurologic dysfunction.

E. Evaluation of Patients for Pulmonary Resection

1. Patients undergoing pulmonary resection have special considerations. The patient's preoperative pulmonary status must be assessed and an attempt made to estimate the postoperative pulmonary function. After a thorough history and physical examination and review of PFT, chest radiograph, and arterial blood gases, a decision must be made about whether the patient has a degree of baseline dysfunction that will preclude removal of any amount of functional lung tissue (Table 2-4).

2. Preoperatively, if there is any question regarding lung tissue to be resected a ventilation–perfusion ($\dot{V}/\dot{Q}$) scan will provide a better estimate of the amount of functioning tissue that will be present

Table 2–4. Contraindications to Pneumonectomy

FVC	<2 L
FEV_1/FVC	<50%
MVV	<50% of predicted
Predicted postoperative FEV_1	<800 ml
PA pressure (on balloon occlusion)	>35 mmHg
PaO_2 (on balloon occlusion)	<45 mmHg

postoperatively. Traditionally, the fraction of lung that would be left after resection has been multiplied by the preoperative FEV_1 to give the "postop FEV_1." A value of less than 800 ml has been considered inoperable secondary to predicted CO_2 retention. To more accurately account for patient size, Gass has recommended using a percent of normal instead of absolute volume of FEV_1. He suggested that a cutoff of 30% of normal should be used as the lower limit for an operative candidate.

3. Other tests include exercise testing with or without maximum oxygen consumption determination and right heart catheterization with balloon occlusion of the PA to be resected.

III. RISK OF POSTOPERATIVE PULMONARY COMPLICATIONS

A. Patients with several conditions are at increased risk for postoperative respiratory complications.

1. Acute or chronic respiratory disease
2. Age greater than 65
3. Obesity
4. Cigarette smoking
5. Upper abdominal or thoracic surgery
6. General anesthesia duration of greater than 3 hours

B. Incidence of Postoperative Complications

1. In one retrospective review, 2.9% to 70% of patients between 1922–1969 had pulmonary complications, with the highest rate occurring after upper abdominal and thoracic surgical procedures (Latemen and coworkers).
2. There is a 3% complication rate in patients with normal PFTs (normal values: Appendix C) versus a 70% rate in patients with abnormal PFTs (Stein and colleagues).

Table 2–5. *Therapies to Decrease Pulmonary Complications*

Preoperative

Patient education
Cessation of smoking
Optimization of nutritional status
Treatment of respiratory tract infection
Maximization of bronchodilator therapy in bronchospastic disease
Prophylaxis for thromboembolic disease in high-risk patients

Intraoperatively

Minimize anesthesia and surgical time
Use of regional anesthesia when possible

Postoperatively

Early ambulation
Respiratory therapy maneuvers (cough and deep breathing, exercise, and incentive spirometry)
Adequate pain control with pain medications or regional block
Nutritional support
Supplemental oxygen as needed

3. Pulmonary complications are decreased by patient instruction in postoperative pulmonary care, minimizing surgical and anesthetic duration, and early ambulation (Table 2-5).

C. Perioperative changes in pulmonary mechanics increase the risk of pulmonary complications.
   1. Diminished sigh and cough attributable in part to surgical pain.
   2. Reflex elimination of diaphragmatic excursion, especially after upper abdominal and thoracic surgery.
   3. Alteration of pulmonary host defenses with colonization of tracheobronchial tree with pathogenic gram-negative organisms.

IV. PREOPERATIVE PREPARATION
   A. Preoperative preparation of these patients can significantly reduce not only the incidence of postoperative complications but also the length of the hospital stay. This preparation is best achieved by both teaching the patient selective respiratory maneuvers to be used postoperatively and providing appropriate preoperative pulmonary therapy. A wide variety of practices have been developed to prevent the familiar postoperative progres-

sion of atelectasis, tachypnea, hypoxia, fever, and pneumonitis.

B. The beneficial respiratory maneuvers to teach patients preoperatively are incentive spirometry and cough and deep breathing techniques, which help maximize alveolar inflation and maintain a normal FRC.

C. Patients should also be instructed to stop smoking for at least 3 weeks prior to the planned operation. Cessation of smoking will improve lung volumes and decrease bronchial secretions and carboxyhemoglobin levels.

D. One should continue the patient's usual medications until the morning of surgery and add aerosolized bronchodilators if the patient has any component of reversible bronchospasm. Steroid coverage should be provided as necessary.

E. Preoperative sedation must be individualized, and narcotics should be given in small doses, if at all, to avoid respiratory depression. Many of these patients will not tolerate any sedation.

V. ANESTHETIC MANAGEMENT

A. Monitoring

Monitoring should include the standard ECG, blood pressure cuff, stethoscope, oxygen analyzer, airway pressure alarm, and temperature probe. Additionally, pulse oximetry, arterial blood gas analysis, end-tidal CO_2 monitor or mass spectrometer, and neuromuscular blockade monitors should be used. If assessment of intravascular volume is needed, the use of the PA catheter would be preferred to the central venous pressure (CVP) catheter because pulmonary hypertension, which is common in patients with COLD, prevents the CVP monitor from reflecting left ventricular end-diastolic volume accurately.

B. Inhaled Anesthetics

1. The presence of COLD does not necessarily dictate a specific anesthetic agent or technique. Different combinations of general anesthetic techniques with or without muscle relaxation have been shown to have no discernible effect on postoperative mortality rates. The volatile anesthetic agents usually cause bronchodilatation, helping decrease airway resistance.

2. Although N_2O is frequently administered during general anesthesia, it should be administered with care, if at all, to the patient at risk for barotrauma or with bullous disease. In addition, the use of N_2O will limit the inspired concentration of O_2 that can be administered during anesthesia, and this may be critical, especially during one-lung ventilation.

3. Narcotics and sedatives must be administered with care, keeping in mind the possibility of severe and prolonged postoperative respiratory depression.

4. Mechanical ventilators

   a. Controlled ventilation is recommended for long operations. In patients with moderate to severe emphysema, large tidal volumes (10–12 ml/kg) with slow inspiratory flow rates will maintain the best matching of ventilation and perfusion. A slow rate of ventilation (6–10 breaths/min) is necessary to prevent air trapping in patients with COLD and to avoid hyperinflation.

   b. Because the endotracheal tube bypasses the natural airway humidification system, the inspired gas should be humidified to prevent drying of secretions. Systemic dehydration should be avoided.

   c. If the $PaCO_2$ has been chronically elevated, the plasma bicarbonate level will also be elevated, and it is important not to correct the hypercarbia abruptly. Sudden normocarbia can result in profound metabolic alkalemia, which may provoke cardiac dysrhythmias and central nervous system (CNS) dysfunction with seizures.

   d. The hazard of barotrauma in these patients must be appreciated, especially if high airway pressures are required to provide adequate ventilation. Positive end-expiratory pressure (PEEP) and pressure retard maneuvers should be used with caution. Intraoperative bronchospasm can become a problem as well (see section on asthma).

C. Regional Anesthesia

   1. Regional anesthesia is ideal in this patient population if it is appropriate for the planned surgical procedure and acceptable to the patient and surgeon.

   2. Regional anesthetics are most appropriate for lower abdominal and extremity procedures.

3. Sensory blocks above T_6 and spinal or epidural anesthesia are not recommended because of the decrease in respiratory muscle function and expiratory reserve volume and the resultant diminished depth of breathing, cough, and clearing of secretions.

VI. POSTOPERATIVE MANAGEMENT

A. Postoperatively, the patient with severe pulmonary disease may require continued intubation and mechanical ventilation, especially if upper abdominal or thoracic surgery has been performed. The presence of a $PaCO_2$ above 50 mmHg postoperatively without a history of CO_2 retention or an FEV_1/FVC below 50% preoperatively is often associated with the need for mechanical ventilation postoperatively.

B. Good postoperative pain control allows the patient to perform breathing exercises adequately.

C. Early ambulation will help decrease atelectasis and perioperative deep venous thrombosis.

VII. SUMMARY OF ANESTHETIC CONSIDERATIONS

Patients at the greatest risk for postoperative pulmonary complications are those with acute or chronic respiratory disease, smoking history, advanced age, and upper abdominal or thoracic surgery. Preoperative instruction in maneuvers such as incentive spirometry and cough and deep breathing techniques to be used postoperatively helps decrease the incidence of postsurgical atelectasis, hypoxia, fever, and pneumonitis in patients with COLD. In addition to becoming adept at breathing exercises, these patients should have pulmonary infections treated and bronchodilator therapy, if needed, established before surgery.

Patients requiring lung resection will need special evaluation to ensure that an FEV_1 of at least 800 ml is left after surgery.

In general, the presence of COLD does not dictate a specific anesthetic agent or technique, although a regional technique would be preferred. Sensory blocks above T_6 and spinal or epidural anesthesia are not recommended because of the decrease in accessory muscle function, with the resultant difficulty with coughing and clearing secretions. Using N_2O must be carefully considered, because it will limit the inspired O_2 concentration, which could increase the possibility of barotrauma if extensive bullous disease is present. Intraoperative mechanical ventilation must be carefully adjusted to ensure adequate expiratory time and to minimize respiratory or metabolic alkalosis. Good postoperative pain control is especially important in those patients who need to ambulate early and perform breathing exercises.

Aspiration

I.   INCIDENCE AND OUTCOME
   A.   Aspiration of gastric contents is one of the most serious complications of anesthesia and accounts for considerable morbidity and mortality in surgical, obstetrical, and intensive care unit patients. The actual incidence of regurgitation and subsequent aspiration is difficult to assess, because the condition is often undiagnosed. Silent regurgitation of small amounts of gastric fluid into the oropharynx reportedly occurs in 4% to 26% of all inductions for general anesthetics. The incidence of subsequent aspiration is probably in the range of 10% to 20%.
   B.   Death occurs in about 30% of cases of significant aspiration of gastric contents, with a range of 3% to 70% depending on the type of material aspirated and the subsequent therapy.

II.   ASPIRATE
   A.   The material aspirated may be particulate or liquid. The aspiration of liquid gastric contents is common.
   B.   The course of clinical events will then depend on the pH, volume, presence of particulate matter, and infective nature of the aspirated material.
      1.   pH
         Severe chemical pneumonitis may occur when the pH is below 2.5. With aspiration of acidic material, mucosal damage occurs within seconds. In addition to bronchospasm and atelectasis, there will be tissue breakdown with alveolar edema, loss of surfactant activity, and hemorrhage.
      2.   Volume
         The critical volume has been stated to be greater than 0.4 ml/kg. As little as 25 ml of liquid with a pH below 2.5 has caused chemical pneumonitis. If a small volume of pH-neutral material is inhaled, the patient may react with some degree of broncho-

spasm and atelectasis. Lung fuction usually returns to baseline within 24 hours in these latter cases.

   3.   Content

If the aspirate contains particulate matter, acute airway obstruction may ensue. Atelectasis develops distal to the obstruction, and, if it is untreated, infection may result in pneumonia and eventual abscess formation. The inhalation of grossly infected material, as in a patient with an intestinal obstruction, results in extremely high mortality rates.

III. SITUATIONS THAT INCREASE THE RISK OF ASPIRATION

   A.   Protective airway reflexes are depressed with general anesthesia, sedation, topical anesthesia of the posterior pharynx, neurologic and muscular diseases, and advanced age.

   B.   The gastric contents can reach the oropharynx by active vomiting or passive regurgitation, which can occur during induction or emergence.

   C.   For passive regurgitation to occur, there must be either increased intragastric pressure or incompetence of the lower esophageal sphincter.

   1.   The sphincter remains competent up to intragastric pressures of 20 cmH_2O. The patient who coughs, strains, or has some degree of respiratory obstruction can develop intragastric pressures up to 60 cm H_2O, causing reflux. Succinylcholine-induced fasciculations can also raise the intragastric pressure sufficiently to cause reflux.

   2.   Incompetence of the lower esophageal sphincter can occur whenever the stomach is distended. Delayed gastric emptying causing increased gastric pressure and distention is common in surgical patients secondary to pain, anxiety, obesity, diabetes, metabolic abnormalities, drug toxicity, parasympathetic agents, ascites, intra-abdominal masses including the gravid uterus, narcotics, or intestinal obstruction. Increased gastric secretion leading to increased gastric pressure is also seen in outpatients and patients with duodenal ulcers. Other patients who may have an incompetent lower esophageal sphincter include those with a hiatal hernia, a nasogastric (NG) tube, collagen vascular disease, or pernicious anemia.

IV. PREOPERATIVE MEASURES TO DECREASE ASPIRATION AND ITS COMPLICATIONS
- **A.** Gastric Emptying
  - **1.** The preoperative use of an NG tube may be most helpful for ensuring an empty stomach.
  - **2.** Usually, having a patient receive nothing by mouth for 8 hours will minimize gastric volume.
  - **3.** Metoclopramide, a cholinomimetic alkaloid, opens the pylorus, stimulates gastric motility, and causes antegrade emptying of the stomach into the duodenum (Table 2-6).
- **B.** Increasing Gastric pH
  - **1.** The gastric pH can be raised simply and effectively with antacids. However, particulate antacids, such as aluminum and magnesium compounds, may cause pneumonitis when aspirated.
  - **2.** A nonparticulate antacid, sodium citrate, may therefore be preferred. It works reliably but it increases gastric volume and lasts only 60 minutes.
  - **3.** H$_2$-receptor antagonists
    - **a.** The H$_2$-antagonists cimetidine and ranitidine inhibit gastric secretion, thereby decreasing volume and acidity. They may be valuable in the patient scheduled for elective surgery.

Table 2–6. *Prophylaxis Against Pulmonary Aspiration*

Sodium citrate

15–30 ml orally 30 min prior to the induction of anesthesia (can use two Alka Seltzer in 30 ml of water). Consider for outpatients, obstetric and emergency patients, and patients at high risk for aspiration.

H$_2$-receptor antagonists

Ranitidine 150 mg orally or 50 mg IV or cimetidine 300 mg orally or IV. Give oral medication 2–3 hours preoperatively; IV 1 hour preoperatively. Consider use in patients at risk to have large gastric volume and low pH such as those with obesity, hiatal hernia, hypersecretion syndromes, or peptic ulcer disease and the critically ill.

Metoclopramide

10 mg orally, IM, or IV. Use to enhance gastric emptying in patients with diabetes, abnormal lower esophageal sphincter tone (connective tissue disease, pernicious anemia, elderly), hiatal hernia. Give 1 hour before surgery.

> **b.** Neither cimetidine nor ranitidine affect the acidity of the secretions already in the stomach at the time of administration. Therefore, the use of the H_2 antagonists alone as prophylaxis prior to emergency surgery is of doubtful benefit. Under these circumstances, an antacid is probably a better prophylactic measure.
>
> **c.** The use of H_2-antagonists intraoperatively in emergency patients can certainly be considered to decrease further secretion and thereby limit acidity and volume postoperatively.
>
> **d.** Cimetidine decreases hepatic blood flow and inhibits microsomal enzymes. This effect will diminish the clearance of the benzodiazepines, propranolol, theophylline, phenytoin, and lidocaine. The same problems exist with the other H_2-antagonists but to a lesser degree.

C. Anticholinergics

> **1.** The anticholinergics, such as glycopyrrolate, have also been used to decrease gastric volume and increase pH. Salem et al. used large doses (7.5–10 μg/kg) of glycopyrrolate and found the frequency of gastric samples with a pH above 2.5 significantly increased over control.
>
> **2.** With the customarily used doses (3 μg/kg), Stoelting found that neither volume nor acidity was modified.
>
> **3.** Despite increasing gastric pH, anticholinergic agents, as well as morphine, meperidine, and diazepam, may increase the risk of aspiration by decreasing the tone of the lower esophageal sphincter.
>
> **4.** Prophylactic use of anticholinergic agents is not recommended because of the inconsistent effect on gastric pH and volume and the alteration of sphincter function.

V. DECREASING ASPIRATION DURING INDUCTION

A. Awake Intubation

> **1.** Awake intubation should be considered in all patients who are at high risk of aspiration and in those patients where intubation is felt to be technically difficult or especially hazardous. Judicious sedation with maintenance of airway reflexes is possible.
>
> **2.** Topical anesthesia for the oropharynx may be helpful, but the vocal cords and trachea should not be anesthetized in this group of patients.

B. Rapid-sequence Intubation
  1. An alternative to an awake intubation is rapid-sequence induction and intubation. This technique begins with preoxygenation with 100% O_2 for 2 to 3 minutes or, alternatively, for at least four or five deep breaths. Thiopental is then administered followed by a muscle relaxant (dose appropriate for age, weight, volume status, and cardiac reserve) while cricoid pressure is applied (Sellick's maneuver). After the patient becomes apneic, endotracheal intubation is performed without prior positive pressure ventilation and with a stylet in the endotracheal tube. The cuff is inflated, proper tube placement is checked by listening for bilateral chest sounds, and only then is cricoid pressure removed.
  2. This type of induction certainly has risks of its own. The overall incidence of difficult or delayed intubation is approximately 5% and may be as high as 10% when a stylet is not used. One of the most important components in this sequence is the proper application of cricoid pressure. Pressure applied properly over the cricoid cartilage will make intubation easier, whereas if pressure is mistakenly applied to the thyroid cartilage, intubation will be more difficult.
  3. If cricoid pressure is appropriately applied, nearly all cases of aspiration should be preventable. This maneuver will overcome esophageal pressures up to 100 cmH_2O, and therefore during active vomiting, one must consider the possibility of esophageal rupture.
  4. If any doubt exists as to the ease of intubation, one must strongly consider an awake intubation.
  5. Patients for whom a rapid-sequence induction has been performed will still be at increased risk for regurgitation and aspiration at the end of the procedure. Therefore, the stomach should be emptied with an NG tube, and only when the patient is fully awake with return of protective laryngeal reflexes should extubation take place.
C. Cuffed Endotracheal Tubes
Endotracheal intubation with a cuffed tube does not ensure that aspiration will not occur in the high-risk patient, but it certainly affords the best possible protection in the anesthetized state.

D. Although there are several available methods to decrease gastric volume, increase gastric pH, and protect the airway, none of them is infallible. Therefore, local or regional anesthesia should be considered when feasible.

VI. THERAPY

    A. Recognition

        1. The recognition of the possibility of aspiration is the first step and may be as simple as seeing gastric contents at the level of the larynx during intubation. Often, however, the aspiration is not witnessed.

        2. Clinically, aspiration is characterized by tachypnea, tachycardia, wheezing, and arterial hypoxemia (PaO_2/FIO_2 <300 mmHg).

        3. There will be a marked decrease in pulmonary compliance secondary to the loss of surfactant activity and edema.

    B. Securing the Airway

        1. Once regurgitation has occurred, the oropharynx and trachea should be suctioned as quickly as possible, both to minimize the volume of aspirate and to stimulate coughing.

        2. An adequate airway must be established immediately and oxygen administered. This is usually by endotracheal intubation.

        3. If particulate matter of significant size has been aspirated, bronchoscopy should be performed.

        4. With acid aspiration, the damage to the mucosa occurs within 30 seconds, and attempts at lavage not only are not efficacious but may lead to further hypoxemia and damage. Bronchial secretions alone will neutralize the acid within minutes.

    C. Ventilation

        1. Treatment is mainly supportive, with maneuvers directed at maintenance of adequate gas exchange and oxygenation.

        2. If the patient is still hypoxemic and breathing spontaneously with supplemental O_2, then continuous positive airway pressure (CPAP) by mask should be applied and titrated to maintain PaO_2 above 80 mmHg and FIO_2 below 0.6 mmHg.

        3. The patient who is not alert or cooperative, who requires CPAP above 10, or for whom mechanical ventilation is otherwise indicated (CO_2 retention, hypoxemia with spontaneous breathing) requires intubation. The addition of PEEP to mechanical ventilation should improve the ability to oxygenate the patient adequately at acceptable levels of FIO_2 by increasing the FRC and reducing intrapulmonary shunt (for further ventilatory management, see the section on ARDS).

D. Antibiotics

1.   Prophylactic antibiotics are not recommended, as this action simply increases the incidence of superinfection with antibiotic-resistant organisms.

2.   Daily Gram staining of the tracheal aspirate and chest radiographs are needed because of the high incidence of secondary infection. Treatment should be instituted when needed on this basis.

3.   Treatment can be readjusted as necessary on the basis of sputum culture and sensitivity reports. Empiric therapy while awaiting final culture results should be directed against anaerobic organisms and oral flora.

E.   Steroids

Recent well-designed studies showed no beneficial effect from the use of steroids in aspiration syndromes. Indeed, the use of steroids in aspiration syndromes or ARDS interferes with the healing process, increases the incidence of secondary infections, and does not improve the survival rate.

VII. SUMMARY OF ANESTHETIC CONSIDERATIONS

Aspiration of large volumes (>0.4 ml/kg) of gastric contents with acidic pH (<2.5) may produce significant intraoperative and postoperative pulmonary complications. To decrease the possibility of aspiration during anesthesia, the patient should not have eaten within 6 hours of induction. Metaclopramide and an NG tube connected to suction can help ensure an empty stomach. Preoperative nonparticulate antiacids and H_2 agonists will increase gastric pH.

If patients needing general anesthesia are at high risk for aspiration, in addition to maneuvers used to ensure gastric emptying and increased gastric pH, they should either be intubated awake or by rapid sequence.

Despite all precautions, aspiration may occur. Most importantly, suctioning and removal of as much of the aspirated material as possible should be done promptly. If hypoxemia is present with FIO_2 above 0.5, PEEP should be applied to help improve oxygenation. Antibiotics may be needed with signs of pulmonary infection. Prophylactic steroid administration is no longer recommended.

Deep Venous Thrombosis and Pulmonary Embolism

I. INCIDENCE
   A. Pulmonary embolism occurs as a complication of venous thrombosis and reportedly is a cause of 50,000 deaths per year in this country. The primary sources of emboli are deep venous thromboses.
   B. Thromboembolic disease is a common problem, occurring in half a million persons per year, with a greater incidence in patients undergoing anesthesia and surgery. The indication for surgery and the choice of anesthetic technique may well influence this incidence.

II. PATHOPHYSIOLOGY
   A. Blood flow stasis, blood vessel injury, and a hypercoagulable state enhance thrombogenesis. Many risk factors can be identified and understood in terms of this triad (Table 2-7). One of the most important risk factors is immobilization, especially after trauma or surgical procedures. The greater the number of associated risk factors, the greater the likelihood of a thromboembolic complication.

Table 2–7. Risk Factors for Thromboembolic Disease

Immobilization*	Oral contraceptive use
Age >65	Prior thromboembolic disease
Malignancy	Sickle cell disease
Pregnancy	Obesity
Congestive heart failure or recent myocardial infarction	Deficiencies of native inhibitors of coagulation (antithrombin III, protein C or S)
Systemic lupus erythematosus	Abnormal activity of the fibrinolytic system
Inflammatory bowel disease	
Polycythemia vera	

*Especially after trauma or after neurosurgical, orthopedic (involving the hip or lower extremity), urologic, gynecologic, and general surgical procedures in patients over 65.

Table 2–8. Risk Groups for Venous Thromboembolism

Group	Incidence of Venous Thrombosis (%)	Site	Incidence of Fatal PE (%)	Prophylaxis
Hip fracture	40–70	Thigh and calf	7–10	Any of the following: dextran, adjusted-
Total hip replacement	40–70	Thigh and calf	4–7	dose heparin, low-dose warfarin,
Total knee replacement	40–70	Thigh and calf	3–7	pneumatic compression
Urologic surgery	15–20	Calf	<5	Pneumatic compression
General and gynecologic surgery	15–20	Calf	1	Low-dose heparin
Neurologic surgery	15–20	Calf	<1	Pneumatic compression
Medical patients	<15	Calf	<1	Low-dose heparin

(From Hyers TM, Hull RD, Weg JG. Chest 1986;89(5):27.)

B. Nearly all pulmonary emboli arise from venous thrombosis of the lower extremities and pelvis. Rarely, pulmonary emboli originate in the upper extremities, usually secondary to long-term intravenous line placement.

C. Deep venous thrombosis (DVT) occurs in 15% to 70% of patients with increased risk factors when they undergo major surgical procedures (Table 2-8). Fatal pulmonary emboli (PE) have been reported in 1% of high-risk patients.

III. MEASURES TO DECREASE THE INCIDENCE OF DVT AND PE

A. Drugs and Devices that Decrease DVT

1. Low-dose heparin (5000 units subcutaneously every 8–12 hours) beginning 2 hours prior to surgery decreases the risk of DVT and PE by greater than 50% for most surgical procedures.

   a. This dose interferes with Factor X activation, does not routinely lengthen the partial thromboplastin time (PTT), and entails a minimally increased risk of bleeding.

            b. The addition of dihydroergotamine, a veno-constrictor, may increase the efficacy of heparin.

            c. Low-dose heparin is not effective in orthopedic surgery (hip and knee) or open prostatectomy because of the release of large quantities of tissue thromboplastin during such operations.

      2. Dextran decreases the risk of DVT and PE in all surgical procedures including orthopedic surgery, but it can increase the risk of bleeding.

      3. External pneumatic compression devices are effective if applied preoperatively.

      4. Graduated compression elastic stockings may decrease the incidence of DVT and PE.

   B. Indications for Prophylaxis

      1. In general, all high-risk patients undergoing urologic, gynecologic, or long operations should receive low-dose heparin or alternative prophylaxis.

      2. Patients at high risk who are undergoing hip or knee surgery should receive dextran, an adjusted heparin dose (to place the PTT at 1.5 times control), or mechanical measures.

      3. All patients undergoing intracranial neurosurgical procedures should have external pneumatic compression devices applied preoperatively.

IV. ANESTHESIA MANAGEMENT

   A. Anesthesia and Thromboembolism

      1. The high incidence of thromboembolism after anesthesia and surgery is largely related to blood flow stasis. Modig et al. showed, in a study of orthopedic patients undergoing total hip replacement, that patients who had the procedure performed under general anesthesia had a 67% incidence of DVT, and 33% of these went on to have a PE. In comparison, patients who had hip replacement performed under continuous epidural anesthesia continued for 24 hours postoperatively had only a 13% and 10% incidence of DVT and PE, respectively.

      2. In another study, McKenzie showed that patients undergoing femoral neck repair under general anesthesia had almost twice the incidence of DVT postoperatively as those having the operation performed with spinal anesthesia. Similar results have been found in patients undergoing open prostatectomy when general anesthesia was compared with an epidural technique.

B. Decreased thrombosis with regional anesthesia may be secondary to reduction of blood flow stasis because of decreased vascular resistance from sympathetic nerve block, decrease in blood viscosity from hemodilution, or a beneficial effect of the local anesthetic on the vascular endothelium.

C. Consideration should be given to measures that decrease the incidence of perioperative thromboembolism: subcutaneous heparin, sequential pneumatic devices, compression stockings, and regional anesthesia.

V. **VENA CAVAL INTERRUPTION AND EMERGENCY PULMONARY EMBOLECTOMY**

    A. Vena Caval Interruption

        1. The procedure may be performed either in the radiology suite or the operating room.

            a. At present, fluoroscopically directed caval filters, mesh, or umbrellas are placed via a transvenous (internal jugular, femoral) approach. This eliminates many of the greater complications associated with transabdominal placement of caval clips. These newer devices also remain patent longer.

            b. General or regional anesthesia usually is not required.

        2. Inferior vena caval interruption usually is performed in the following instances:

            a. An absolute contraindication to anticoagulation in a patient with known proximal DVT or PE.

            b. Recurrent PE in a patient receiving adequate anticoagulation.

            c. Life-threatening complications such as bleeding and heparin-induced thrombocytopenia during adequate anticoagulation.

            d. At the time of emergency embolectomy.

    B. Emergency Pulmonary Embolectomy

        1. Presentation

            a. These patients usually have not responded to routine anticoagulation or thrombolytic therapy.

            b. The size of the PE and the degree of outflow obstruction leading to acute hemodynamic decompensation differ depending on the associated pathology, underlying cardiac reserve, and the extent of chronic right ventricular hypertrophy.

    c. These patients are often hypotensive, severely hypoxemic, hypercarbic, and acidotic and may have severe right-sided heart failure. They may be undergoing CPR while they are being prepared for surgery.

  2. Therapy

    a. Initial therapy may include fluid resuscitation, intubation with oxygen supplementation and assisted or controlled ventilation, and inotropic support.

    b. Sedatives, analgesics, and anesthetic agents should be administered with great care until hemodynamic stability is obtained.

    c. Patients should be monitored with an arterial line. A PA catheter is desirable for hemodynamic monitoring, but placement may be difficult because of acutely elevated PA pressure or occlusion.

    d. Although emergency embolectomy is a rare procedure, rapid resuscitation and use of cardiopulmonary bypass have improved salvage rates in a number of larger medical centers.

VI. SUMMARY OF ANESTHETIC CONSIDERATIONS

Patients undergoing surgery are often at risk for DVT and subsequently for PE. Several measures effective in decreasing the incidence of perioperative DVT are subcutaneous heparin, intravenous dextran, and external pneumatic compression devices. Also, the incidence of DVT is reduced in patients receiving regional anesthesia compared with those having general anesthesia. This effect may be secondary to the reduction of blood flow stasis from decreased arterial and venous resistance, decreased blood viscosity from hemodilution, and local anesthetic effect on vascular endothelium.

A large PE may cause significant pulmonary hypertension and systemic hemodynamic instability and hypoxia. Prior to emergency pulmonary embolectomy, patients usually require intubation and ventilation with high concentrations of oxygen. Both fluid resuscitation and inotropic support are usually necessary also. These patients will benefit from continuous blood pressure monitoring and PA catheterization. Any anesthesia is poorly tolerated and must be titrated carefully.

Chest Trauma

I.   HISTORY AND PHYSICAL EXAMINATION
   A.   History
      1.   Despite the need for rapid treatment, a history must be obtained to identify factors that might influence the anesthetic management. Information on the patient's preinjury state of health, drug therapy, allergies, anesthetic experience, and previous surgery should be obtained from family or friends if the patient is unable to communicate.
      2.   In a series of 1000 anesthetics for trauma surgery, the overall mortality rate, 5.3%, increased to 7.2% in patients with existing disease and to 10% in patients with a history of significant cardiovascular or CNS disease.
   B.   Physical Examination
      1.   Extent of injuries, especially airway patency, adequacy of breathing, level of consciousness, amount of hemorrhage, cardiovascular status, and presence of acute intoxication must be quickly established.
      2.   After initial control of the airway and hemodynamic stabilization, a more thorough physical examination of the head and neck, chest, abdomen, long bones, spine, and pelvis should be performed.
      3.   Thoracic examination
         a.   The physical examination of the patient with chest trauma should commence with an overview, looking at the shape of the thoracic wall and the symmetry of expansion.
         b.   Auscultation may reveal wheezing, rhonchi, rales, or lack of breath sounds.
         c.   Palpation of the trachea will indicate displacement or crepitus in the presence of severe intrathoracic or neck injuries.
         d.   Rib fractures, subcutaneous emphysema, open chest wounds, or tympanitic areas should lead to more aggressive evaluation for associated barotrauma or pneumothorax.
         e.   The chest radiograph is important and should be examined closely preoperatively. Flail sternum or a fractured sternum can be noted on chest radiograph, as can barotrauma, parenchymal injury, cardiac trauma, and other associated injuries. The possibility of a dissecting

aortic aneurysm should be considered in the presence of a widened mediastinum or apical capping (blood in the pulmonary apices).

II. TYPES OF THORACIC INJURIES
  A. Flail Chest
    1. A flail chest results from loss of structural continuity between the chest wall and the flail segment. This will occur secondary to the fracture of ribs in at least two places, costochondral separation, or sternal fracture.
    2. Paradoxical movement of the flail segment may be noted, with inward motion of the chest wall during inspiration. If the patient has minimal breathing effort and lung compliance is normal, this paradoxical motion may be difficult to discern. With an increased breathing effort secondary to obstruction, pulmonary contusion, atelectasis, or cadiac failure, there will be more obvious paradoxical motion.
    3. Historically, initial therapy was directed at stabilization of the flail segment by external fixation with straps, sandbags, or towel clips or by internal fixation with intramedullary wiring. Now, intubation and mechanical ventilation is felt to be the treatment of choice. The actual bony injury is not as important as the associated pulmonary contusion, atelectasis, and pulmonary infection secondary to hypoventilation.
  B. Pulmonary Contusion
    1. Pulmonary contusion can be defined as edema and hemorrhage into the lung parenchyma secondary to blunt trauma. Pulmonary contusive injuries may result from a direct blow or from contrecoup action. They often are associated with bone fractures, cardiac contusion, and vascular injuries but may occur in the absence of thoracic wall injury.
    2. The patient will present with a history of blunt trauma, have moist rales on auscultation, produce blood-tinged secretions, and have relative hypoxemia as evidenced by an increased alveolar–arterial oxygen difference while receiving supplemental oxygen.
    3. The initial chest radiograph may be unimpressive in 40% of patients, but the contusion may appear over the next 6 to 24 hours. It will then appear as an area(s) of increased density with ill-defined margins

that do not conform to lobar or segmental anatomy. If significant blood is lost at the time of the injury, hypoperfusion may temporarily limit the apparent extent of the pulmonary trauma. Failure to discern a correlation between the severity of the contusion on chest radiography and the magnitude of hypoxemia is commonly reported.

4. The mortality rate associated with severe pulmonary contusion ranges from 14% to 40%. One of the major risk factors for death is the presence of other significant injuries: whereas the mortality rate for simple pulmonary contusion is approximately 5%, one additional major extrathoracic injury increases the mortality rate to 24%, and a second injury increases it to 42%.

C. Esophageal Injury

1. Esophageal injury is a catastrophic event that occurs not only with trauma but also with NG tube placement, endoscopy, vomiting, coughing, CPR, and surgery.

2. The chest radiograph may reveal pneumomediastinum, subcutaneous emphysema, or pleural effusion, often with an air–fluid interface.

3. An aggressive diagnostic approach is necessary, including endoscopy and barium swallow. The mortality rate approaches 2% per hour, with as many as 65% of the deaths occurring in the first 24 hours secondary to a progressive purulent mediastinitis.

D. Cardiac Injury

1. Traumatic injuries of the heart include penetration, rupture, contusion, tamponade, coronary vessel laceration or thrombosis, valvular injury, damage to the conduction system, or aneurysm formation.

2. Chest radiography, angiography, echocardiography, or nuclear imaging may be necessary to make the diagnosis.

III. PERIOPERATIVE PULMONARY COMPLICATIONS

A. Hypoxemia

1. Continuous positive airway pressure by mask

a. In the awake patient whose hypoxemia is refractory to oxygen by nasal cannula or mask, CPAP for 24 to 72 hours may obviate intubation.

b. With the use of a CPAP mask, it is imperative

that the patient be sufficiently alert and cooperative and able to remove the mask should regurgitation occur secondary to gastric distention.

    c. Mask CPAP should be used with caution in patients with head trauma, especially if they have cerebrospinal fluid leaks or deteriorating levels of consciousness, CO_2 retention, or possible esophageal or gastrointestinal injuries.

    d. If moderate levels of mask CPAP (5–10 cmH_2O) are unable to restore acceptable oxygenation at an FIO_2 of less than or equal to 0.5, the patient is likely to require intubation and mechanical ventilation with PEEP.

  2. The therapy and anesthetic management of severe pulmonary contusion is essentially identical to that for ARDS (see following section).

B. Noncardiogenic Pulmonary Edema

  1. Fluid restriction and diuretic therapy is advocated by many clinicians as a mainstay of therapy for pulmonary contusions. This view is based on experimental work that showed anatomic and physical extension of the contusion after rapid administration of crystalloid to animals with experimentally produced pulmonary contusion. Anything that increases intravascular hydrostatic pressure will increase extravasation of fluid into the area of contusion.

  2. Although fluid restriction theoretically appears ideal, it often is difficult to achieve safely in the traumatized patient. Compromise of the cardiovascular system secondary to fluid restriction and diuretic use may produce significant deterioration in other organ systems.

  3. Patients with severe contusion usually require invasive monitoring. An arterial line and Foley catheter are standard. If the patient's intravascular volume is in question, a PA catheter is warranted. It permits quantitation of preload, cardiac output, mixed venous PO_2, intrapulmonary shunt fraction, and calculation of pulmonary and systemic vascular resistances. In addition, a patient requiring greater than 10 cmH_2O of PEEP may benefit from a PA catheter to optimize PEEP while maintaining cardiac performance.

    C. Infection
- **1.** Pulmonary infection is the most common complication after pulmonary contusion. The blood and fluid that extravasate into the alveoli and interstitial spaces are an excellent culture medium. Lung abscesses and emphysema may develop.
- **2.** Development of traumatic cysts and benign cavities has been reported.
- **3.** Delayed ARDS is a potentially fatal complication in this patient population.

    D. Barotrauma
- **1.** Barotrauma is defined as the presence of inappropriate air within the thorax, soft tissues, or abdominal cavity secondary to dissection along various tissue planes after damage to the tracheobronchial tree or esophagus.
- **2.** The diagnosis must be considered in all patients with blunt or penetrating trauma, as well as after central intravenous access procedures and in patients requiring high airway pressures during positive pressure ventilation.
- **3.** The presentation can be subtle, and therefore the condition must be carefully sought prior to an anesthetic. Small collections of air, especially if under tension within the pleural space, mediastinum, or pericardium, can have rapid and devastating sequelae.

IV. ANESTHESIA AND CHEST TRAUMA
    A. Oxygenation
- **1.** All patients with chest trauma should receive supplemental oxygen in the perioperative period.
- **2.** Flail chest will worsen the oxygenation problems associated with any other lung problems because of the paradoxical movement of the chest wall. Patients having regional anesthesia may require intubation and PEEP to avoid hypoxemia.
- **3.** During general anesthesia for nonthoracic surgery, the development of tension pneumothorax from pulmonary laceration or bronchial injury should be considered with the sudden onset of hypotension, loss of pulmonary compliance, or decreased ventilating volume.

    B. Monitoring
- **1.** With the possibility of cardiac and pulmonary injury, an intra-arterial catheter must be used for con-

tinuous blood pressure monitoring and for drawing samples for blood gas analysis.

    2. Many patients will be hemodynamically unstable on arrival in the operating room, receiving both fluid resuscitation and inotropic drugs. A PA catheter will be helpful in providing more objective information to guide therapy.

C. Maintenance Anesthesia

    1. The degree of trauma can be as varied as the patients who sustain it. Therefore, there is no absolute standard anesthesia approach.

    2. Any anesthetic agent selected should have minimal cardiac depressant or vasodilating properties.

    3. Nitrous oxide should be avoided, because it can limit the amount of oxygen delivered, and it can worsen any barotrauma.

D. Postoperative Care

    1. Patients with minor chest trauma may be extubated shortly after surgery.

    2. Patients with significant pulmonary contusions or flail chest should be left intubated postoperatively until they are capable of ventilating and oxygenating without mechanical support or high levels of FIO_2.

V. SUMMARY OF ANESTHETIC CONSIDERATIONS

Oxygenation after chest trauma may be difficult. In addition to mechanical ventilation and oxygen, PEEP may be necessary. No standard anesthetic approach is best for all these patients. The most important concern is to avoid anesthetic agents that have cardiac depressant or vasodilatory effects. Invasive monitoring is an important aspect for all anesthetics given to patients with significant chest trauma.

Adult Respiratory Distress Syndrome

I. INCIDENCE AND OUTCOME

A. There are 150,000 to 200,000 new cases of ARDS per year in this country.

B. This syndrome often affects patients without primary pulmonary pathology or insult, occurs frequently in young patients, and, unfortunately, has few if any well-defined markers associated with its development. The incidence increases with multiple associated risk factors (Table 2-9).

Table 2–9. Diseases Associated with Development of ARDS

Sepsis	Disseminated intravascular coagu-
Pulmonary aspiration	lation
Pulmonary contusion	Pneumonia
Multiple emergency transfusions	Pancreatitis (severe, associated
(greater than 10 units in 48	with hypotension)
hours)	Near drowning
Multiple long bone or major	Head injury
fractures	

    C. ARDS most frequently develops within 48 to 72 hours of the initial insult, although its development may be delayed as long as 7 to 10 days.

    D. The overall mortality rate is between 50% and 65% despite aggressive therapy. Of note is that this devastating prognosis has not been altered, despite advances in medical therapy, since the syndrome was first defined and formally recognized in 1967.

    E. Nonsurvivors either die acutely (within several days of the onset) secondary to intractable respiratory failure and acidosis or survive weeks to months only to expire from progressive multisystem organ failure, most commonly associated with sepsis.

    F. Patients who survive ultimately regain near-normal or normal respiratory function and make surprisingly complete recoveries. Frequently, survivors resume their original lifestyles within 6 to 12 months of hospital discharge.

II. PATHOPHYSIOLOGY

    A. Etiology

    ARDS is a final common disease process that can be secondary to multiple etiologies through either direct alveolar injury such as aspiration or inhalation injuries or indirect endothelial damage secondary to, among others, sepsis or activation of the clotting or complement cascade.

    B. Cellular Response

        1. The exudative phase is characterized initially by a nonhydrostatic pulmonary edema secondary to endothelial injury and alteration of gas exchange with damage to Type I and II epithelial cells.

        2. This phase is followed by a proliferative phase with re-epithelialization. Further reparative processes result in either recovery of lung function or progression to a fibrotic phase, with deposition of collagen and resultant protracted respiratory failure.

C. Pulmonary Effects

Important physiologic sequelae of ARDS include decreased FRC and decreased pulmonary compliance with arterial hypoxemia (PaO_2 <50 mmHg with FIO_2 >0.5 mmHg) and hypercarbia secondary to increased dead space ventilation (Vd/Vt). The diffuse pulmonary edema responsible for the initial physiologic sequelae is secondary to abnormal capillary permeability and not to increased pulmonary hydrostatic pressure.

III. THERAPY

A. The overall management goal of the ARDS patient is reestablishment of tissue oxygen delivery and nutrition with reversal of any underlying cause of pulmonary injury in order to provide time for the lungs to heal.

B. Respiratory Management

    1. Ventilation

        a. Large minute volumes (up to 30–40 L/min), frequently requiring high respiratory rates, are utilized to overcome the increased dead space and provide adequate arterial oxygenation (PaO_2 >55 mmHg). A relative hypocarbia ($PaCO_2$ 25–35 mmHg) is often produced.

        b. As ARDS worsens and Vd/Vt increases, hypercarbia may develop despite maximal ventilatory support.

        c. Close monitoring of peak and mean airway pressure, compliance, and respiratory ratio are performed to minimize air trapping and barotrauma.

        d. Various alternatives to conventional ventilation, such as high-frequency, jet, and oscillatory ventilation, have not as yet been shown to be more efficacious than conventional mechanical ventilation.

    2. Oxygenation

        a. The use of the lowest concentration of O_2 without causing tissue hypoxemia is advocated to avoid the potential of pulmonary oxygen toxicity as well as the possibility of absorption atelectasis with resultant worsening of the shunt fraction. Hyperoxia itself may be a cause of the ARDS or worsen the syndrome if excessive concentrations of O_2 are administered for protracted periods.

    b. Oxygen toxicity is minimized by keeping an FIO_2 of 0.5 or less as soon as clinically possible while maintaining an O_2 saturation of at least 85% to 90%. PEEP, inspiratory hold, and reverse I:E ratio are used to improve oxygenation by alveolar recruitment and improving $\dot{V}/\dot{Q}$ matching. These maneuvers will usually allow FIO_2 to be decreased but may cause barotrauma from increasing mean and peak airway pressure.

    c. Even though PEEP is frequently successful in decreasing FIO_2 requirements, there are no controlled studies that prove that these therapeutic maneuvers improve survival from ARDS, nor have they been shown to be effective in high-risk patients to prevent the development of ARDS. A potential serious side effect of PEEP and positive pressure ventilation is pulmonary barotrauma. Cullen and Caldera have shown that the incidence of this is surprisingly low in critically ill patients, however.

IV. COMPLICATIONS OF OXYGEN THERAPY

    A. Oxygen Toxicity

        1. Oxygen administration at high concentrations (>50%) can be toxic to pulmonary endothelial and epithelial cells. Protracted exposure to high concentrations is a potential cause of ARDS.

        2. Gas exchange, lung metabolic function, and pulmonary defense may all be affected. It appears that the concentration and duration of hyperoxia, as well as patient age, associated pathology, nutritional and endocrine status, drug therapy, and prior oxidant and hyperoxic exposure, all play a role in the potential for increased toxicity.

        3. Agents that interact with O_2 and enhance oxygen toxicity are bleomycin, nitrofurantoin, amiodarone, cyclophosphamide, and irradiation.

    B. Pathophysiology

        1. Free radical metabolites of oxygen such as superoxide, hydrogen peroxide, and the hydroxyl radical are believed to be the cause of pulmonary oxygen toxicity. These toxic substances are generated during the normal reduction of O_2 to H_2O in proportion to the inspired concentration of oxygen delivered to the patient.

2. Free radicals can inactivate crucial enzymes, cause lipid peroxidation, damage membranes, depolymerize mucopolysaccharides, cause DNA scission, and activate phospholipase.

3. Phospholipase activation results in metabolism of arachidonic acid and formation of inflammatory substances such as leukotrienes and prostaglandins. These deleterious changes can result in an amplified process that can cause severe acute lung injury and even death.

C. Prevention

1. The lung has several potent defenses, including antioxidant enzymes and antioxidant substances (Table 2-10).

2. Medical therapy includes drugs that enhance natural antioxidants, supply exogenous antioxidants via liposomes or propylene glycol entrapment, or act directly as antioxidants (dimethylthiourea (DMTU) or dimethylsulfoxide).

3. Increasingly routine use of in-line oxygen analyzers, analysis of respired gases by mass spectroscopy, and determination of hemoglobin saturation via pulse oximetry and arterial blood gas measurements ensure the adequacy of oxygen delivery. This monitoring, along with the maintenance of reasonable hemoglobin levels and cardiac output, allows the safe intraoperative and postoperative limitation of inspired oxygen concentrations.

Table 2–10. Antioxidant Defenses of the Lung

Enzymes	*Nonenzymatic*
Superoxide dismutase	Vitamins A, C, E
Glutathione peroxidase	Glutathione
Catalase	Thiol-containing amino acids
Glucose-6-phosphate dehydrogenase	Thioesters
	Polyunsaturated fatty acids
	Ceruloplasmin
	Iron-binding proteins

V. PERIOPERATIVE MANAGEMENT

    A. Hemodynamic Monitoring

        1. The other serious concern with the use of PEEP is the adverse effect it has on the hemodynamic stability of the patient, with a potentially deleterious effect on O_2 delivery. PEEP can decrease cardiac output by decreasing venous return, by altering the normal geometry of the heart to diminish intraventricular volume, and possibly by causing the release of a negative inotropic substance. Aggressive hemodynamic monitoring is helpful in the titration of PEEP to optimize O_2 delivery without hemodynamic compromise.

        2. Arterial cannulation is used to monitor blood pressure and blood gases.

        3. Right heart catheterization with the Swan-Ganz catheter is frequently used to evaluate the effect of PEEP on the intravascular volume and cardiac output. Measured mixed venous oxygen saturation and calculated venous admixture or shunt, as well as other derived measures used to estimate cardiac function, can be obtained with right heart catheterization. High levels of PEEP ($>10\,cmH_2O$) may interfere with PA catheter values. Caution should be used in interpreting isolated PA catheter data after starting PEEP, especially if they are markedly different from prior recent data and physical findings.

    B. Transport

    Transport of these critically ill patients is often extremely difficult and can be life threatening. Specific attention should be directed toward reproducing the level of ICU support during transport to and from the operating room as well as intraoperatively. Additional diagnostic or therapeutic interventions should be anticipated and performed when possible prior to surgery. During transfer, resuscitation equipment, including a laryngoscope, endotracheal tube with stylet, an adequate oxygen supply, an Ambu bag with the required amount of PEEP, resuscitative drugs, and transport monitoring equipment (pulse oximetry, ECG, and blood pressure) must be available.

    C. Intraoperative Care

        1. These patients often require transport of the ventilator used in the ICU to the operating room. Adequate ventilation should be documented as soon as possible after arrival there by inspection, ausculation, pulse oximetry, end-tidal gas analysis, and measurement of arterial blood gases. Ideally, in the operating room, these patients require no more than the level of respiratory support provided in the ICU.

2. Appropriate infusion controllers are mandatory to ensure proper delivery of vasoactive drugs, fluids, and total parenteral nutrition.

3. Monitoring of the ECG, temperature, O_2 saturation via pulse oximetry, airway pressure, urine output, and intra-arterial blood pressure should be undertaken.

4. If possible, a PA catheter should be utilized in patients undergoing protracted surgery or procedures with large fluid shifts or fluid requirements. Trend monitoring of the hemodynamic data, along with clinical observation, will allow more thorough evaluation of the patient's response to anesthetic agents, blood loss, fluid replacement, and hemodynamic interventions.

VI. ANESTHESIA

A. The ultimate goal of anesthesia in these patients is to supply necessary analgesia, sedation, and amnesia while maintaining an often all-too-marginal physiological state.

B. Regional anesthesia can be used if it is appropriate for the procedure, acceptable to the patient, and without intolerable risk of side effects for patients who frequently have associated hemodynamic lability, sepsis, and coagulopathy. Patients may not tolerate the various positions required for the regional technique or the sympathectomy that occurs with various blocks.

C. Intravenous Agents

1. Drugs such as benzodiazepines, ketamine, or etomidate in small and repeated doses can be given slowly to induce anesthesia.

2. Maintenance anesthesia with narcotics such as fentanyl, sufentanil, and alfentanil may then be administered.

3. Altered drug distribution and metabolism should be taken into account in patients with associated multisystem organ dysfunction. Patients may have a significantly altered volume of drug distribution as

well as rate of drug metabolism related to associated pathology.

D. Inhalational Agents

1.   Use of N_2O is avoided in the majority of these patients so as to provide a high FIO_2 and to avert side effects such as expansion of air in a closed space (as with a pneumothorax or small-bowel obstruction), hemodynamic depression when used with narcotics or volatile anesthetics, and potential adverse effects on neurologic function in patients who may be severely malnourished.

2.   Volatile anesthetics can be used, but only with careful monitoring of effect on cardiac performance as well as the potential effect on hypoxic pulmonary vasoconstriction and $\dot{V}/\dot{Q}$ matching. Low concentrations of volatile agents should be administered initially with careful monitoring of vital signs.

3.   Muscle relaxants may be needed to optimize surgical conditions and gas exchange.

E.   After adequate analgesia, sedation and relaxation are provided, and physiologic alterations related to surgical manipulation are treated pharmacologically. This may include treatment with vasopressors, inotropes, or vasodilators.

F.   Postanesthetic Management

After the surgical procedure is completed, careful transfer back to the ICU is undertaken, reversing the steps of the original transport. After arrival in the ICU, an oral report is given to the bedside care providers, and adequacy of ventilation and cardiac function is again documented. Postoperative analgesia is provided as needed with IV narcotics or regional nerve blockade with local anesthesia or narcotics.

VII.   SUMMARY OF ANESTHETIC CONSIDERATIONS

Patients with ARDS require high FIO_2 and minute ventilation for oxygenation. This makes the transport of these patients very difficult, as any break in the ventilatory support, even for seconds, can result in hypoxemia. Extensive invasive monitoring is required. High levels of PEEP ($>10\,cmH_2O$) can compromise hemodynamic stability. Frequently, fluid challenges and inotropic agents are required to maintain minimally acceptable blood pressure.

Sympathectomy from regional anesthesia such as spinal or epidural blocks is poorly tolerated. Sepsis, a frequent cause of ARDS, also causes bacteremic coagulopathies, which are contraindications for regional anesthesia.

Intravenous anesthetics often have a more intense and long-acting effect because of the altered volume of distribution and liver and kidney dysfunction. High requirements for oxygen preclude the utilization of N_2O. Muscle relaxants are frequently required to optimize surgical conditions and gas exchange in agitated patients who are unable to tolerate much anesthesia. Postoperative transport of these patients to the ICU is complicated by invasive lines and the need to maintain uninterrupted high minute ventilation and PEEP.

Recommended Reading

Asthma

Bierman MI, Brown M, Muren O, et al. Prolonged isoflurane anesthesia in status asthmaticus. Crit Care Med 1986;14:832.

Downes H, Hirshman CA. Lidocaine aerosols do not prevent allergic bronchoconstriction. Anesth Analg 1981;60:28.

Downes H, Hirshman CA, Leon DA. Comparison of local anesthetics as bronchodilator aerosols. Anesthesiology 1983;58:216.

Dueck R. Anesthesia for the asthmatic patient. Semin Anesth 1987;4:2.

Fairshter RD, Wilson AF. Relationship between site of airflow limitation and localization of the bronchodilator response in asthma. Am Rev Respir Dis 1980;122:27.

Fowkes FGR, Lunn JN, Farrow SC, et al. Epidemiology in anesthesia III: mortality risk in patients with coexisting physical disease. Br J Anaesth 1982;54:819.

Hirshman CA, Downes H, Farbood A, et al. Ketamine block of bronchospasm in experimental canine asthma. Br J Anaesth 1979;51:713.

Hirshman CA, Edelstein G, Peetz S, et al. Mechanism of action of inhalational anesthesia on airways. Anesthesiology 1982;56:107.

Kingston HGG, Hirshman CA. Anesthetic management of patients with bronchospastic disease. Clin Anesthesiol 1983;1:377.

Kingston HGG, Hirshman CA. Perioperative management of the patient with asthma. Anesth Analg 1984;63:844.

Pare PD, Lawson LM, Brooks LA. Patterns of response to inhaled bronchodilators in asthmatics. Am Rev Respir Dis 1983;127:680.

Parnass SM, Feld JM, Chamberlin WH, et al. Status asthmaticus treated with isoflurane and enflurane. Anesth Analg 1987; 66:193.

Pratter MR, Hingston DM, Irwin RS. Diagnosis of bronchial asthma by clinical evaluation: an unreliable method. Chest 1983;84:42.

Roizen MF, Stevens WC. Multiform ventricular tachycardia due to the interaction of aminophylline and halothane. Anesth Analg 1978;57:738.

Schwartz SH. Treatment of status asthmaticus with halothane. JAMA 1984;251:2688.

Shnider SM, Papper EM. Anesthesia for the asthmatic patient. Anesthesiology 1961;22:886.

Stirt JA, Berger JM, Roe SD. Safety of enflurane following administration of aminophylline in experimental animals. Anesth Analg 1981;60:871.

Chronic Obstructive Lung Disease

Bartlett RH, Gazzaniga AB, Geraghty TR. Respiratory maneuvers to prevent postoperative pulmonary complications: a critical review. JAMA 1973;224:1017.

Bromage PR, Camporesi E, Chestnut D. Epidural narcotics for postoperative analgesia. Anesth Analg 1980;59:473.

Celli BR, Rodriguez KS, Snider GL. A controlled trial of intermittent positive pressure breathing, incentive spirometry, and deep breathing exercises in preventing pulmonary complications after abdominal surgery. Am Rev Respir Dis 1984;130:12.

Chodoff P, Margand PMS, Knowles CL. Short term abstinence from smoking: its place in preoperative preparation. Crit Care Med 1975;3:131.

Cousins MJ, Mather LE. Intrathecal and epidural administration of opioids. Anesthesiology 1984;61:276.

Craig DB. Postoperative recovery of pulmonary function. Anesth Analg 1981;60:46.

Gass GD, Olsen GN. Preoperative pulmonary function testing to predict postoperative morbidity and mortality. Chest 1986;89:127.

Gold MI, Schwam SJ, Goldberg M. Chronic obstructive pulmonary disease and respiratory complications. Anesth Analg 1983;62:975.

Gracey DR, Divertie MB, Didier EP. Preoperative pulmonary preparation of patients with chronic obstructive pulmonary disease. Chest 1979;76:123.

Gross JB, Zebrowski ME, Carel WD, et al. Time course of ventilatory depression after thiopental and midazolam in normal subjects and in patients with chronic obstructive pulmonary disease. Anesthesiology 1983;58:540.

Knill RL, Gelb AW. Ventilatory responses to hypoxia and hypercapnia during halothane sedation and anesthesia in man. Anesthesiology 1978;49:244.

Latimer RG, Dickman M, Clinton Day W, et al. Ventilatory patterns and pulmonary complications after upper abdominal surgery determined by preoperative and postoperative computerized spirometry and blood gas analysis. Am J Surg 1971;122:622.

Milledge JS, Nunn JF. Criteria of fitness for anesthesia in patients with chronic obstructive pulmonary disease. Br Med J 1975;3:670.

Pietak S, Weenig CS, Hickey RF, et al. Anesthetic effects on ventilation in patients with chronic obstructive pulmonary disease. Anesthesiology 1975;42:160.

Ready LB, Oden R, Chadwick HS, et al. Development of an anesthesiology based postoperative pain management service. Anesthesiology 1988;68:100.

Rehder K. Anesthesia and the respiratory system. Can Anaesth Soc J 1979;26:451.

Rehder K, Sessler AD, Marsh HM. General anesthesia and the lung. Am Rev Respir Dis 1975;112:541.

Rodriguez R, Gold MI. Enflurane as a primary anesthetic agent for patients with chronic obstructive pulmonary disease. Anesth Analg 1976;55:806.

Stein M, Konta G, Sum M, et al. Pulmonary evaluation of surgical patients. JAMA 1962;181:760.

Tarhan S, Moffit EA, Sessler AD, Douglas WW, Taylor WF. Risk of anesthesia and surgery in patients with chronic bronchitis and chronic obstructive pulmonary disease. Surgery 1973;74:720.

Tisi GM. Preoperative evaluation of pulmonary function: validity, indications and benefits. Am Rev Respir Dis 1979;119:293.

Tisi GM. Preoperative identification and evaluation of patients with lung disease. Med Clin North Am 1987;71:399.

Weil JV, McCullough RE, Klines JS, Sodal IE. Diminished ventilatory response to hypoxia and hypercapnia after morphine in normal man. N Engl J Med 1975;292:1103.

Yeager MP, Glass DD, Neff RK, et al. Epidural anesthesia and analgesia in high risk surgical patients. Anesthesiology 1987;66:729.

Aspiration

Burgess GE III, Cooper JR, Marino RJ, et al. Laryngeal competence after tracheal extubation. Anesthesiology 1979;51:73.

Carlsson C, Islander G. Silent gastroesophageal regurgitation during anesthesia. Anesth Analg 1981;60:655

Cohen SE, Jasson J, Talafre ML, et al. Does metoclopramide decrease the volume of gastric contents in patients undergoing cesarean section? Anesthesiology 1984;61:604.

Dewan DM, Floyd HM, Thistlewood JM, et al. Sodium citrate pretreatment in elective cesarean section patients. Anesth Analg 1985;64:34.

Francis RN, Kwik RSH. Oral ranitidine for prophylaxis against Mendelson's syndrome. Anesth Analg 1982;61:130.

Gates S, Huang T, Cheney FW. Effects of methylprednisolone on resolution of acid aspiration pneumonitis. Arch Surg 1983;118:1262.

Hodgkinson R, Glassenberg R, Joyce III TH, et al. Comparison of cimetidine with antacid for safety and effectiveness in reducing gastric acidity before elective cesarean section. Anesthesiology 1983;59:86.

Joyce TH III. Prophylaxis for pulmonary acid aspiration. Am J Med 1987;83(suppl 6A):46.

Lam AM, Grace DM, Manninen PH, et al. The effects of cimetidine and ranitidine with and without metoclopramide on gastric volume and pH in morbidly obese patients. Can Anaesth Soc J 1986;33:773.

Lam AM, Grace DM, Phil D, et al. Prophylactic intravenous cimetidine reduces the risk of acid aspiration in morbidly obese patients. Anesthesiology 1986;65:684.

Maltby JR, Sutherland AD, Sale JP, et al. Preoperative oral fluids: is a five hour fast justified prior to elective surgery? Anesth Analg 1986;65:1112.

Manchikanti L, Colliver JA, Marrero TC, et al. Assessment of age-related acid aspiration risk factors in pediatric, adult, and geriatric patients. Anesth Analg 1985;64:11.

Manchikanti L, Colliver JA, Marrero TC, et al. Ranitidine and metoclopramide for prophylaxis of aspiration pneumonitis in elective surgery. Anesth Analg 1984;63:903.

Manchikanti L, Grow JB, Colliver JA, et al. Bicitra and metoclopramide in outpatient anesthesia for prophylaxis against aspiration pneumonitis. Anesthesiology 1985;63:378.

Rao TLK, Madhavareddy S, Chinthagada M, et al. Metoclopramide and cimetidine to reduce gastric fluid pH and volume. Anesth Analg 1984;63:1014.

Salem MR, Wong AY, Mani M, et al. Premedicant drugs and gastric juice pH and volume in pediatric patients. Anesthesiology 1976;44:216.

Sellick BA. Cricoid pressure to control regurgitation of stomach contents during induction of anesthesia. Lancet 1961;2:404.

Sellick BA. Rupture of the esophagus following cricoid pressure? Anaesthesia 1982;37:213.

Solanki DR, Suresh M, Ethridge HC. The effects of intravenous cimetidine and metoclopramide on gastric volume and pH. Anesth Analg 1984;63:599.

Stoelting RK. Response to atropine, glycopyrrolate, and Riopan of gastric fluid pH and volume in adult patients. Anesthesiology 1978;48:367.

Deep Venous Thrombosis and Pulmonary Embolism

Brown DI, Bodary AK, Kirby RR. Anesthetic management of pulmonary thromboendarterectomy. Anesthesiology 1984;61:197.

Consensus conference. Prevention of venous thrombosis and pulmonary embolism. JAMA 1986;256:744.

Dismuke SE, Wagner EH. Pulmonary embolism as a cause of death: the changing mortality in hospitalized patients. JAMA 1986;15:2039.

Goldhaber SZ. Pulmonary Embolism and Deep Venous Thrombosis. Philadelphia: WB Saunders, 1985.

Mattox KL, Feldtman RW, Beall AC. Pulmonary embolectomy for acute massive pulmonary embolism. Ann Surg 1982;6:726.

McKenzie PJ, Wishart HY, Gray I, et al. Effects of anesthetic technique on deep venous thrombosis: a comparison of subarachnoid and general anesthesia. Br J Anaesth 1985;57:853.

Modig J, Borg T, Karlstrom G, et al. Thromboembolism after total hip replacement: role of epidural and general anesthesia. Anesth Analg 1983;62:174.

Pearl RG. Pulmonary embolism. Semin Anesth 1987;4:153.

Pingleton SK, et al. Prevention of pulmonary emboli in a respiratory intensive care unit: efficacy of low dose heparin. Chest 1981;6:647.

Rubenstein E. Thromboembolism. In: Rubenstein E, Federman D, eds. Medicine. New York: Scientific American, 1987;18:1.

Chest Trauma

Bogetz MS, Katz JA. Airway management of the trauma patient. Semin Anesth 1985;4:114.

Bogetz MS, Katz JA. Recall of surgery for major trauma. Anesthesiology 1984;61:6.

Bowe EA, Klein EF Jr. Pulmonary contusion. Semin Anesth 1985;4:145.

Clemmer TP, Fairfax WR. Critical care management of chest injury. Crit Care Clin 1986;2:759.

Maunder RJ, Pierson DJ, Hudson LD. Subcutaneous and mediastinal emphysema: pathophysiology, diagnosis and management. Arch Intern Med 1984;144:1447.

Theye RA, Perry LB, Brzica SM. Influence of anesthetic agent on the response to hemorrhagic hypotension. Anesthesiology 1974;40:32.

Trunkey D. Trauma. Sci Am 1983;249(2):28.

Watson CB, Norfleet EA. Anesthesia for trauma. Crit Care Clin 1986;2:717.

Weiskopf RB, Fairley HB. Anesthesia for major trauma. Surg Clin North Am 1982;62:31.

Adult Respiratory Distress Syndrome

Ashbaugh DG, Bigelow DB, Petty TL, et al. Acute respiratory distress in adults. Lancet 1967;2:319.

Bauman WR, Jung RC, Koss M, et al. Incidence and mortality of adult respiratory distress syndrome: a prospective analysis from a large metropolitan hospital. Crit Care Med 1986;14:1.

Bernard GR, Luce JM, Sprung CL, et al. High dose corticosteroids in patients with adult respiratory distress syndrome. N Engl J Med 1987;317:1565.

Cheney FW, Huang TW, Gronka R. The effects of 50% oxygen on the resolution of pulmonary injury. Am Rev Respir Dis 1980; 122:373.

Connors AF Jr, McCaffree DR, Gray BA. Evaluation of right heart catheterization in the critically ill patient population without acute myocardial infarction. N Engl J Med 1983;308:263.

Cross CE, Halliwell B, Borish ET, et al. Oxygen radicals and human disease. Ann Intern Med 1987;107:526.

Cullen DJ, Caldera DL. The incidence of ventilator-induced pulmonary barotrauma in critically ill patients. Anesthesiology 1979;50:185.

Davis WB, Rennard SI, Bitterman PB, et al. Pulmonary oxygen toxicity: early reversible changes in human alveolar structure induced by hyperoxia. N Engl J Med 1983;309:878.

Deneke SM, Fanburg BL. Normobaric oxygen toxicity of the lung. N Engl J Med 1980;303:76.

Eisenberg PR, Jaffe AS, Schuster DP. Clinical evaluation compared to pulmonary artery catheterization in the hemodynamic assessment of critically ill patients. Crit Care Med 1984;12:549.

Fowler AA, Hamman RF, Good JT, et al. Adult respiratory distress syndrome: risk with common predispositions. Ann Intern Med 1983;98:593.

Fowler AA, Hamman RF, Zerbe GO, et al. Adult respiratory distress syndrome: prognosis after onset. Am Rev Respir Dis 1985; 132:472.

Frank L, Massaro D. Oxygen toxicity. Am J Med 1980;69:117.

Froese AB, Bryan AC. High frequency ventilation. Am Rev Respir Dis 1987;135:1363.

Hudson LD. Causes of the adult respiratory distress syndrome: clinical recognition. Clin Chest Med 1982;3:195.

Ingbar DH, Matthay RA. Pulmonary sequelae and lung repair in survivors of the adult respiratory distress syndrome. Crit Care Clin 1986;2:629.

Jackson RM. Pulmonary oxygen toxicity. Chest 1985;88:900.

Marini JJ. Hemodynamic monitoring with the pulmonary artery catheter. Crit Care Clin 1986;2:551.

Montgomery AB, Stager MA, Carrico CJ, Hudson LD. Causes of mortality in patients with the adult respiratory distress syndrome. Am Rev Respir Dis 1985;132:485.

Pepe PE. The clinical entity of adult respiratory distress syndrome: definition, prediction, prognosis. Crit Care Clin 1986;2:377.

Pepe PE, Potkin RT, Holtman Reus D, Hudson LD, Carrico CJ. Clinical predictors of the adult respiratory distress syndrome. Am J Surg 1982;144:124.

Petty TL. Indicators of risk, course, and prognosis in adult respiratory distress syndrome (ARDS) [editorial]. Am Rev Respir Dis 1985;132:471.

Pick RA, Handler JB, Murata GH, Friedman AS. The cardiovascular effects of positive end expiratory pressure. Chest 1982;82:345.

Sibbald WJ, Bone RC. The adult respiratory distress syndrome in 1987: is it a systemic disease? Soc Crit Care Med 1987;8:279.

Springer RR, Stevens PM. The influence of PEEP on survival of patients in respiratory failure: a retrospective analysis. Am J Med 1979;66:196.

Weisman IM, Rinaldo JE, Rogers RM. Positive end expiratory pressure in adult respiratory failure. N Engl J Med 1982;307:1381.

Wiedemann HP, Matthay MA, Matthay RA. Cardiovascular–pulmonary monitoring in the intensive care unit 1. Chest 1984;85:537.

Wiedemann HP, Matthay MA, Matthay RA. Cardiovascular–pulmonary monitoring in the intensive care unit 2. Chest 1984;85:656.

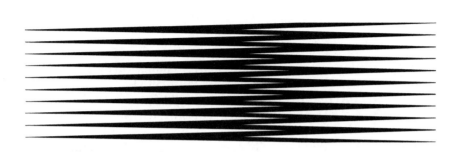

Acid–Base Disturbances
and Electrolyte Disorders

Jonathan Kay

Acid–Base Disturbances

The Henderson-Hasselbach equation describes the relations among pH, HCO_3, and $PaCO_2$ for the blood buffering system:

$$pH = pK + \log \frac{(HCO_3)}{(0.03 \times PaCO_2)}$$

There usually is a direct correlation between changes in the pH and the HCO_3, whereas pH correlates inversely with $PaCO_2$.

I. ESTIMATING CHANGES IN $PaCO_2$ AND HCO_3 WITH META-BOLIC AND RESPIRATORY ALTERATIONS
   A. Simple Metabolic Disorders
      1. Metabolic changes are reflected in alterations in HCO_3. Alveolar ventilation changes in an attempt to normalize pH.
      2. For simple metabolic disturbances, the expected respiratory compensation is predictable.
         a. Calculated $PaCO_2$ compensation for metabolic acidosis:

$$PaCO_2 = (1.5 \times HCO_3) + 8 \pm 2$$

         b. Calculated $PaCO_2$ compensation for metabolic alkalosis:

$$PaCO_2 = (0.9 \times HCO_3) + 9 \pm 2$$

   B. Simple Respiratory Disorders
      1. The change in alveolar ventilation is reflected in the change in $PaCO_2$. In turn, the degree of pH and HCO_3 response to ventilation is dependent on the degree of $PaCO_2$ change and its duration.
      2. In simple respiratory disorders, compensatory changes in HCO_3 may be predicted from the formulae below for both acute and chronic alveolar ventilation.

Change in PaCO₂	Change in HCO₃
Acute 10 mmHg increase	increase 1 mEq/L
Acute 10 mmHg decrease	decrease 2 mEq/L
Chronic 10 mmHg increase	increase 3 mEq/L
Chronic 10 mmHg decrease	decrease 5 mEq/L

C. Acid–Base Nomogram

Numerous nomograms present the information in the formulae graphically; that is, the expected value for one variable given the others in the Henderson-Hasselbach equation in simple disorders (e.g., Figure 3-1). Deviations from these expected values represent superimposed complex acid–base disturbances.

II. RESPIRATORY ACIDOSIS

A. There are four general categories of disorders that cause respiratory acidosis:

    1. Reduced central nervous system (CNS) function secondary to drugs or disease.

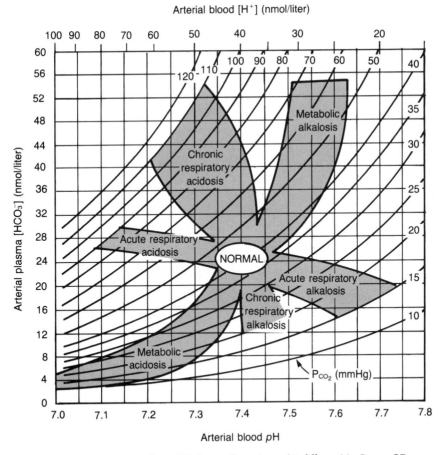

Figure 3-1 Nomogram for acid–base disorders. *(Goldberg M, Green SB, Moss ML, et al. Computer-based instruction and diagnosis of acid–base disorders. JAMA 1973; 273:270.)*

      2. Depressed neuromuscular function secondary to drugs or disease.

      3. Intrinsic pulmonary disease that increases shunt or dead space.

      4. Increased metabolic production of CO_2.

B. Pathophysiology of Compensation

      1. Increased respiratory drive

          a. The increase in the partial pressure of CO_2 causes a direct increase in the concentration of plasma hydrogen ions. Carbon dioxide readily crosses lipid membranes and causes a rapid decrease in pH of the cerebrospinal fluid (CSF) and blood. The low CSF and plasma pH stimulates medullary chemoreceptors in the fourth ventricle and carotid bodies, respectively, to increase ventilation.

          b. Gradually, plasma bicarbonate increases, and bicarbonate is transported across the blood–brain barrier to restore CSF pH. The stimulus to ventilation then decreases.

      2. The kidney responds to the increase in $PaCO_2$ by augmenting the excretion of hydrogen ions and the reabsorption of bicarbonate into the plasma. The maximum renal response takes 72 hours.

C. Treatment

      1. The underlying disorder should be corrected.

      2. Rapid restoration by increasing ventilation, although tempting, is dangerous, especially in patients with chronic CO_2 retention. Rapid restoration of normocapnia can reduce the brain and body level of CO_2 much more rapidly than HCO_3 can cross the blood–brain barrier or the kidney can reduce the production of serum bicarbonate. The resulting acute metabolic alkalosis can cause electrolyte imbalance, neuromuscular irritability, and seizures.

III. RESPIRATORY ALKALOSIS

A. Respiratory alkalosis is the result of alveolar hyperventilation.

B. The etiology of respiratory alkalosis is diverse.

      1. Iatrogenic: overly enthusiastic mechanical ventilation (common cause)

      2. Self induced: hysteria or anxiety

      3. Decreased barometric pressure

      4. CNS injury

5. Arterial hypoxemia
6. Pulmonary vascular disease
7. Sepsis
8. Elevated body temperature
9. Pregnancy
10. Salicylate overdose.

C. Pathophysiology of Compensation
   1. Compensation in respiratory alkalosis is the reverse of the events in respiratory acidosis. Reduction in the partial pressure of CO_2 decreases the stimulus to breathe, which is mediated by carotid body and medullary chemoreceptors.
   2. Bicarbonate is actively transported out of the CSF, eventually restoring the pH to normal.
   3. Blood and tissue buffers react with bicarbonate to produce CO_2. Lactate levels increase as the pH-dependent generation of lactate from glycolysis increases. Lastly, renal tubular reabsorption of hydrogen ions increases. All these changes tend to offset the increase in pH.

D. Treatment
   1. The underlying cause should be corrected.
   2. If patient is being mechanically ventilated, reduction of minute ventilation may be appropriate (not in patients with elevated intracranial pressure).

IV. METABOLIC ACIDOSIS
The concept of an "anion gap" is useful in this disorder. The number of unmeasured anions is defined by:

$$\text{Anion gap} = Na^+ - (Cl^- + HCO_3^-)$$

A normal anion gap is less than 12 mEq/dl.

A. Etiology
   1. Non-anion gap acidosis
       a. Hypokalemic acidosis
           1) Renal tubular acidosis (proximal or distal) is the result of a buffer deficiency (phosphate, ammonia)
           2) Diarrhea
           3) Posthypocapnic acidosis
           4) Carbonic anhydrase inhibitors (acetazolamide, mafenamide)
           5) Ureteral diversions (ureterosigmoidostomy, ileal bladder, ileal ureter).

  b. Normal to hyperkalemic acidosis
    1) Early renal failure
    2) Hydronephrosis
    3) Addition of HCl, NH_4Cl, arginine-HCl, or lysine-HCl
    4) Sulfur toxicity
    5) Mineralocorticoid deficiency
    6) Renal disease: secondary to systemic lupus erythematosus, interstitial nephritis, amyloidosis, sickle cell nephropathy.

 2. Elevated anion gap acidosis
  a. Causes
    1) Renal failure
    2) Ketoacidosis (starvation, diabetes mellitus, alcohol intoxication, glycogenolysis, defects in gluconeogenesis)
    3) Lactic acidosis
    4) Toxins (methanol, ethylene glycol, salicylates, paraldehyde).

  b. Elevated anion gap acidosis is further subdivided into four types by Frommer. Type A is the most important for the anesthesiologist to recognize, as it is the most frequently encountered.

    Type A: Secondary to tissue hypoxia; for example, exercise, seizures, shock, cardiac arrest, cardiogenic pulmonary edema, severe hypoxemia, severe anemia, asthma, and carbon monoxide poisoning.

    Type B_1: Secondary to diseases sometimes associated with lactic acidosis but not always attributable to tissue hypoxia; for example, hepatic disease, Reye's syndrome, sepsis, some malignancies, diabetes mellitus, alcoholic ketoacidosis, short-bowel syndrome, iron deficiency, pancreatitis, and renal failure.

    Type B_2: Secondary to drugs or toxins; for example, phenformin and other biguanide hypoglycemic agents, fructose, sorbitol, xylitol, glucose, epinephrine, norepinephrine, ritodrine, ethanol, cyanide, sodium nitroprusside, salicylates, acetaminophen, propylene glycol, ethylene glycol, methanol, isoniazid, streptozotocin, nalidixic acid, papaverine, butane, ether, halothane, iron, and carbon monoxide.

Type B_3: Secondary to inborn errors of metabolism; for example, glucose 6-phosphatase deficiency (glycogen storage disease Type I or von Gierke's disease), fructose 1,6-diphosphatase deficiency, pyruvate carboxylase deficiency, pyruvate dehydrogenase deficiency, and defects in oxidative phosphorylation.

    4. In severe metabolic acidosis, elevated serum lactate levels (normal up to 1.8 mmol/L) are associated with a poor outcome. Lactate levels are a reasonable index of therapeutic efficacy in patients with shock.

B. Pathophysiology of Compensation

    1. As plasma bicarbonate levels drop from the buffering of nonvolatile acids, there is enhanced excretion of hydrogen ions in the form of ammonium by renal tubular cells.

    2. Alveolar ventilation increases in response to the hydrogen ion stimulation of the carotid body.

    3. Buffers in bone are mobilized, causing bone loss in the chronic metabolic acidosis in renal failure.

C. Treatment

    1. The underlying cause must be identified and treated as rapidly as possible.

    2. If myocardial depression or dysrhythmias occur, bicarbonate is indicated (usually a pH less than 7.25). The following equation may be used to estimate initial bicarbonate replacement:

$$HCO_{3\,required} = 0.4 \text{ kg body wt} \times (HCO_{3\,desired} - HCO_{3\,actual})$$

Initially, half the calculated amount is given over 5 minutes. Further replacement should be determined by monitoring both pH and HCO_3.

V. METABOLIC ALKALOSIS

A. The cause of metabolic alkalosis is generally a loss of nonvolatile acid from the extracellular fluid.

B. The following are causes of metabolic alkalosis:

    1. Vomiting, gastric suction, and diuretics (most common causes)

    2. Chloride-wasting diarrhea

3. Villous adenoma
4. Hyperaldosteronism
5. Cushing's syndrome (i.e., from corticosteroid use)
6. Bartter's syndrome
7. Alkali ingestion
8. Lactate or citrate conversion to bicarbonate after extensive administration of lactated Ringer's solution or blood.

C. Pathophysiology of Compensation
Compensatory responses include decreased renal excretion of hydrogen ions and alveolar hypoventilation.

D. Treatment of Metabolic Alkalosis
1. Urinary chloride is usually less than 10 mEq/L in metabolic alkalosis caused by volume depletion. Sodium and potassium are lost in the attempt to correct metabolic alkalosis and should be replaced. In many cases, volume resuscitation with normal saline and KCl supplementation are key steps in therapy.
2. Rarely, central intravenous infusion of hydrogen ions as ammonium chloride or 0.1N hydrochloric acid is needed.
3. Acetazolamide (Diamox), a carbonic anhydrase inhibitor, can be used to correct metabolic alkalosis. However, because it is a diuretic, it must be avoided in patients who may be intravascularly depleted.

VI. SUMMARY OF ANESTHETIC CONSIDERATIONS
Understanding the interrelations among pH, $PaCO_2$, and HCO_3 helps define acid–base abnormalities. The cause of simple acid–base disorders and whether the usual physiologic compensation has occurred can be determined by the equations in this section. This knowledge will help in the perioperative interpretation of arterial blood gas results and in the selection of therapeutic maneuvers.

Recommended Reading

Cogan MG, Liu FY, Berger BE, Sebastian A, Rector FC Jr. Metabolic alkalosis. Med Clin North Am 1983; 67:903.
Dubose TD Jr. Clinical approach to patients with acid–base disorders. Med Clin North Am 1983; 67:799.
Frommer SP. Lactic acidosis. Med Clin North Am 1983; 67:815.

Kaehny WD. Respiratory acid–base disorders. Med Clin North Am 1983; 67:915.

Mehta PM, Kloner RA. Effects of acid–base disturbance, septic shock, and calcium and phosphorus abnormalities on cardiovascular function. Crit Care Clin 1987; 3:747.

Oh MS, Carroll HJ. Electrolyte and acid–base disorders. In: Chernow B, ed. The pharmacologic approach to the critically ill patient. 2nd ed. Baltimore: Williams & Wilkins, 1988:803.

Riley LJ Jr, Ilson BE, Narins RG. Acute metabolic acid–base disorders. Crit Care Clin 1987; 3:699.

Stoelting RK, Dierdorf SF, McCammon RL. Acid–base disturbances. In: Stoelting RK, Dierdorf SF, eds. Anesthesia and co-existing disease. 2nd ed. New York: Churchill Livingstone, 1988:251.

Electrolyte Disorders

Electrolyte disorders commonly impact upon anesthetic management. These problems may be subtle, as in the mental status changes associated with the gradual onset of hyponatremia, or dramatic, as in the ventricular irritability associated with severe hypokalemia. Knowledge of the clues to the diagnosis and the ability to manage these problems promptly are critical to the safe practice of anesthesia.

Normal values for electrolytes and body water are listed in Table 3-1.

I. SODIUM

Normal values are 138 to 142 mEq/L.

    A. Hyponatremia

    Hyponatremia may occur with reduced, normal, or increased intravascular volume. Pseudohyponatremia and true hyponatremia must be distinguished.

        1. Pseudohyponatremia

        Pseudohyponatremia is a spurious reduction in serum sodium attributable to a measurement error. In these cases, serum sodium is normal when measured by an ion-specific electrode, and osmolarity is likewise normal. Pseudohyponatremia can occur with hyperlipidemia, hyperproteinemia, or increased plasma viscosity.

        2. True hyponatremia

        True hyponatremia signifies a proportionate decrease in plasma osmolarity. Cellular overhydration

Table 3–1.   Normal Values for Body Water and Electrolytes

	Plasma and Whole Blood Concentrations (mEq/L)*	Intracellular Concentrations (mEq/L)*
Na^+	138–142	5–15
K^+	3.8–5	135–155
Cl^-	98–105	4–10
HPO_4^{3-}	1–2 (3–4.5 mg/dl)	30–45
Ca^{2+}	4.5–5.3 (9–10.5 mg/dl) ionized = 1.17–1.3 mmol/L	2–4
Mg^{2+}	1.5–2.5	25–30

	Body Water (liters)		Body Weight (%)	
	60-kg woman	70-kg man	60-kg woman	70-kg man
Total body water	29	39	49	54
Intracellular water	15	22	26	31
Extracellular water	13	17	23	23
Interstitial water	9	12	19	9

*Values may vary slightly from lab to lab.
(From Shoemaker WC. Fluid and electrolytes in the adult. Critical Care Medicine 1982; 3:iii(N):7.)

occurs because of a shift of water into cells, resulting in neuromuscular dysfunction, convulsions, and death if this shift is abrupt. Cellular overhydration is independent of extracellular volume, because the shift of water across the membrane depends only on the osmotic gradient. Paradoxically, accumulation of a substance such as mannitol that is restricted to the extracellular fluid can cause hyponatremia by increasing extracellular osmolarity and hence causing a shift of water from the intracellular to the extracellular space. In such circumstances, cells are dehydrated despite hyponatremia.

3.   Etiology of true hyponatremia
   a.   Increased water intake; e.g., primary polydipsia
   b.   Reduced water excretion
      1)   Reduced delivery of fluid to the distal

nephron because of low intravascular volume. Increased levels of antidiuretic hormone (ADH) are usually present as well (e.g., heart failure, nephrotic syndrome, hepatic cirrhosis, gastrointestinal sodium loss, sweating, diuretic therapy or renal salt wasting, adrenal insufficiency, hypothyroidism).

2) Advanced renal failure

3) Inappropriate secretion of ADH (SIADH) (e.g., tumors, pulmonary disease, CNS disorders, and drugs such as chlorpropamide, barbiturates, morphine, and indomethacin).

4) Physical and emotional stress; nausea; pain

5) Endocrine abnormalities (e.g., glucocorticoid deficiency, myxedema)

6) Reset osmostat

7) Idiopathic.

4. Pathophysiology

  a. Four basic mechanisms are responsible for hyponatremia.

    1) A shift of water from the cell to the intravascular space caused by accumulation of extracellular solutes other than sodium.

    2) Retention of excess water in the body because the kidney is unable to excrete water.

    3) Urinary loss of sodium.

    4) Shift of sodium into cells.

  b. The appropriate response to hyponatremia is renal excretion of excess water. Failure of the kidney to excrete the water may be attributable to glomerular disease in which ultrafiltrate production is decreased; excess ADH, which will inhibit the production of free water; or decreased renal perfusion.

  c. The term "inappropriate ADH secretion" is reseved for hyponatremia associated with normal or increased effective intravascular volume. The diagnostic criteria are:

Urinary sodium greater than 10 mg/dl
Serum urea nitrogen less than 10 mg/dl

Serum creatinine less than 1 mg/dl
Serum urate less than 4 mg/dl
Absence of adrenal insufficiency.

Note that urine osmolarity is not critical to the diagnosis.

    d.   Mild hyponatremia may also be caused by a "resetting of the osmostat" at a lower than usual level in association with increased thirst and polydipsia, such as is frequently found in institutionalized patients receiving phenothiazines.

5.   Treatment

    a.   In most cases, water restriction will correct hyponatremia.

    b.   Salt should be given to patients with hyponatremia secondary to salt depletion (diuretic therapy or salt-wasting nephropathy).

    c.   Water should be removed in states with normal or increased sodium content (osmotic diuretics or furosemide along with 3% hypertonic saline infused at a rate below 1 ml/kg per hour).

    d.   The treatment of acute symptomatic hyponatremia (usually Na<115 mEq/L) will require the administration of sodium. Correction of serum sodium should not exceed a rate of 1 to 2 mEq/L per hour in a monitored setting. There is no advantage to correcting beyond 125 mEq/L. The amount of sodium required (in mEq) is given by the formula:

$$Na_{required} = TBW \times (Na_{desired} - Na_{actual})$$

where TBW = total body water.

    e.   Central pontine myelinolysis is a danger, as is congestive heart failure, in the rapid correction of hyponatremia. A safe rate of correction is less than 2 mEq/L per hour.

    f.   Chronic hyponatremia should be treated with water restriction if possible. Alternatively, pharmacologic agents that interfere with urine concentration may be used, such as lithium or demeclocycline. In the future, specific vasopressin antagonists may be available.

B. Hypernatremia

Hypernatremia may occur with reduced, normal, or increased intravascular volume.

1. Clinical features

    a. Unlike hyponatremia, in which osmolarity may or may not be abnormal, hypernatremia always implies abnormality, namely hyperosmolarity.

    b. Extracellular fluid volume may be low, normal, or high, depending on the cause of the hypernatremia.

    1) Whether hypernatremia is attributable to sodium retention or water loss usually can be determined from the history and the volume status. If the serum sodium is 170 mEq/L and the patient is normotensive and has no orthostatic drop, it is unlikely that the hypernatremia is caused entirely by water loss. In order to elevate the serum sodium to 170 mEq/L by water loss alone, 20% of the body water must be lost, which is improbable in a patient with an intact thirst mechanism because a sodium elevation of just a few milliequivalents per liter induces drinking.

    2) Measurement of central venous pressure or pulmonary artery occlusion pressure may help resolve the question of intravascular volume

    c. The pathogenesis of hypernatremia is varied (Table 3-2). Often, several causes will be present.

2. Treatment

    a. In substantial water deficit with mild to moderate hypernatremia, 0.9% or 0.45% saline is given initially to restore intravascular volume. More hypotonic fluids (0.2% saline or 5% dextrose in water) are substituted after the cardiovascular system is stabilized.

    1) In acute symptomatic hypernatremia, the serum sodium concentration should be reduced by 6 to 8 mEq/L in the first 4 hours, followed by a more gradual decline

Table 3–2.   Causes of Hypernatremia

Loss of Water	Gain of Sodium

Reduced water intake
  Defective thirst mechanism
  Unconsciousness
  Inability to drink
  Lack of access
Increased water loss
  Gastrointestinal loss
    (vomiting, osmotic diarrhea)
  Cutaneous loss
    (sweating and fever)
  Respiratory loss
    (hyperventilation)
  Renal loss (diabetes insipidus,
    osmotic diuresis)
	Increased intake
	  Hypertonic saline infusion
	  Ingestion of sea water
	  Hypertonic sodium
	    bicarbonate infusion
	Renal salt retention, usually in
	  response to primary water
	  deficit

(From Oh MS, Carroll HJ. Electrolyte and acid–base disorders. In: Chernow B, ed. The pharmacologic approach to the clinically ill patient, 2nd ed. Baltimore: Williams & Wilkins, 1988:807.)

          of 1 mEq/L per hour with hypotonic fluid administration.

2)   The amount of water needed to correct hypernatremia fully is predicted by the following formula:

$$\text{Water deficit} = \text{TBW} \times \frac{\text{Na}_{actual}}{\text{Na}_{desired}}$$

where TBW = total body water.

b.   If excess sodium and fluid is the problem, the combination of diuretics and 5% dextrose in water is appropriate, taking care to reduce serum sodium gradually.

c.   In chronic hypernatremia from diabetes insipidus, oral chlorpropamide, thiazide diuretics, or exogenous arginine vasopressin may be used.

II.   POTASSIUM

Normal values are 3.8 to 5.0 mEq/L.

A.   Hypokalemia

    1.   Clinical considerations

Because potassium is largely intracellular, the plasma may not reflect the total body potassium stores. Furthermore, the serum potassium concentration is affected by pH changes: a change in pH of 0.1 may cause as much as a

0.5 to 0.8-mEq/dl change in serum potassium in the opposite direction.

    a.   Hypokalemia may be caused by increased intracellular uptake, urinary excretion, or loss from the gastrointestinal (GI) tract (Table 3-3).

Table 3–3. Causes of Potassium Disturbances

Hypokalemia

Shift into the cell
    Correction of acidosis
    Administration of insulin and glucose
    Alkalosis
    Hypokalemic periodic paralysis
    Barium poisoning
    Increased catecholamines secondary to acute stress
Reduced intake
Increased loss
    Renal
        Primary hyperaldosteronism
        Secondary hyperaldosteroinism (e.g., diuretic therapy, malignant hypertension, Bartter's syndrome, renal artery stenosis)
        Mineralocorticoids other than aldosterone (e.g., licorice, fluoroprednisolone ointment, carbenoxolone)
        Miscellaneous (hypercalcemia, Liddle's syndrome, magnesium deficiency, L-dopa, renal tubular acidosis, acute myelocytic or monocytic leukemia, poorly reabsorbable anions)
    Gastrointestinal (vomiting, nasogastric suction, diarrhea)
    Fistula drainage

Hyperkalemia

Pseudohyperkalemia (thrombocytosis, massive leukocytosis, use of tourniquet with fist exercise, in vitro hemolysis)
True hyperkalemia
    Extravascular shift
        Severe acidosis (especially inorganic acidosis)
        Catabolic states
        Periodic paralysis
        Succinylcholine
        Cationic amino acids
    Excessive ingestion (rare if renal function is normal)
    Decreased renal excretion
        Hypoaldosteronism, Addison's disease, selective hypoaldosteronism (hyporeninemic hypoaldosteronism, heparin, congenital adrenal enzyme deficiencies, angiotensin-converting enzyme inhibitors)
        Tubular unresponsiveness to aldosterone; congenital salt-losing nephropathy
        Potassium-sparing diuretics
        Severe dehydration

(From Oh MS, Carroll HJ. Electrolyte and acid–base disorders. In: Chernow B, ed. The pharmacologic approach to the clinically ill patient, 2nd ed. Baltimore: Williams & Wilkins, 1988:809, 810.)

b. Potassium losses from the GI or genitourinary tract are mediated or worsened by increased mineralocorticoid activity. Metabolic alkalosis commonly accompanies hypokalemia because bicarbonate is such a poorly reabsorbable anion and aldosterone is elevated in volume-contracted states. The mechanism for hypokalemia associated with hypercalcemia is unclear. The association of hypomagnesemia with hypokalemia may reflect elevated aldosterone levels.

2. Treatment

    a. Anesthesiology mythology has deemed a potassium concentration of less than 3 mEq/L (3.5 mEq/L with digoxin therapy) too low for a safe anesthetic because of the increased risk of dysrhythmias. Recent studies dispute this myth. Acute administration of potassium will temporarily increase the serum K^+ concentration but does not replete the large intracellular loss of the ion. Serum potassium of less than 2.5 mEq/L is much more likely to be associated with cardiac dysrhythmias.

    b. Chronic reduction in serum potassium of 1 mEq/L has been estimated to represent a total body deficit of 100 to 200 mEq. Replacement of more than 0.5 mEq/kg per hour is considered unsafe without ECG monitoring.

    c. Altered distribution of potassium from hyperventilation and changes in acid–base status are under the control of the anesthesiologist. An effort should be made to avoid hyperventilating hypokalemic patients.

    d. Infusion of glucose-containing solutions and catecholamine surges can worsen hypokalemia and should be avoided.

    e. The ECG should be monitored for T-wave changes as a guide to the serum potassium concentration.

    f. The addition of 10 to 20 mEq of potassium to each liter of fluid to be infused is reasonable replacement therapy for patients with moderate hypokalemia (3–3.5 mEq/L).

    g. The potassium-depleted heart may be more vulnerable to the effects of digoxin, calcium, and catecholamines and more easily depressed by volatile anesthetics. The potential for prolonged neuromuscular blockade also exists.

B. Hyperkalemia

   1. Clinical considerations

   True hyperkalemia is related to extravascular shifts or decreased renal excretion (Table 3-3). Pseudohyperkalemia is an increase in potassium only in the local blood vessel or in vitro and has no physiological consequences.

   2. Treatment

      a. Ideally, potassium should be below 5.5 mEq/L before elective surgery. Patients with dialysis-dependent renal failure, burns, or intense catabolism may have very rapid rises in potassium; therefore, the serum potassium concentration should be checked shortly before anesthetic induction.

      b. If the potassium is less than 5.5 mEq/L and there is no indication of cardiac toxicity on the ECG, the treatment of hyperkalemia should be directed at the underlying cause(s).

      c. When cardiac toxicity exists (usually at concentrations of >7 mEq/L), manifested by peaked T waves, ventricular dysrhythmia, or prolongation of the PR or QRS complexes, emergency therapy is indicated (Table 3-4). Also important is avoidance of factors that can worsen hyperkalemia (e.g., use of succinylcholine, metabolic acidosis, and hypoventilation).

III. CALCIUM

Normal values are 9.0 to 10.5 mg/dl or 2.2 to 2.6 mM/L; ionized normal values are 1.17 to 1.31 mM/L.

   A. General Considerations

      1. Calcium circulates in the blood in three forms: an ionized fraction (50%), a protein-bound fraction (40%), and a diffusible but nonionized form (10%). Many factors influence the total serum calcium value (pH, serum albumin) as well as the distribution. The active form is the ionized fraction. The ionized value should therefore be measured and followed to direct therapy.

      2. The regulation of calcium involves a complex interplay of many organ systems, including the GI tract,

Table 3–4.   Treatment of Hyperkalemia

Therapy	Dose	Onset	Duration	Complication/ Limitations
Membrane Stabilization				
Calcium gluconate or Calcium chloride	10 to 20 ml IV 10% solution	Immediate	~1hr	Hypercalemia Digitalis glycosides
Redistribution				
Sodium bicarbonate	50 to 100 mEq IV	5 to 10 min	1 to 2 hr	Alkalosis Volume overload
Insulin/glucose	10 to 20 units regular insulin/ IV/50 g glucose IV	30 min	4 to 6 hr	Hypoglycemia Hyperglycemia
Enhanced Elimination				
Loop diuretics Lasix Bumetanide	40 mg IV 1 mg IV	30 min	Throughout diuresis	Volume depletion
Kayexalate	25 to 50 g PO or PR with 70% sorbitol	Several hours	Hours	Patient intolerance
Dialysis Hemodialysis Peritoneal dialysis		Minutes	Throughout dialysis	Dialysis

(Weisberg LS, Szerlip HM, Cox M, et al: Disorders of potassium homeostasis in critically ill patients. Crit Care Clin 3(4):849, 1987)

liver, kidney, bone, and parathyroid glands. The diet supplies the basic substrate in combination with the skin.

3. Cardiovascular signs of calcium imbalance of most importance to the anesthesiologist are hypotension, cardiac insufficiency, bradycardia, dysrhythmias (ventricular fibrillation), and the failure of pressors that rely on calcium to modulate their effects (digoxin, catecholamines, glucagon).

    4. Of particular importance to the anesthesiologist is the tetany and laryngospasm that can arise after neck surgery. Ionized calcium should be checked every 12 hours in patients at risk.

B. Hypocalcemia

    1. Many causes of hypocalcemia have been identified (Table 3-5).

    2. Clinical manifestations

        a. Cardiovascular

            Hypotension
            Cardiac insufficiency
            Bradycardia
            Dysrhythmias
            Insensitivity to catecholamines and digitalis

        b. ECG

            QT- and ST-interval prolongation
            T-wave inversion

        c. Respiratory

            Laryngeal spasm
            Apnea
             Bronchospasm

        d. Neuromuscular

            Tetany
            Chvostek's and Trousseau's signs
            Muscle spasm
            Paresthesias
            Seizures
            Weakness
            Extrapyramidal manifestations

        e. Psychiatric

            Anxiety
            Dementia
            Depression
            Irritability
            Psychosis
            Confusion

        f. Miscellaneous

            Coarse, dry, scaly skin
            Brittle nails
            Thin brittle hair
            Cataracts

Table 3–5.   Causes of Calcium Disturbances*

Hypocalcemia

Hypoparathyroidism
  Primary
  Secondary
    After neck surgery
    Radioiodine
    Metastasis
    Hemochromatosis
  Neonatal
Hypomagnesemia or hyper-
  magnesemia
Hyperphosphatemia
  Iatrogenic
  Tumor lysis
  Rhabdomyolysis
Chelators
  Blood
  Albumin
  Radiocontrast medium
Vitamin D deficiency
  Dietary
  Malabsorption
  Renal insufficiency
  Pseudohypoparathyroidism
Pancreatitis
Sepsis
Hungry bone syndrome
Fat embolism syndrome
Toxic shock syndrome
Burns
Drugs: Albumin, aminogly-
  cosides, calcitonin, cisplatin,
  citrate, EDTA, estrogens, eth-
  ylene glycol, heparin, loop di-
  uretics, magnesium, mithra-
  mycin, phenobarbitol, pheny-
  toin, phosphates, protamine,
  radiocontrast medium

Hypercalcemia

Malignancy
Hyperparathyroidism
Immobilization
Iatrogenic administration
Renal causes
  Chronic renal failure
  Recovery from acute renal
    failure
  After renal transplantation
Posthypocalcemic hypercalcemia
Hypocalciuric hypercalcemia
  Familial
  Hypoparathyroidism
  Lithium
  Thiazides
  Adrenal insufficiency
  Bartter's syndrome
Granulomatous syndromes
  Sarcoidosis
  Histoplasmosis
  Coccidioidomycosis
  Tuberculosis
Hyperthyroidism
Acquired immune deficiency
  syndrome (AIDS)
Phosphorus depletion syndrome
Multiple endocrine neoplasia
  (MEN) syndromes
Pheochromocytoma
Acromegaly
Drugs: Calcium, estrogens or pro-
  gestins for malignancy, lithium,
  theophylline, thiazides, vitamin
  D or A

*Tables 3–5 through 3–14 are reproduced with permission from Zaloga GP, Chernow B. The divalent ions: calcium, magnesium, and phosphorus. In: Chernow B, ed. The pharmacologic approach to the critically ill patient. 2nd ed. Baltimore, Williams & Wilkins, 1988.

3. Treatment

    a. Treatment should be given if the ionized calcium level is less than 1.5 mM/L. Normal values may vary from lab to lab.

    b. Concurrent values of phosphorus and magnesium should be checked and corrected if low.

    c. Any respiratory or metabolic alkalosis should be corrected rapidly, as it can depress ionized calcium level.

    d. The ECG findings should not be relied on to confirm hypocalcemia. Such findings are neither sensitive nor specific for the condition.

    e. The profoundly hypocalcemic patient should not be extubated, as the neuromuscular junction is affected.

    f. Elemental calcium 100–200 mg (Table 3-6) should be administered over 10 minutes followed by a maintenance infusion of 1 to 2 mg/kg per hour until measured ionized calcium levels are constantly over the minimum normal value (varies between hospitals).

C. Hypercalcemia

  1. Causes

    a. Among the commonest causes seen by the anesthesiologist are hyperparathyroidism, malignancy, and immobilization (Table 3-5).

    b. Anesthesiologists must recognize the potential for the multiple endocrine neoplasia (MEN)

Table 3–6. Calcium Preparations

	Size (ml)	Elemental Ca^{2+} Contents (mg)
Parenteral		
Calcium gluconate (10%)	10	93 (4.6 mEq)
Calcium gluceptate	5	90 (4.5 mEq)
Calcium chloride (10%)	10	272 (13.6 mEq)
Oral		
Calcium carbonate (e.g., Os-cal 500)	Tablets	500
Calcium gluconate	Tablets	500
Calcium lactate	Tablets	650
Calcium glubionate (e.g., Neo-calglucon)	Syrup	115/5 ml

syndromes associated with hyperparathyroidism. MEN I = hyperparathyroidism, tumors of pancreatic islet cells, and anterior pituitary adenomas; MEN II = hyperparathyroidism, medullary carcinoma of the thyroid, and pheochromocytoma; MEN III (rare) = hyperparathyroidism, medullary carcinoma of the thyroid, pheochromocytoma, and mucosal neuromas.

2. Signs and symptoms
Of particular importance to the anesthesiologist are marked volume depletion, CNS depression, digitalis sensitivity, impaired renal function (especially tubular dysfunction), and peptic ulcer disease. Specific features are noted in Table 3-7.

3. Treatment
    a. While addressing the underlying cause of the hypercalcemia, general measures that will

Table 3–7. Clinical Features of Hypercalcemia

Cardiovascular

Hypertension
Arrhythmias
Digitalis sensitivity
Catecholamine resistance
QT shortening

Urinary

Nephrocalcinosis
Nephrolithiasis
Tubular dysfunction
  Renal tubular acidosis
  Impaired Na^+ reabsorption
  Free water loss
Glomerular disorders
Interstitial nephritis

Gastrointestinal

Peptic ulcers
Pancreatitis
Constipation
Anorexia
Nausea/vomiting

Neuromuscular

Weakness, atrophy
Hyporeflexia

Neuropsychiatric

Depression
Personality change
Psychomotor retardation
Memory impairment
Psychosis
Disorientation
Obtundation
Coma
Seizures
EEG abnormalities

Skeletal

Osteopenia
Osteitis fibrosa cystica

Miscellaneous

Skin necrosis
Corneal calcification
Conjunctivitis
Pruritus
Decreased bronchial clearance
  of secretions
Hypomagnesemia

help reduce the calcium level are applied: hydration with 0.9% saline, correction of hypokalemia, dietary calcium restriction, and, if possible, mobilization of the patient. Careful volume assessment and hydration are the most important anesthetic considerations. More details of therapy are given in Table 3-8.

Table 3–8. Alternatives in the Treatment of Hypercalcemia

General Measures

Hydration
Remove offending drugs
Dietary Ca^{2+} restriction
Treat underlying disorder
Mobilization

Increase Renal Ca^{2+} Excretion

Saline: 2–3 L over 3–6 hours to maintain urine output >200–300 ml/ hour
Furosemide: 10–40 mg IV every 2–4 hours
Dialysis

Decrease Bone Resorption

Calcitonin: 1–2 MRC U/kg IV or IM every 6 hours
Mithramyin: 25 μg/kg IV over 4 hours every 2–7 days
Glucocorticoids: Hydrocortisone 3 mg/kg per day into divided doses given every 6 hours or prednisone 40–60 mg/day
Indomethacin: 25 mg orally every 6 hours
Etidronate disodium: 7.5 mg/kg per day IV in 250 ml of saline over 2 hours for 1–4 days or 5–10 mg/kg per day orally
Cisplatin: 100 mg/m² over 24 hours
Gallium nitrate: 200 mg/m² per day by continuous infusion for 5–7 days

Ca^{2+} Chelators

Phosphates
  Oral: 500–1000 mg every 6 hours
  IV: 50 mM PO_4 over 8–12 hours
  Rectal: Phosphosoda 5 ml every 6 hours; Fleet enema 100 ml twice daily
EDTA: 10–50 mg/kg over 4 hours
Sodium citrate
Sodium sulfate

Ca^{2+} Antagonists

Verapamil 5–10 mg IV
Nifedipine 10–20 mg sublingually

Parathyroid Hormone Antagonists

WR-2721 430–910 mg/m² over 20–60 minutes

    b. Therapy of concurrent hypomagnesemia and hypokalemia is important, as these conditions frequently complicate hypercalcemia.

    c. Cisplatin is most useful in the hypercalcemia of malignancy.

    d. Glucocorticoids are most efficacious in the hypercalcemia of granulomatous disease (sarcoidosis). Although somewhat effective in patients with multiple myeloma or lymphoid malignancies, steroids are ineffective in patients with hyperparathyroidism.

    e. Propranolol is effective in hypercalcemia associated with pheochromocytoma.

    f. Verapamil has been used for the cardiac toxicity of hypercalcemia (supraventricular dysrhythmias).

IV. MAGNESIUM

    A. Clinical Features

Like potassium, magnesium is primarily an intracellular cation. Serum values thus do not necessarily reflect total body levels. Normal values are 1.4 to 2.0 mEq/L or 1.7 to 4.2 mg/dl.

    1. Magnesium is critically important to the functioning of enzyme systems, metabolic pathways, muscle contraction, and oxidative phosphorylation, including the splitting of high-energy phosphate bonds. Magnesium is also involved in the regulation of parathyroid hormone (PTH). Hypermagnesemia and severe hypomagnesemia decrease PTH secretion, whereas mild hypomagnesemia stimulates PTH secretion.

    2. Fifty-five percent of serum magnesium is in the ionized fraction, which is the physiologically active form. The ionized form is not currently clinically measurable.

    B. Hypomagnesemia

    1. Causes

Important causes for the anesthesiologist to appreciate are ethanol withdrawal, hyperalimentation, and diuretic use (Table 3-9).

    2. Signs and symptoms

    a. Neuronal irritability and tetany are the most important signs (Table 3-10). Also of importance to the anesthesiologist are muscle weak-

Table 3–9.   Causes of Magnesium Disturbances

Hypomagnesemia

Gastrointestinal Losses

Reduced absorption
  Malabsorption
  Laxative abuse
  Fistulas
  Long-term nasogastric suction
Reduced intake
  Malnutrition
  Hyperalimentation
  Long-term IV therapy

Drug-Induced Losses

Diuretics
  Furosemide
  Thiazides
  Mannitol
  Glucose
  Urea
Aminoglycosides
Amphotericin B
Cisplatin
Carbenicillin
Thyroid hormone
Digoxin
Calcium
Ethanol
Insulin*
Saline
Citrate (blood)
Catecholamines*

Renal Losses

Renal disease
  Glomerulonephritis
  Tubular disorders
  Interstitial nephritis
  Diuretic phase of acute tubular
    necrosis
Hypercalcemia
Hyperaldosteronism
Hyperthyroidism
PO_4 deficiency
Diabetic ketoacidosis
SIADH

Miscellaneous Losses

Lactation
Pregnancy
Severe sweating
Hungry bone syndrome*
Burns
Sepsis
Hypothermia
Cardiopulmonary bypass
Administration of glucose, amino
  acids, and insulin*
Mg^{2+}-free dialysis
Refeeding after starvation*

Hypermagnesemia

Iatrogenic
  Administration of Mg^{2+} to pa-
    tients with pre-eclampsia and
    eclampsia may result in
    symptomatic hypermag-
    nesemia, with important car-
    diac and neurologic sequelae
    for both mother and child
Magnesium-containing antacids
  (these should not be used in
  renal failure)
Parenteral nutrition
Enemas
Hypothyroidism
Addison's disease
Lithium intoxication
Familial hypocalciuric
  hypercalcemia

*Causes redistribution of Mg^{2+}.

Table 3–10. Clinical Manifestations of Hypomagnesemia

Cardiovascular

Heart failure
Arrhythmias
Coronary artery spasm
Vasospasm
Hypertension
Digitalis sensitivity
Decreased pressor response
ECG: Prolonged PR and QT interval, ST depression, tall peaked T waves (early), Broadening and decreased amplitude of T waves (late), wide QRS (late)

Gastrointestinal

Dysphagia
Anorexia
Nausea
Abdominal cramps

Neuromuscular

Tetany
Muscle spasm, tremor
Seizures
Confusion, disorientation
Obtundation, coma
Ataxia, nystagmus
Apathy
Depression
Paresthesias
Irritability
Weakness
Psychosis

Miscellaneous

Hypokalemia
Hypocalcemia
Hypophosphatemia

ness, paresthesias, decreased respiratory muscle strength, CNS depression (coma), disorientation, cardiovascular depression, coronary artery spasm, dysrhythmias, and hypotension.

b. Most symptomatic patients also have hypocalcemia and hypokalemia, which complicate the clinical picture and should be treated concurrently.

c. Hypomagnesemia may potentiate digitalis intoxication.

3. Treatment

a. Mild deficiency (1–1.5 mg/dl) can be treated with oral magnesium supplementation.

b. Severe hypomagnesemia (<1 mg/dl) warrants intravenous therapy with an initial dose of 600 mg of elemental magnesium over 3 hours followed by a maintenance dose of 600 to 900 mg over 24 hours. Intravenous replacement should not exceed 15 mg/min. Close monitoring of neurologic status (if patellar reflexes are depressed, the magnesium should be stopped), respiratory status, ECG, blood pressure, and renal function is necessary during rapid replacement of magnesium.

    c.   Replacement therapy in renal insufficiency also requires very close monitoring to avoid magnesium toxicity.

    d.   Concomitant therapy of hypocalcemia should be with the chloride salt, because the sulfate salt can chelate magnesium.

    e.   Intractable ventricular arrhythmias associated with hypomagnesemia may respond to replacement therapy, especially in the setting of myocardial infarction. Coexisting hypokalemia should be aggressively treated in this setting. Suppression of cardiac arrhythmias after heart surgery may be facilitated by magnesium replacement.

    f.   Magnesium therapy may help relieve stridor and dyspnea related to bronchospasm because of the inhibitory action of the ion on smooth-muscle contraction and mast-cell histamine release.

C.   Hypermagnesemia

    1.   The etiologies (Table 3-9) and clinical signs and symptoms (Table 3-11) are numerous.

    2.   Treatment

        a.   Definitive therapy of hypermagnesemia includes stopping all magnesium-containing

Table 3–11. Clinical Manifestations of Hypermagnesemia

	Serum Mg^{2+} Level (mg/dl)
Normal	1.7–2.4
Decrease in deep tendon reflexes (DTR)	4–5
ECG changes (*e.g.*, prolonged PR, QRS, ST)	4–6
Bradycardia	4–7
Hypotension	5–7
Somnolence	6–8
Respiratory insufficiency	10–12
Heart block	15
Respiratory paralysis	18
Cardiac arrest	15–24

drugs. Saline and diuretic administration may be indicated.

    b.   In renal failure, the treatment includes dialysis, which is an efficient way to remove magnesium.

    c.   Uncorrected hypermagnesemia frequently complicates anesthesia management by increasing neuromuscular sensitivity, which augments the potency and increases the duration of both nondepolarizing and depolarizing muscle relaxants.

V.   **PHOSPHORUS**

Normal values are 3.0 to 4.5 mg/dl or 1 to 2 mEq/L. Phosphorus is the principal intracellular anion. It is required for carbohydrate, protein, and fat metabolism, as it is the source of the high-energy bonds in ATP and phosphocreatine. These high-energy compounds are critical for the maintenance of cellular integrity, muscle contraction, neurologic function, hormonal secretion, and cell division.

    A.   Clincal Features

        1.   The normal values are different for children (4.0–7.1 mg/dl) and adults (3.0–4.5 mg/dl).

        2.   Serum phosphorus is regulated primarily by the kidneys. Nearly complete proximal reabsorption is modulated by a maximum tubular reabsorption (like glucose), which, in turn, is dependent on PTH levels. Acute hypocalcemia and acute hypomagnesemia worsen hypophosphatemia by increasing the renal excretion of phosphorus by promoting PTH secretion.

        3.   Insulin causes glucose and phosphorus to move intracellularly, which is the mechanism for the decline in serum phosphorus during carbohydrate loading or refeeding.

    B.   Hypophosphatemia

        1.   Etiology

            a.   Respiratory and metabolic alkalosis stimulate intracellular glycolysis, which consumes phosphorus.

            b.   Epinephrine and glucagon also stimulate the utilization of glucose, which accelerates phosphorus utilization.

            c.   Recovery after renal transplantation

            d.   Treatment of diabetic ketosis or hyperosmolar nonketotic coma

      e. Carbohydrate loads

      f. Other causes (Table 3-12).

2. Signs and symptoms

      a. Cardiac dysfunction from depleted intracellular phosphate stores, which can cause hypotension and impaired catecholamine responsiveness.

      b. Impaired neurologic function, including coma and seizures

      c. Impaired platelet function

      d. Rhabdomyolysis with muscle weakness

      e. Decreased tissue oxygenation because of a left-shifted hemoglobin–oxygen dissociation curve

      f. Additional features (Table 3-13).

3. Treatment

      a. Drugs that cause hypophosphatemia (diuretics, phosphorus-binding antacids, intravenous glucose) are stopped whenever possible.

      b. Parenteral phosphorus solutions are hypertonic and should be either diluted before use or given by central line.

      c. Calcium should not be given through the same intravenous access because it may precipitate with the phosphorus.

      d. Therapy is empiric, as phosphorus is primarily an intracellular anion.

         1) For severe disease (<1 mg/dl) of recent origin, 0.6 mg (0.02 mmol)/kg per hour is suggested.

         2) For more chronic conditions of multifactorial origin, 0.9 mg (0.03 mmol)/kg per hour is appropriate.

         3) Monitoring the level of phosphorus every 6 to 12 hours is mandatory. Monitor more frequently if renal impairment is present.

         4) Repletion should be done over 5 to 7 days to replace intracellular stores and maintenance, begun orally if possible, of 1200 mg/day. A list of phosphorus preparations are found in Table 3-14.

      e. Hypomagnesemia is common and should be treated concurrently.

Table 3–12. Causes of Phosphate Disturbances

Hypophosphatemia	Drug Induced	Renal Losses	Hyperphosphatemia
Transcellular Shift	Anabolic steroids	Renal tubular defects (e.g., myeloma, heavy metals, renal tubular acidosis, Fanconi syndrome)	*Reduced Renal Excretion*
Recovery from malnutrition*	Antacids*		Renal insufficiency
Carbohydrate loading*	Calcitonin		Hypoparathyroidism
Recovery from hypothermia*	Corticosteroids	Hyperparathyroidism	PTH resistance
Recovery from burns*	Diuretics	Hypomagnesemia	Hyperthyroidism
Acute alkalosis*	Epinephrine	Hypokalemia	Acromegaly
Alcoholism*	Glucagon	Acidosis	Diphosphonates
Diabetic ketoacidosis*	Insulin*	Pregnancy	Tumoral calcinosis
Sepsis	Sodium bicarbonate	Vitamin D deficiency or resistance	
Salicylate poisoning	Saline diuresis	Reye's syndrome	*Increased PO$_4$ or Vitamin D Intake*
Hungry bone syndrome	Salicylates	Recovery from acute tubular necrosis	Ingestion of PO$_4$ (e.g., laxatives)
Anabolic steroids		After renal transplant	Intravenous PO$_4$
		Diuresis	PO$_4$ enemas
Gastrointestinal Losses		Oncogenic hypophosphatemia	Vitamin D
Malabsorption			
Emesis		*Miscellaneous*	*Increased PO$_4$ Entrance into Extracellular Fluid*
Diarrhea		Hemodialysis	Acidosis
Long-term nasogastric suction		Inadequate PO$_4$ in IV fluids	Chemotherapy
PO$_4$-binding resins			Rhabdomyolysis
Vitamin D deficiency			Sepsis
			Malignant hyperpyrexia
			Fulminant hepatitis
			Severe hypothermia
			Hemolysis

*Most common causes of severe hypophosphatemia (PO$_4$ <1 mg/dl).

238

Table 3–13. Clinical Features of Hypophosphatemia

General
- Weakness
- Malaise
- Myocardial insufficiency
- Impaired pressor responses
- Respiratory insufficiency
- Rhabdomyolysis
- Hepatocellular damage

Hematologic
- Hemolysis
- Platelet dysfunction
- Leukocyte dysfunction

Skeletal
- Osteomalacia
- Fractures
- Increased bone resorption

Metabolic
- Impaired glucose tolerance
- Impaired gluconeogenesis
- Impaired phospholipid synthesis
- Hypercalciuria
- Hypermagnesemia

Neurologic
- Ataxia
- Confusion
- Obtundation
- Coma
- Delirium
- Dysarthria
- Encephalopathy
- Muscle weakness
- Irritability
- Myopathy
- Paresthesias
- Seizures
- Tremor

Gastrointestinal
- Anorexia
- Nausea
- Vomiting

    f.   Risks of therapy include hyperphosphatemia, hypocalcemia, hypotension, hyperkalemia (with potassium phosphate), hypomagnesemia, hyperosmolarity, metastatic calcification (if calcium × phosphorus product exceeds 60 mg/dl), and renal failure.

C. Hyperphosphatemia

    1. Important causes for the anesthesiologist to recognize are malignant hyperpyrexia, renal insufficiency, and rhabdomyolysis (see Table 3-12).

    2. Signs and symptoms
Ectopic calcification is the main adverse consequence of hyperphosphatemia. It is more likely to occur in an alkalotic environment and when the calcium–phosphorus product is greater than 60 mg/dl.

    3. Treatment

        a. Alkalosis must be avoided, as it favors calcification.

Table 3–14. Phosphorus Preparations

Preparation	PO_4 Content (mg)*	Daily Dose
Enteral		
Whole milk	1/ml	1200 ml
Skim milk	0.9/ml	1330 ml
Neutro-Phos†	250/capsule	1–2 TID
Potassium PO_4 (K-Phos)	125/tablet	3–4 TID
	250/tablet	1–2 TID
Parenteral		
Potassium PO_4	93/ml (4 mEq/ml K^+)	1000 mg
Sodium PO_4	93/ml (4 mEq/ml Na^+)	1000 mg
Neutral Sodium PO_4	2.8/ml (0.16 mEq/ml Na^+)	1000 mg
Neutral Sodium Potassium PO_4	3.1/ml (0.16 mEq/ml Na^+; 0.02 mEq/ml K^+)	1000 mg

*31 mg PO_4 = 1 mmol PO_4.
†Also available as a solution.

b. Phosphorus in the diet or in parenteral fluids must be eliminated and excretion in the urine promoted (if renal function is present) with furosemide or acetazolamide.

c. Phosphorus excretion by the GI tract can be promoted by giving phosphorus-binding antacids.

VI. SUMMARY OF ANESTHETIC CONSIDERATIONS

Electrolyte abnormalities are associated with many clinical diseases and with therapy. The normal ranges for serum electrolyte levels are narrow, and abnormal levels, especially if developed over time, can be adequately corrected only over many hours. Often, several electrolyte abnormalities present at the same time and have similar clinical presentations. Because the clinical picture can be nonspecific or confusing, correction of electrolyte deficiencies or excesses is best monitored by measuring serum levels. If surgery cannot be postponed for treatment of electrolyte disorders, it must be remembered not only that preoperative initiation of therapy is important but that continued treatment intraoperatively and postoperatively is necessary. Serum levels must be closely followed, especially because anesthetics often obscure signs and symptoms of abnormalities.

Recommended Reading

Sodium

Arieff AI. Hyponatremia, convulsions, respiratory arrest, and permanent brain damage after elective surgery in healthy women. N Engl J Med 1986; 314:1529.

Cadnapaphornchai P. Disordered sodium metabolism: sodium retention states. Crit Care Clin 1987; 3:779.

Mettauer B, Rouleau JL, Bichet D, et al. Sodium and water excretion abnormalities in congestive heart failure: determinant factors and clinical implications. Ann Intern Med 1986; 105:161.

Oh MS, Carroll HJ. Electrolyte and acid–base disorders. In: Chernow B, ed. The pharmacologic approach to the critically ill patient. 2nd ed. Baltimore: Williams & Wilkins, 1988:803.

Raine AE, Erne P, Burgisser E, et al. Atrial natriuretic peptide and atrial pressure in patients with congestive heart failure. N Engl J Med 1986; 315:533.

Rossi NF, Cadnapaphornchai P. Disordered water metabolism: hyponatremia. Crit Care Clin 1987; 3:759.

Potassium

Oh MS, Carroll HJ. Electrolyte and acid–base disorders. In: Chernow B, ed. The pharmacologic approach to the critically ill patient. 2nd ed. Baltimore: Williams & Wilkins, 1988:803.

Weisberg LS, Szerlip HM, Cox M. Disorders of potassium homeostasis in critically ill patients. Crit Care Clin 1987; 3:835.

Calcium

Davis AM. Hypocalcemia in rhabdomyolysis. JAMA 1987; 257:626.

Desai TK, Carlson RW, Geheb MA. Hypocalcemia and hypophosphatemia in acutely ill patients. Crit Care Clin 1987; 3:927.

Mehta PM, Kloner RA. Effects of acid base disturbance, septic shock, and calcium and phosphorus abnormalities on cardiovascular function. Crit Care Clin 1987; 3(4):747–58.

Zaloga GP, Chernow B. Hypocalcemia in critical illness. JAMA 1986; 256:1924.

Zaloga GP, Chernow B. The multifactorial basis for hypocalcemia during sepsis: studies of the parathyroid hormone–vitamin D axis. Ann Intern Med 1987; 107:36.

Zaloga GP, Chernow B. Divalent ions: calcium, magnesium, and phosphorus. In: Chernow B, ed. The pharmacologic approach to the critically ill patient. 2nd ed. Baltimore: Williams & Wilkins, 1988:603.

Magnesium

Abraham AS, Rosenmann D, Kramer M, et al. Magnesium in the prevention of lethal arrhythmias in acute myocardial infarction. Arch Intern Med 1987; 147:753.

Kafta H, Langevin L, Armstrong PW. Serum magnesium and potassium in acute myocardial infarction: influence on ventricular arrhythmias. Arch Intern Med 1987; 147:465.

Zaloga GP, Chernow B. Divalent ions: calcium, magnesium, and phosphorus. In: Chernow B, ed. The pharmacologic approach to the critically ill patient. 2nd ed. Baltimore: Williams & Wilkins, 1988:603.

Phosphorus

Aubier M, Murciano D, Lecocguic Y, et al. Effect of hypophosphatemia on diaphragmatic contractility in patients with acute respiratory failure. N Engl J Med 1985; 313:420.

Hessov I, Jensen NG, Rasmussen A. Prevention of hypophosphatemia during postoperative routine glucose administration. Acta Chir Scand 1980; 146:109.

Kingston M, Al-Siba'i MB. Treatment of severe hypophosphatemia. Crit Care Med 1985; 13:16.

Mehta PM, Kloner RA. Effects of acid base disturbance, septic shock, and calcium and phosphorus abnormalities on cardiovascular function. Crit Care Clin 1987; 3:747.

Varsano S, Shapiro M, Taragan R, Bruderman I. Hypophosphatemia as a reversible cause of refractory ventilatory failure. Crit Care Med 1983; 11:908.

Zaloga GP, Chernow B. Divalent ions: calcium, magnesium, and phosphorus. In: Chernow B, ed. The pharmacologic approach to the critically ill patient. 2nd ed. Baltimore: Williams & Wilkins, 1988:603.

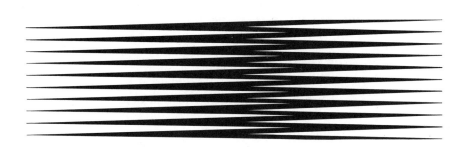

Renal Disorders

Jonathan Kay

The mortality rate for patients with acute renal failure is between 40% and 70%. The anesthesiologist can play a crucial role in reducing this rate by early detection, prevention, and appropriate management of this complication in the perioperative period.

Patients with chronic renal failure present difficulties in monitoring and pharmacodynamics during the surgical interventions they frequently require. They tend to have severe rapid cardiopulmonary deterioration.

I. BASIC RENAL PHYSIOLOGY

A. Excretory Function

1. For balance (i.e., the steady state) to prevail for any substance excreted by the kidneys, this equation must be true:

$$\text{Intake} + \text{production} = \text{output} + \text{retention}$$

Assuming retention is minimal for most excreted substances, the equation becomes:

$$\text{Intake} + \text{production} = \text{output}$$

Taking into account nonrenal excretion leads to the final form:

$$\text{Intake} + \text{production} - \text{nonrenal excretion} = \text{output}$$

2. The kidney is responsible for the metabolism of protein, nucleic acids, and lipids as well as for the excretion of many drugs and drug metabolites.

B. Regulation of Renal Function

1. The kidney receives 25% of the cardiac output (1250 ml/min), of which 10% is filtered (125 ml/min or 180 L/day). Ninety-nine per cent of this filtrate is reabsorbed, so that normal urine output is about 1.8 L/day.

Renal blood flow is described by the equation:

$$\text{Flow} = \frac{\text{renal perfusion pressure}}{\text{renal vascular resistance}}$$

Because renal perfusion pressure = mean arterial pressure − renal venous pressure:

$$\text{Flow} = \frac{\text{MAP} - \text{renal venous pressure}}{\text{renal vascular resistance}}$$

2. Normally, 90% of the blood flow is to the cortex and 9% to the medulla. The regulation of blood flow to the kidney is under the dynamic control of catecholamines, the angiotensin system, arginine vasopressin (ADH), atrial natriuretic factor (ANF), and prostaglandins, as outlined below.

3. Adrenergic receptors are found throughout the kidney. Alpha-receptors are located on or near tubular cells and inhibit sodium reabsorption. Beta-receptor stimulation causes renin release and mild renal vasodilation. Dopaminergic-receptor stimulation causes renal vascular vasodilation.

4. The renin–angiotensin–aldosterone system is intimately involved in the regulation of renal function.

   a. Renin (a renal enzyme) catalyzes the hydrolysis of angiotensinogen (hepatic origin) to angiotensin I. Angiotensin I is metabolized by angiotensin-converting enzyme to angiotensin II. Renin is the rate-limiting step in these two reactions. Renin is stimulated by decreased afferent arteriolar tone, beta-adrenergic stimulation, or decreases in solute delivery to the macula densa. The levels of renin are inversely proportional to sodium excretion.

   b. Angiotensin II causes intense vasoconstriction and stimulates aldosterone production and thirst. Angiotensin II potentiates norepinephrine release and inhibits renin release (feedback inhibition).

   c. Aldosterone secretion is stimulated by hyperkalemia, angiotensin II, and ACTH. The acute release of aldosterone causes increased distal sodium reabsorption, redistribution of potassium into cells, and increased potassium excretion.

   d. The actions of ANF reduce intravascular volume. The release of ANF is stimulated by atrial myocyte stretch. ANF increases the glomerular filtration rate (GFR) by increasing glomerular capillary pressure and increases the filtration fraction and ultrafiltration coefficient. ANF also antagonizes the vasoconstriction from angiotensin II and the actions of renin and aldosterone.

C. Glomerular Filtration

    1. Glomerular filtration is described in the following equation:

$$GFR = kf^*(Pgc - Pt) - r(COPgc - COPt)$$

where kf^* = ultrafiltration coefficient, Pgc = glomerular capillary pressure, Pt = interstitial pressure, r = reflection coefficient, COPgc = glomerular capillary osmotic pressure, and COPt = interstitial osmotic pressure. The kf^* is related to the filtration area and the permeability of the glomerular capillary network. It is decreased by vasoconstricting substances such as vasopressin and angiotensin II.

    2. The relation described in the equation implies that filtration is the difference between the hydrostatic pressure gradient and the colloid osmotic pressure gradient. As filtration occurs along the nephron, COPgc increases, which in turn will reduce the net ultrafiltration pressure. This process is time dependent, so that reducing glomerular plasma flow implies a higher COPgc and hence a lower net ultrafiltration pressure.

D. Tubular Functions

    1. The proximal tubule reabsorbs 60% to 75% of the glomerular filtrate. It reabsorbs virtually all filtered bicarbonate, amino acids, glucose, potassium, and phosphate. Organic acids and bases are secreted proximally. Ammonia diffuses into the tubular lumen and is proteinated and trapped as ammonium.

    2. The collecting duct is responsible for the final urine concentration, mediated by ADH. The normally wide range of urine concentration (50–1200 mOsm) is possible only when all nephron segments are functional.

    3. The distal tubule reabsorbs that sodium not reabsorbed by the proximal tubule. Potassium and hydrogen are exchanged for the sodium. Calcium and phosphate are reabsorbed.

    4. Of note is the relation between tubular and glomerular function, called tubuloglomerular feedback. As the rate of delivery of solute to the distal tubule increases, GFR falls because of a reduction in glomerular capillary flow.

II. ACUTE RENAL FAILURE

    A. Etiology

        Acute renal failure (ARF) is usually multifactorial and results from a dynamic interaction between glomerular and tubular elements. Frequently, a drop in glomerular perfusion pressure begins the assault, with subsequent ischemic or toxic tubular injury as perpetuating factors. The manifestations of the first insult may be delayed by hours or days and hence may be hard to ascribe to specific intraoperative events. Vigilance is required at all times to maintain optimal perfusion.

    B. Diagnosis and Therapy of Oliguria

        1. Definition

            Anuria is defined as less than 100 ml of urine per day, and oliguria is defined as less than 400 ml/day or less than 0.25 ml/kg per hour.

        2. Obstruction to urine flow

            Obstruction must always be ruled out in any case of ARF, oliguric or nonoliguric. Partial obstruction can cause nonoliguric ARF. Ultrasonography provides the fastest and most accurate diagnosis of obstruction.

        3. Prerenal versus intrinsic renal disease causing oliguria

            a. It is important to differentiate prerenal from "intrinsic" or parenchymal renal failure, also called acute tubular necrosis (ATN) or acute vasomotor nephropathy. The differences in urine indices are outlined in Table 4-1.

            b. Microscopic analysis of urine sediment looking specifically for muddy brown renal failure casts that should be done before diuretic administration.

            c. The drawbacks to the indices listed in Table 4-1 include the fact that there are many exceptions to the rules. For example, the indices are invalidated by diuretic use in the preceding 4 to 6 hours. Most importantly, they require precious time to obtain, time that might be better spent aggressively limiting the most probable insult. Recognizing that ARF usually results from hypoperfusion and that successful prophylaxis against ARF reduces the mortality rate, the algorithm in Figure 4-1 may be used.

Table 4–1. Discrimination of Prerenal and Parenchymal ARF

Test	Calculation
Tubular sodium resorption	
Urine sodium concentration (U_{Na})	Direct measurement
Renal failure index (RFI)	$\dfrac{U_{Na}}{U/P_{Cr}}$
Fractional excretion of sodium (FE_{Na})	$\dfrac{U/P_{Na}}{U/P_{Cr}} \times 100$
Tubular water resorption	
Urine specific gravity	Direct measurement
Urine osmolality (U_{Osm})	Direct measurement
Urine–serum osmolality ratio (U_{Osm}/P_{Osm})	Direct measurement
Free water clearance (C_{H_2O})	Urine flow rate $-$ C_{Osm} $$C_{Osm} = \frac{(U_{Osm} \times U \text{ flow rate})}{P_{Osm}}$$
Urine–serum creatinine ratios (U/P_{Cr})	Direct measurement
Urine–serum urea ratio (U/P_{urea})	Direct measurement

*Some investigators use 3 as the cutoff value.

4. Treatment (see Fig. 4-1)

    a. Patients at risk for ARF include elderly patients with cardiac compromise (including cardiopulmonary bypass) and those with hepatic dysfunction, renal compromise, and diabetes, especially if they have recently received intravenous contrast medium.

    b. Fluid challenges are frequently the initial therapy; however, further volume may be hazardous if the patient has a history of congestive heart failure or the pulmonary status is already compromised.

    c. Although an intravascular volume represented by a pulmonary artery occlusion pressure (PAOP) of 15 mmHg is frequently optimal for cardiac performance, fluid as well as medical therapy should be individualized on the basis

Expected Results		
Functional	*Parenchymal*	**Discrimination**
20 mEq/L	40 mEq/L	Poor
<1	>1	Good
<1	>1*	Good
>1.020	<1.010	Poor
>500 mOsm/L	<350 mOsm/L	Poor
>2	<1.1	Fair
Negative values	Positive values	Good
>40	<20	Fair
>20	<10	Fair

(Adapted from Donegan JH. Manual of anesthesia for emergency surgery. New York: Churchill Livingstone, 1988.)

of the specific calculation of left ventricular stroke work index (LVSWI). Some patients with sepsis maximize LVSWI with significantly lower PAOP (10–12 mmHg), and some with cardiac disease will require higher PAOP (18–20 mmHg). The LVSWI is a function of the four determinants of myocardial oxygen consumption (blood pressure, preload, heart rate, and, indirectly, contractility):

$$LVSWI = (MAP - PAOP) \times \frac{CI}{HR} \times 0.014$$

where CI = cardiac index; and HR = heart rate. Other indices of tissue perfusion besides LVSWI may prove useful in the patient with multisystem organ failure who develops intra-

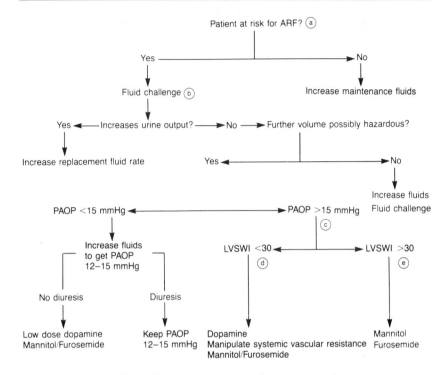

Figure 4-1 Flow chart for management and treatment of perioperative oliguria. (See section II, B, 4 of the outline, parts a through f.)

operative oliguria (e.g., serum lactate, mixed venous oxygen saturation, and oxygen consumption).

d. Patients with high PAOP and low LVSWI need to have their myocardial performance improved with inotropes and possibly manipulation of systemic vascular resistance and their renal perfusion improved with low-dose dopamine.

e. Patients with both a high PAOP and a high LVSWI may increase their urine output in response to mannitol, low-dose dopamine to improve the distribution of flow, or a single large dose of a loop diuretic.

f. Several caveats apply to attempting to promote solute excretion in patients with perioperative oliguria.

1) Such attempts should be made only after

aggressive and early optimization of pre-load and perfusion as outlined in the algorithm.

2) Solute excretion promotion is of greatest value in cases of acute pigmenturia (hemoglobinuria/myoglobinuria) that accompany rhabdomyolysis.

3) A single large dose of furosemide (5–10 mg/kg intravenously) in conjunction with dopamine (2–5 µg/kg per min) has occasionally converted oliguric to nonoliguric renal failure, which is much easier to manage in the intensive care unit. There is no evidence that a small test dose of a potent loop diuretic decreases the morbidity or the mortality rate, especially as many of these patients have tenuous volume status.

4) Early use of mannitol is theoretically attractive because it increases GFR, "flushes" tubular debris and may reduce tubular swelling. Its use must be monitored carefully to avoid excess diuresis, hyperosmolarity, or acute volume overload.

C. Common Problems in ARF Management

1. Metabolic acidosis

Acidosis from ARF is usually not a problem until creatinine clearance drops below 10 ml/min. Lactic acidosis from hypoperfusion may worsen acidosis. A pH below 7.25 is corrected with $NaHCO_3$:

$$HCO_{3\ required} = 0.4\ Wt\ (kg) \times (25 - HCO_{3\ actual})$$

One-half of this total is traditionally given and arterial blood gases then remeasured for reassessment of bicarbonate need. The hypotension and the cause of the acidosis must be treated aggressively.

2. Hyperkalemia

Emergency therapy for a serum K^+ exceeding 6.0 mEq/L includes modest hyperventilation to a $PaCO_2$ of 30 mmHg, correcting any significant metabolic acidosis with bicarbonate (see equation), calcium chloride (2–3 g over 5–10 min) to help stabilize membranes, and insulin–glucose (0.15 units of regular insulin IV/kg lean body weight and half an ampul of 50% glucose). Glucose levels must be followed every 15 minutes; an additional half ampul of 50% glucose may be required to prevent hypoglycemia. Sodium polystyrene sulfonate (Kayexalate), a cation-exchange resin, by enema or gastric tube is used to reduce the total body potassium load and takes time to work. The dose is 0.5 to 1 g/kg with 50 ml of sorbitol. The resin may be contraindicated when the gastrointestinal tract is nonfunctional. Hemodialysis is necessary if other therapeutic maneuvers are unsuccessful in reducing serum K^+ to a safe level.

3. Fluid overload
   a. Efforts to optimize preload and GFR frequently result in fluid overload, as ARF intensifies and the ability of the failing kidneys to excrete salt and water diminishes.
   b. Judicious use of intravenous vasodilators to reduce PAOP and optimize cardiac output and careful titration of positive end expiratory pressure will help maintain oxygenation.
   c. Continuous arteriovenous hemofiltration (CAVH) is a very effective method of removing excess fluid. It is a process whereby water and solute are transported convectively from the blood through a semipermeable membrane by hydrostatic pressure. The hydraulic driving pressure, produced by the systemic arterial pressure or the addition of a blood pump, produces continuous ultrafiltration of serum across the membrane. The addition of negative pressure to the ultrafiltrate line permits up to 2–3 L/hr to be removed. The filtrate is equivalent in solute composition to plasma (unlike dialysis, discussed below, in which the solute composition in the patient is changed).

D. Fluids of Choice
   1. Crystalloid low in sodium and without potassium is the initial fluid of choice for maintenance. Physiologic saline is used for replacement. Electrolytes, ionized calcium, magnesium, and phosphorus are closely monitored and corrected as necessary.
   2. No clearcut advantage and some controversial disadvantages are associated with colloid use in ARF.

However, colloid should be considered when the colloid osmotic pressure (albumin) is low and the PAOP is high, especially when pulmonary edema is present. Colloid as fresh frozen plasma should be used when prolongation of prothrombin time and partial thromboplastin time persist. Red cells should be used when hemoglobin drops below about 10 g/dl.

E. Dialysis

    1. Indications

    Indications for dialysis in ARF include volume overload that threatens oxygenation, reduced myocardial contractility that is unresponsive to inotropes or afterload reducers, uncontrollable hyperkalemia exceeding 6.0 mEq/L, severe metabolic acidosis, encephalopathy presumed secondary to the azotemia, or bleeding diathesis.

    2. Methods

        a. Definition

        1) Dialysis is the transport of solute down an osmotic gradient across a semipermeable membrane. Solutes such as urea and potassium that accumulate in the blood in renal failure move across the membrane into a chemically prescribed dialysate.

        2) Dialysis is capable of removing, maintaining, or adding substances to the patient, depending on the concentration of the substance in the dialysate compared with that in the patient. Substances are removed if the dialysate contains little or none of the substance compared with the patient's plasma (potassium, urea nitrogen, creatinine). Substances are maintained if the dialysate and plasma have the same concentration. Substances may be added to the plasma if the dialysate contains a higher concentration than the plasma (phosphorus).

        3) Transport across the dialysate membrane is described by the equation below. Clearance of solute by dialysis is inversely proportional to its molecular weight from 0 to 100,000.

$$JS = DA(CB - CD)$$

where JS = solute flux, D = diffusion coefficient of the membrane for that solute, A = area of the membrane, CB = solute concentration in blood, and CD = solute concentration in dialysate.

b. Peritoneal dialysis

1) The hyperosmolar solutions glucose 1.5% (347 mOsm/L) or 4.25% (983 mOsm/L) remove water at a rate of 130 and 750 ml/hour, respectively.

2) The efficiency of dialysis is a function of the blood flow to the peritoneal membrane (diabetics with poor circulation of the membrane get notoriously poor peritoneal dialysis), the volume and composition of the dialysate, the surface area of the peritoneal membrane, and the permeability of the tissue between the blood and the dialysate.

c. Hemodialysis

1) Acute temporary hemodialysis is done through specially designed double-lumen central venous catheters. One lumen serves to draw blood from the patient into the dialysis machine, and the other is used to return cleansed blood from the machine to the patient.

2) Dialysis catheters provide excellent central venous access. They should be handled in a strictly sterile manner when used for central pressure measurement or fluid and drug administration. Some of these catheters are softer than regular PVC central venous catheters. Rarely, they erode through large veins, resulting in hemodynamic or respiratory compromise.

III. ANESTHESIA AND PERIOPERATIVE MANAGEMENT OF ACUTE AND CHRONIC RENAL FAILURE

A. Preoperative Evaluation

1. Central nervous system

Careful documentation of central nervous system (CNS) deficits is mandatory. Changes in mentation can be caused by the same process that was responsible for the renal failure (sepsis, hemorrhage, hypotension) or by the gross metabolic derangements that may accompany renal failure (hyponatremia, accumulation of toxic "middle molecules," BUN >100 mg/dl). Premedication should be reduced appropriately or withheld in proportion to the deficits. Postoperative airway protection may be necessary until the CNS status has improved.

2. Airway management
Coagulation abnormalities are common when the BUN exceeds 80 mg/dl. Awake nasal intubation is relatively hazardous. Well-lubricated nasal dilators and intranasal vasoconstrictors should be considered if nasal intubation is absolutely necessary.

3. Pulmonary management
   a. Review of a recent chest radiograph is desirable to look for signs of congestive failure or aspiration (both common and often "asymptomatic" in encephalopathic patients).
   b. Noncardiogenic pulmonary edema is common because of the low colloid osmotic pressure in the patient with hypoalbumenic renal failure. Baseline arterial blood gases or at least an arterial hemoglobin saturation by pulse oximetry is very useful because of occasional unexpected low values prior to any anesthetic intervention.

4. Cardiovascular management
   a. Intravascular volume assessment is crucial in these patients. Common potential causes of hypovolemia include too-vigorous diuresis and fluid restriction, bleeding, and gastrointestinal losses from vomiting or diarrhea. Hypervolemia is common because of the inability of the patient with renal failure to excrete salt and water and of dietary indiscretion or inadequate dialysis.
   b. Because of the rapidity with which renal failure can change volume status, central venous pressure or pulmonary artery catheterization may be necessary for fluid management.
   c. Recent evidence suggests that transesophageal echocardiography is the modality of choice to assess left ventricular volume directly rather

than depending on the PAOP, which is an indirect reflection of this volume.

5. Gastrointestinal management

Gastrointestinal bleeding is common in renal failure from platelet dysfunction and mucosal barrier breakdown. H_2-blocker therapy, magensium-free antacids, or mucosal barrier protectants should be considered. The dose adjustment for cimetidine is given in Table 4-2. The dose for ranitidine for patients with a creatinine clearance below 50 ml/minute is 50 mg orally every 18 to 24 hours.

6. Genitourinary management

Any tubes used to divert the urinary tract should be checked preoperatively to ensure their integrity and freedom from obstruction.

7. Metabolic and endocrine management

a. Elevated phosphorus and decreased calcium levels result from the inability of the failing kidney to excrete phosphorus. The use of calcium to raise the blood pressure is contraindi-

Table 4-2. Cimetidine Dosage in Patients with Impaired Renal Function

Estimated Creatinine Clearance* (ml/min/1.73 m²)	Dose of 300 mg per
>40 (mild)	6 hours
20-40 (moderate)	8 hours
0-20 (severe)	12 hours

*Calculated as follows:

Men:

$$Cl_{cr} = \frac{140 - age}{serum\ creatinine} \times \frac{weight\ (kg)}{72}$$

Women:

$$Cl_{cr} = \frac{140 - age}{serum\ creatinine} \times \frac{weight\ (kg)}{72} \times 0.85$$

(Johnson DA, Cattau EL. Pharmacologic approach to gastrointestinal disease in critical illness. In Chernow B, ed. The pharmacologic approach to the clinically ill patient. 2nd ed. Baltimore: Williams & Wilkins, 1988:325.)

cated when the calcium–phosphorus product exceeds 60, because intravascular precipitation may result.

b. Treatment of acidosis with $NaHCO_3$ is common. Treatment is reasonably titrated to pH 7.30 in normocapnic patients with renal failure.

c. Succinylcholine is contraindicated when serum potassium exceeds 5.5 mEq/L, as a rise of at least 0.7 mEq/L is associated with its use. Restoration of normal pH and potassium status may not be possible in these cases without dialysis, especially in catabolic patients.

B. Premedication

1. Benzodiazepines

a. Diazepam has active and long-lasting metabolites (>24 hours) in renal failure.

b. Midazolam has virtually no active metabolites. The half-life is minimally prolonged in renal failure, and the drug is thus quite useful when carefully titrated.

2. Narcotics (see also Section C4)

a. Meperidine is more lipophilic than morphine, is 60% protein bound, and is metabolized to compounds that are less potent respiratory depressants, which are renally excreted. It can cause convulsions in high concentrations. It cannot be removed by dialysis.

b. Morphine can cause excessive respiratory depression in renal failure because of brain levels of the metabolites. Such brain levels are pH dependent and increase with respiratory alkalosis. Morphine is not removed by dialysis.

3. Anticholinergics
Both atropine and glycopyrrolate are excreted 20% to 50% unchanged in the urine. The dose should be reduced accordingly.

4. Other drugs
A list of drugs for which renal excretion is important and which are commonly used in anesthetic practice is found in Table 4-3.

C. Anesthetic Agents

1. Pharmacokinetics in renal failure
Highly protein-bound drugs will have more target-organ effect because of decreased protein binding

Table 4–3. Drugs Employed or Encountered in Anesthesia Practice for Which Renal Excretion Is a Significant Elimination Pathway

Digoxin	Acetazolimide	Vancomycin
Barbital	Chlorothiazide	Penicillin G
Amphetamine	Amiloridine	Carbenicillin
Pancuronium	Chlorpropamide	Ampicillin
d-Tubocurarine	Metocurine	Cephaloridine
Gallamine	Colistin	Cephlexin
Metocurine	Polymyxin B	Lincomycin
Hexamethonium	Kanamycin	Sulfonamides
Neostigmine	Gentamicin	Cycloserine
Pyridostigmine	Streptomycin	Methotrexate
Atropine	p-Aminosalicylic acid	
Diazoxide	Neomycin	

(Modified from Prescot LF: Mechanisms of renal excretion of drugs [with special reference to drugs used by anesthetists]. Br J Anaesth 1972;44:246.)

and low total protein levels. For example, a drug that is normally 95% protein bound may be only 90% bound in renal failure, which results in a 100% increase in the free drug (from 5% to 10%). The decreased protein binding is probably secondary to endogenous organic acids that accumulate in uremia and which can bind to proteins, thereby displacing protein-bound drugs. Drugs in this class include cardiac glycosides, benzodiazepines, anticonvulsants, hypoglycemic agents, and d-tubocurarine. Serum concentrations may be unreliable, especially in volume-overloaded patients with a large volume of distribution.

2. Induction agents
   a. Sodium thiopental may have an exaggerated effect in renal failure because of decreased protein binding and possibly a compromised blood–brain barrier.
   b. Ketamine has sympathomimetic effects. The rise in blood pressure and pulse may be deleterious in this population, which tends to be hypertensive and has a high incidence of coronary disease.

      c.   Midazolam is a useful induction agent because of a short elimination half-life and few active metabolites.

3.   Neuromuscular blocking agents

      a.   Specific agents

            1) Succinylcholine is contraindicated if serum potassium is above 5.5 mEq/L because a rise of 0.7 to 1.0 mEq/L is typically observed after a dose.

            2) Gallamine is 85% to 100% excreted by the kidneys. The half-life is 16 hours in complete renal failure.

            3) Metocurine is 60% renally excreted. Prolonged paralysis occurs in renal failure.

            4) Pancuronium is 10% to 20% renally excreted. An active metabolite may accumulate in renal failure. The half-life is at least 4 to 8 hours in renal failure.

            5) *d*-Tubocurarine is 40% renally eliminated. The alternate route of elimination is bile.

            6) Vecuronium is 10% to 25% eliminated by the kidney. Its action is not prolonged in renal failure even with relatively large doses, but the duration will be prolonged with coexisting hepatic insufficiency.

            7) Atracurium is enzymatically degraded independent of renal or hepatic function. It is thus an excellent choice in renal failure. Histamine release occurs with doses exceeding 0.5 mg/kg, especially when given rapidly.

      b.   Recurarization

          Paralysis may recur after reversal of neuromuscular blockade because the duration of neostigmine's effect is less than the duration of the relaxant. Edrophonium (0.5–1.0 mg/kg) is excreted by the kidney and may be an ideal reversal agent in renal failure.

      c.   Prolongation of neuromuscular blockade

          Neuromuscular blockade is potentiated by some antibiotics (aminoglycosides decrease the prejunctional release of acetylcholine) and diuretics (both mannitol and furosemide displace some of the neuromuscular drugs from binding sites).

4. Narcotics

a. Meperidine

Ninety per cent of meperidine is demethylated or hydrolyzed in the liver. Less than 5% is excreted unchanged in urine. Urinary excretion is pH dependent (lower pH favors excretion of unchanged compound). One metabolite (normeperidine) has an elimination half-life of 15 to 40 hours and has CNS stimulatory effects, manifest as myoclonus or seizures, in renal failure patients receiving meperidine for a long time.

b. Morphine

Fifty-five per cent of morphine is conjugated, and less than 10% is excreted unchanged in urine. The principal metabolite is inactive. Renal failure patients have a higher plasma concentration than normal persons, which can result in the reported increased sensitivity to the drug (volume of distribution is smaller in renal failure).

c. Fentanyl

Eighty-five per cent of fentanyl appears in the urine and feces as inactive metabolites. Less than 8% is recovered unchanged in the urine. The relatively slow elimination half-life (185–219 min) is secondary to a large volume of distribution. This effect is exaggerated in renal failure.

d. Sufentanil

Less than 1% of sufentanil appears unchanged in the urine. There are some weakly active metabolites, which have been reported to cause prolonged respiratory depression in patients in renal failure.

e. Alfentanil

Less than 1% of alfentanil is excreted unchanged in the urine. There are no active metabolites, and alfentanil has a small volume of distribution.

5. Inhalational agents

All of the currently used agents (isoflurane, enflurane, and halothane) decrease GFR and renal plasma flow while increasing renal vascular resistance and filtration fraction (Table 4-4). These effects may be mediated by the adrenergic nervous system and its effects on the redistribution of flow, but carefully controlled studies in intact man are lacking. The deleterious effects can be partially offset by preinduction hydration.

6. Regional blockade in renal failure

Platelet dysfunction and residual heparin from hemodialysis increase the likelihood of bleeding associated with regional anesthesia. Although there is reduced protein binding in renal failure, this effect, which would enhance local anesthetic potency, is more than offset by the increased hepatic clearance from the hyperdynamic circulation. Of interest in this regard is the reduction in the duration of supraclavicular blocks by 40% in renal failure. The duration of axillary blocks is unchanged.

D. Common Problems in Renal Failure

1. Vascular access

Patients with renal failure have an increased tendency to bleed because of platelet dysfunction (and

Table 4–4. *Average Effects of Anesthesia and Surgery**

	Flow Rate (ml/min)	Sodium (mEq/L)	Sodium Excretion (mEq/min)	Urea (mg/dl)	Osmolarity (mOsm/L)
Plasma	750→500	140	105→70	10	290
Filtrate	125→100	140	17→14	10	290
Proximal tubule	44→35	140	6→5	15	290
Henle's loop	25→20	70	1.7 →1.5	50	100
Distal tubule	20→10	10→1.0	0.20→0.01	100	290
Final urine	0.5	100→20	0.20→0.01	500	800

*A decrease in renal blood flow and GFR and an increase in ADH and aldosterone secretion are assumed.

(Prough DS. Perioperative management of acute renal failure. Advances in Anesthesia 1988; 5:135.

immediately postdialysis from residual heparin). Central and arterial catheterization thus is more hazardous. If clinical bleeding not secondary to anticoagulant medication is obvious, desmopressin (0.3 μg/kg) intravenously over 30 minutes should be considered just prior to line placement to improve platelet function. The presence of an arteriovenous fistula for dialysis precludes using that extremity for all but emergency access. The judicious placement of a central venous catheter using strictly aseptic technique and the Seldinger method frequently is justified. The axillary artery may be used in preference to the radial, which may be needed for fistula access.

2. Volume assessment and fluid management
   a. The patient's predialysis and postdialysis weights are usually reasonable guides to volume status.
   b. The central venous pressure or PAOP may be less reliable than transesophageal echocardiography in the assessment of left ventricular volume. Ventricular compliance changes very rapidly in this group of patients with stiff left ventricles, hypertension, and coronary disease.
   c. Colloids for fluid replacement may be justified when colloid osmotic pressure is low and filling pressures are high. A gradient between colloid osmotic pressure and PAOP of less than 7 mmHg puts patients at risk for pulmonary edema. Potassium-free solutions should be used and serum potassium closely monitored perioperatively.
   d. Fresh frozen plasma should be considered when the prothrombin time is prolonged and volume is needed.

3. Cardiopulmonary compromise
   a. The rapid onset of pulmonary edema (both cardiogenic and hydrostatic) is common. Patients with renal failure have an elevated cardiac output, which tends to offset their chronic anemia. Obtunding this protective mechanism with beta-blockade to treat perioperative hypertension may precipitate congestive heart failure.

    b. The patient should be prepared for the possibility of invasive monitoring and postoperative mechanical ventilation. Intensive dialysis may be necessary to facilitate weaning from mechanical ventilation. Extubation should occur only after strict criteria are met to assure metabolism of anesthetics and adequate gas exchange (respiratory rate <30, vital capacity >15 ml/kg, negative inspiratory force more negative than -25 cmH$_2$O).

  4. Metabolic problems

    a. Hypocalcemia (primarily attributable to decreases in vitamin D production and gastrointestinal calcium absorption) is typical. The use of calcium to increase blood pressure perioperatively is associated with an increased risk of intravascular calcification if the calcium–phosphorus product exceeds 60.

    b. Hypothyroidism is difficult to diagnose. Measurement of the TSH level or a TRH stimulation test may be required for the diagnosis because of the common occurrence of "euthyroid sick" values on routine testing.

    c. Diabetes is more common when steroids are used for patients with a kidney allograft.

E. Renal Failure and Dialysis

  1. Chronic ambulatory peritoneal dialysis

  Chronic ambulatory peritoneal dialysis (CAPD) uses the peritoneum as the dialysis membrane. The catheter is tunneled percutaneously. Four fluid exchanges per day are usually performed with a dwell time of 4 to 8 hours each. The patient's weight when the peritoneum is empty is the dry weight. This form of dialysis is considered less likely to disturb the patient's hemodynamics than is hemodialysis.

  2. Chronic hemodialysis

    a. An arteriovenous fistula is most commonly used (radial artery to cephalic vein). Alternative sites are a Gortex graft connecting the brachial artery to the basilic vein or the femoral artery to the femoral vein.

    b. Dialysis access should be protected with careful positioning and padding during surgery.

The access should be confirmed as functional before allowing the patient to emerge from anesthesia, especially if hypotension has occurred during surgery. Revision of the graft thus can be done immediately if necessary.

c. Patients may become acutely unstable hemodynamically while on dialysis. Hypotension may occur from rapid or excessive fluid withdrawal, complement activation, or metabolic acidosis from use of acetate dialysate.

d. Hypoxemia may occur secondary to a variety of causes. Leukostasis, complement activation, and acute correction of metabolic acidosis leading to hypoventilation are some of the presumed causes.

IV. SUMMARY OF ANESTHETIC CONSIDERATIONS
Anesthesiologists must be aware of the factors predisposing to ARF (hypovolemia, myoglobinuria, aminoglycoside toxicity) and learn how to minimize such insults. Obstruction should be ruled out by ultrasound. The urine indices that may help discriminate parenchymal renal failure (ATN) from prerenal failure include a fractional excretion of sodium greater than 1 and a positive free-water clearance. Overall, body perfusion should be optimized by monitoring therapeutic maneuvers with left ventricular stroke work index, serum lactate levels, and mixed venous saturation rather than blood pressure only. Management of the complications of ARF includes careful (often invasive) assessment of intravascular volume, treatment of hyperkalemia ($NaHCO_3$, hyperventilation, calcium, insulin–glucose, Kayexalate), and correction of acidosis. Patients in chronic renal failure present with the above problems as well as with more difficult venous and arterial access; hemodynamic instability; calcium, magnesium, and phosphorus imbalance; and a tendency to pulmonary edema.

Recommended Reading

Abreo K, Moorthy AV, Osborne M. Changing patterns and outcome of acute renal failure requiring hemodialysis. Arch Intern Med 1986;146:1338.

Alpert RA, Roizen MF, Hamilton WK, et al. Intraoperative urinary output does not predict postoperative renal function. Anesthesiology 1983;59:A157.

Atlas SA, Volpe M, Sosa RE, Laragh JH, Camargo MJ, Maack T. Effects of atrial natriuretic factor on blood pressure and the renin–angiotensin–aldosterone system. Fed Proc 1986;45:2115.

Brown CB, Ogg CS, Cameron JS. High dose furosemide in acute renal failure: a controlled trial. Clin Nephrol 1981;15:90.

Byrick RJ. Acute renal failure: update. Can Anaesth Soc J 1986; 33(3 pt 2):S9.

Cahill CJ. Prevention of postoperative renal failure in patients with obstructive jaundice: the role of bile salts. Br J Surg 1983; 70:590.

Carvalho AC. Bleeding in uremia: a clinical challenge. N Engl J Med 1983;308:38.

Collins AJ, Keshaviah P, Ilstrup KM, Shapiro F. Clinical comparison of hemodialysis and hemofiltration. Kidney Int 1985; 17(suppl):S18.

Eneas JF, Schoenfeld PY, Humphreys MH. The effect of infusion mannitol–sodium bicarbonate on the clinical course of myoglobinuria. Arch Intern Med 1979;139:801.

Hyneck ML. Current concepts in clinical therapeutics: drug therapy in acute renal failure. Clin Pharm 1986;5:892.

Janson PA, Jubelirer SJ, Weinstein MJ, Deykin D. Treatment of the bleeding tendency in uremia with cryoprecipitate. N Engl J Med 1980;303:1318.

Kron IL, Harman PK, Nolan SP. The measurement of intra-abdominal pressure as a criterion for abdominal re-exploration. Ann Surg 1984;199:28.

Kron IL, Joob AW, Van Meter C. Acute renal failure in the cardiovascular surgical patient. Ann Thorac Surg 1985;39:590.

Leunissen KM, Hoorntje SJ, Fiers HA, Dekkers WT, Mulder AW. Acetate versus bicarbonate hemodialysis in critically ill patients. Nephron 1986;42:146.

Lien J, Chan V. Risk factors influencing survival in acute renal failure treated by hemodialysis. Arch Intern Med 1985;145:2067.

Luft FC. Acute renal failure: contemporary management. Indiana Med 1985;78:672.

Makhoul RG, Gewertz BL. Renal prostaglandins. J Surg Res 1986; 40:181.

Mann HJ, Fuhs DW, Hemstrom CA. Acute renal failure. Drug Intell Clin Pharm 1986;20:421.

Mason J. The pathophysiology of ischemic acute renal failure: a new hypothesis about the initiation phase. Renal Physiol 1986;9:129.

Mazze RI, Sievenpiper TS, Stevenson J. Renal effects of enflurane and halothane in patients with abnormal renal function. Anesthesiology 1984;60:161.

Myers BD, Moran SM. Hemodynamically mediated acute renal failure. N Engl J Med 1986;314:97.

Pru C, Kjellstrand CM. The FENa test is of no prognostic value in acute renal failure. Nephron 1984;36:20.

Rasmussen HH, Pitt EA, Ibels LS, McNeil DR. Prediction of outcome in acute renal failure by discriminant analysis of clinical variables. Arch Intern Med 1985;145:2015.

Ron D, Taitelman U, Michaelson M, Bar-Joseph G, Bursztein S, Better OS. Prevention of acute renal failure in traumatic rhabdomyolysis. Arch Intern Med 1984;144:227.

Shin B, Mackenzie CF, McAslan TC, Helrich M, Cowley RA. Postoperative renal failure in trauma patients. Anesthesiology 1979; 51:218.

Wait RB, White G, Davis JH. Beneficial effects of verapamil on postischemic renal failure. Surgery 1983;94:276.

Wilkes BM, Mailloux LU. Acute renal failure: pathogenesis and prevention. Am J Med 1986;80:1129.

Zarich S, Fang LS, Diamond JR. Fractional excretion of sodium. Arch Intern Med 1985;145:108.

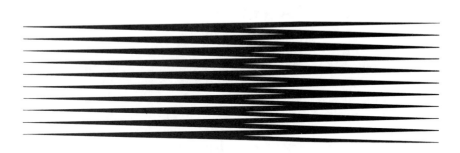

Nervous System Disorders

≡ Cerebrovascular Disease

Patricia H. Petrozza
Donald S. Prough

Intracranial Aneurysms

I. INCIDENCE
In North America, 28,000 persons annually manifest symptoms of a subarachnoid hemorrhage (SAH) from a previously undiagnosed cerebral aneurysm. Too frequently, the clinical diagnosis is delayed, while mortality rates in those referred to neurosurgical care remain distressingly high secondary to vasospasm, recurrent hemorrhage, and medical and surgical complications. With optimal medical and surgical treatment, only one-third of the original 28,000 patients will return to their previous occupations.

II. CLINICAL CLASSIFICATION
   A. Operative outcome correlates well with the clinical grade given to a patient with a ruptured aneurysm on admission to the hospital and at the time of surgery. The Hunt system of clinical grading and the surgical mortality rates are described in Table 5-1.
   B. The presence of serious systemic diseases such as severe arteriosclerosis or the demonstration of vasospasm on cerebral arteriography serve to place a patient in the next less-favorable category.

III. PERIOPERATIVE MANAGEMENT
   A. Rebleeding and cerebral vasospasm are the most significant causes of clinical deterioration after SAH. Although recurrent hemorrhage is almost uniformly fatal, 65% of the patients in a recent large series who survived an episode of cerebral vasospasm had an eventual good or excellent outcome.
   B. Vasospasm
      1. Symptoms
      The symptoms of vasospasm usually begin insidiously 5 to 7 days after the initial hemorrhage. Patients may exhibit symptoms, such as drowsiness and stupor, of a global reduction in cerebral blood flow (CBF), after which many suffer focal manifestations of cerebral ischemia. Classic vasospastic symptoms develop in about half of those patients who have angiographically evident vasospasm.

Table 5–1. Hunt's Clinical Grades for Subarachnoid Hemorrhage

	Criteria	Surgical Mortality Rate (%)
Grade I	Asymptomatic or minimal headache and slight rigidity	0–5
Grade II	Moderate to severe headache, nuchal rigidity, but no neurologic deficit other than cranial nerve palsy	2–10
Grade III	Drowsiness, confusion, or mild focal deficit	10–15
Grade IV	Stupor, mild to severe hemiparesis, possible early decerebrate rigidity, moribund appearance	60–70
Grade V	Deep coma, decerebrate rigidity, moribund appearance	70–100

The original classification has been revised to include a Grade 0 for patients who have unruptured aneurysm and a Grade Ia for patients with a stable residual neurologic deficit who are past the period of acute cerebral reaction.

2. Treatment
    a. Vasodilators
       Attempts to prevent or treat cerebral vasospasm have been made with at least 90 vasodilating drugs or drug combinations, most not effective. Nimodipine, a calcium channel-blocking agent, in a randomized, placebo-controlled cooperative study, lowered the incidence of subsequent vasospasm and ischemic deficits.
    b. Fluid and inotropes
       Although most other attempts to improve CBF with vasodilators have been disappointing, augmentation by an increase in systemic blood pressure and cardiac output shows promise. Currently, pulmonary arterial and systemic arterial catheters are inserted in patients who develop neurologic deficits secondary to vasospasm, and cardiac output is increased by augmenting intravascular volume. On occasion,

vasoactive drugs such as dopamine are added to increase cardiac output further. However, hypertension must be avoided if the aneurysm has not yet been clipped.

C. Rebleeding

Within the first 2 weeks after an initial SAH, approximately 19% of patients rebled. To avoid the extremely high mortality and morbidity rates from a second hemorrhage, the prevention of rebleeding is approached in three ways.

1. First, some neurosurgeons advocate early surgical isolation of the aneurysm.

2. Second, efforts are made to reduce the transmural pressure exerted on the aneurysm wall. Transmural pressure, defined as the systemic mean arterial pressure minus the intracranial pressure (MAP − ICP), is controlled by reducing the patient's anxiety or agitation through adequate sedation with barbiturates or benzodiazepines. If further blood pressure reduction is necessary, antihypertensive drugs such as hydralazine or methyldopa are frequently added.

3. Third, antifibrinolytic agents such as epsilon-aminocaproic acid are given to delay lysis of the clot surrounding the hemorrhage site. However, the resultant decrease in the rebleeding rate appears to be accompanied by an increased incidence of ischemic complications.

D. Systemic Effects of Subarachnoid Hemorrhage

1. Electrocardiographic (ECG) abnormalities such as U waves, ST-segment depression and elevation, T-wave inversion or flattening, and prolonged QT intervals have long been recognized as manifestations of SAH.

2. These nonspecific ECG changes do not increase the operative morbidity. Occasionally, dysrhythmias are noted, and microscopic evidence of focal areas of necrosis in the myocardium has been seen at autopsy.

3. Elevations of serum and urine catecholamines, as well as increased myocardial uptake of epinephrine, have been noted in patients who have sustained an SAH acutely. Circulating blood volume is reduced in many patients and may be a manifestation of sympathetic nervous system hyperactivity.

E. Diagnostic Tests
   1. Once the diagnosis of SAH is suspected because of the patient's clinical presentation and CT scan, cerebral angiography is undertaken. Injected views of both carotid arteries and at least one vertebral artery are obtained.
   2. The participation of an anesthesiologist is frequently requested to provide adequate sedation, monitoring of circulatory and respiratory status, and treatment of any contrast reactions. Small amounts of narcotics and sedatives are usually effective in these cases. Occasionally, endotracheal intubation with general anesthesia is required in the uncooperative patient.

F. Timing of Surgery
Controversy surrounds the timing of surgery after SAH to eliminate cerebral aneurysms. Early exclusion of the aneurysm from the circulation reduces the incidence of rebleeding and allows more aggressive cardiac output augmentation in patients at risk for cerebral vasospasm. However, surgical conditions are compromised when microscopic surgery is performed within the first 72 hours after hemorrhage because the clot over the aneurysm is poorly organized, and brain edema is prevalent. The Cooperative Aneurysm Study demonstrated that early surgery reduces the rebleeding rate but does not improve the overall morbidity and mortality rates, primarily because of the frequent postoperative development of vasospasm.

IV. ANESTHETIC MANAGEMENT
   A. Goals
   An anesthetic for the surgical manipulation of an intracranial aneurysm must stabilize and maintain the patient's cardiovascular and cerebral perfusion. Careful attention to systemic blood pressure and the appropriate use of measures that decrease ICP reduce the occurrence of large changes in the transmural pressure across an aneurysmal wall. To minimize the risk of postoperative neurologic deficits, the reduction or prevention of cerebral edema must be addressed with the knowledge that autoregulation is impaired in a brain affected by an SAH.
   B. Preoperative Preparation
   1. The proposed anesthetic procedures, possibility of transfusion, and the postanesthetic recovery period should be skillfully and succinctly explained to the patient and family.

     2. To avoid blood pressure elevation attributable to emotional stress, a more detailed explanation of the possibility of intraoperative aneurysmal rupture and need for controlled hypotension might be provided to the patient's family in a separate site.

     3. Patients in Hunt Grades 0 to 2 should receive a small amount of an oral sedative such as a benzodiazepine before surgery. Additional sedation can be given when the patient arrives in the operating room. Patients with more severe deficits rarely require preoperative sedation.

C. Monitors

     1. Once the patient arrives in the surgical preparation area, a reliable intravenous infusion with a T-connector, as well as an arterial catheter, is placed. Additional sedation is given if necessary.

     2. The patient should then have a central venous (CVP) or pulmonary artery catheter placed through either the antecubital fossa or an internal jugular route.

     3. Other routine monitors such as a pulse oximeter, ECG (V5 lead), precordial stethoscope, and peripheral nerve stimulator are applied prior to induction.

D. Induction

     1. A smooth anesthetic induction is essential. Agents that decrease CBF, cerebral metabolism, and ICP, such as thiopental, methohexital, midazolam, or etomidate, are appropriate. Thiopental is the most popular agent, whereas etomidate is used infrequently because of the adrenal suppression associated with this drug.

     2. For muscle relaxation prior to intubation, most nondepolarizing muscle relaxants are appropriate, as they do not increase ICP and maintain cardiovascular stability. Curare is rarely employed because of histamine release.

     3. While awaiting the onset of relaxation, narcotics (fentanyl 5 μg/kg) may be infused to blunt the hypertensive response to endotracheal intubation.

     4. To further reduce hypertension caused by laryngoscopy, 1.5 mg/kg of lidocaine is administered intravenously approximately 1.5 minutes before the anticipated intubation.

E. Intubation

     1. When peripheral nerve stimulation demonstrates

complete relaxation, a small amount of additional thiopental is given, and laryngoscopy is performed. If necessary, additional thiopental and narcotics are administered to control the blood pressure response to laryngoscopy.

2. Rarely, hypertension during induction necessitates the use of intravenous sympathetic-blocking agents such as esmolol, a beta$_1$-blocking agent, or labetalol, a combination alpha–beta-adrenergic blocking agent, or direct vasodilators such as nitroglycerin or nitroprusside.

3. Once correct positioning of the endotracheal tube is confirmed, the tube is taped on the side of the mouth opposite to the operative site, and an oral gastric tube and esophageal stethoscope are added, as is a capnograph, a temperature monitor, and, if available, a mass spectrometer.

4. Nitrous oxide and small amounts of isoflurane, as well as additional increments of intravenous narcotics, are usually administered at this time, particularly to stabilize the patient's blood pressure before the application of a surgical head holder.

F. Maintenance Anesthesia

1. A maintenance technique utilizing a nitrous/narcotic base and the addition of isoflurane (<1.0 MAC) provides good brain relaxation and a stable hemodynamic course.

   a. Some clinicians question the use of N_2O where the possibility for ischemia exists, because this agent, in recent animal experiments involving cerebral ischemia, has been associated with poor outcome.

   b. Conversely, evidence exists that isoflurane may provide protection in the event of cerebral ischemia because of its ability to produce an isoelectric EEG in clinically useful concentrations.

2. Although N_2O and isoflurane both increase CBF, halothane and enflurane cause much larger increases at similar anesthetic levels.

G. Fluid Management

1. Glucose administration during surgery is avoided, as cerebral ischemic injury may be aggravated in the presence of elevated glucose levels.

2. Initially, the patient should have a normal or low

intravascular volume. Water deficits resulting from the patient's NPO status are not replaced. Maintenance crystalloid is given, and colloid is infused to replace blood loss.

3. If the brain is particularly edematous, diuretics such as furosemide and mannitol may be necessary.

4. Lumbar CSF drainage is frequently utilized to obtain good operating conditions. The drain is opened slowly after consultation with the surgeon, usually as the dura is incised.

5. Following the placement of the aneurysm clip, volume expansion to offer prophylaxis against cerebral vasospasm may be initiated.

H. Ventilation

Particularly in the case of early (within 72 hours) surgery following an SAH, arterial $PaCO_2$ is maintained between 30 and 35 mmHg to facilitate operative conditions. Concern regarding the aggravation of cerebral ischemia by hypocarbia, particularly when induced hypotension is employed, may necessitate maintenance of $PaCO_2$ at more normal levels. Some centers employ EEG or somatosensory evoked potential (SSEP) monitoring to detect ischemia.

I. Induced Hypotension

1. As the surgeons approach the aneurysm, many anesthesiologists induce hypotension. Nitroprusside is the most frequently used agent.

2. As the dura is opened, the infusion of sodium nitroprusside is begun very slowly with incremental increases of the drug to maintain the patient's MAP (measured at the level of the foramen magnum) at approximately 50 to 70 mmHg during surgical dissection. In patients with poorly controlled chronic hypertension, a higher MAP should be maintained.

3. When nitroprusside is used and there are no contraindications to β-blockers, 1 to 3 mg of intravenous propranolol may facilitate management by antagonizing the effects of nitroprusside-induced reflex tachycardia and renin release.

4. Sodium nitroprusside should be administered with a calibrated pump, and blood gases should be checked frequently, not only to assess the development of a metabolic acidosis, but also to detect changes in arterial oxygenation secondary to the

induced hypotension and inhibition of the hypoxic pulmonary vasoconstriction reflex.

5. Tachyphylaxis develops with the use of sodium nitroprusside. To minimize cyanide and thiocyanate toxicity, the nitroprusside infusion rate should not exceed 8.0 µg/kg per minute.

6. Induced hypotension can also be produced by labetalol or esmolol in conjunction with potent inhalational agents or by these inhalational agents alone.

7. Intraoperative aneurysm rupture
   If an aneurysm ruptures intraoperatively, induced hypotension must be maintained, and occasionally made more profound, during efforts to replace lost blood volume. On occasion, carotid compression will be necessary to control bleeding.

J. Emergence from Anesthesia
After the surgical clip ligation of the aneurysm, the patient's blood pressure is allowed to return to preinduction levels while the aneurysm is observed for bleeding under the surgical microscope. At the end of the case, smooth extubation is the goal following the application of the head dressing and the removal of the patient from the pin head holder. The use of 0.5 to 1.0 mg/kg of lidocaine intravenously can decrease coughing in this situation. For patients who preoperatively are Grade III or worse, postoperative ventilation may be employed until neurologic status improves.

V. POSTOPERATIVE CARE
Blood pressure monitoring is continued in transit to the postanesthesia care unit (PACU) or ICU. The level of consciousness is assessed frequently. Intravascular volume expansion is usually continued in the early postoperative course utilizing the CVP or the pulmonary artery occlusion pressure as a guide. For patients with persistent vasospasm despite optimizing preload, cerebral perfusion pressure may be increased using vasoconstrictors or positive inotropic agents.

VI. SUMMARY OF ANESTHETIC CONSIDERATIONS
Patients with unruptured cerebral aneurysms or ruptured aneurysms with subarachnoid hemorrhage must have their blood pressure strictly controlled. Large increases in blood pressure can cause rupture or rebleeding. Antihypertensive agents, frequently beta-blockers or calcium channel antagonists are used. Also, sedation with benzodiazepines and bar-

biturates is used to reduce anxiety and agitation that can stimulate the sympathetic system. It is important to continue these medications up to the time of surgery. Additional sedation should be given for preoperative anxiety or invasive monitor placement.

Patients who rebleed and have cerebral vasospasm rarely need sedatives, and often, to maintain cerebral perfusion, the patient will be receiving large volumes of fluid or inotropic agents, which should be continued until the time of induction.

Drugs used for induction should be titrated to avoid any change in blood pressure. Extra boluses of intravenous induction agents such as thiopental plus intravenous lidocaine just prior to laryngoscopy will minimize the hypertensive response to intubation. One of the goals of maintenance anesthesia is to produce good brain relaxation and hemodynamic stability. A nitrous oxide–narcotic base with isoflurane up to one MAC is often used. As the aneurysm is approached, surgeons may request hypotensive anesthesia. This can be accomplished with titrating isoflurane, nitroprusside, or a sympathetic blocking agent alone or in combination. Intraoperative monitoring must include arterial catheterization and a CVP catheter. If vasoconstrictor drugs are used, or if there is underlying cardiac disease, pulmonary artery catheterization is usually indicated.

The goal of postoperative care is to prevent vasospasm with vasodilators and sedatives. Patients may develop persistent vasospasm despite vasodilators and optimized preload, in which case cerebral perfusion pressure may be increased with vasoconstrictors or positive inotropic agents.

Arteriovenous Malformations

I.   INCIDENCE AND PRESENTATION
   A.   Tortuous cerebral arteries emptying directly into cerebral veins without normal intervening capillaries are termed "arteriovenous malformations" (AVMs).
   B.   In more than 50% of cases, hemorrhage is the first sign of the nearly 2000 AVMs identified each year. Seizures are a frequent manifestation, occurring in approximately 33% of patients, while another 10% have a combination of intermittent hemorrhage and seizures. Rarely, an AVM produces a "steal syndrome" by diverting a large fraction of the cerebral blood flow through the lesion and render-

ing the rest of the ipsilateral hemisphere ischemic. Occasionally, a large AVM precipitates high-output cardiac failure because of the high flow through it. The peak incidence of bleeding occurs between the ages of 15 and 20.

C. In general, because surgical mortality and morbidity rates are low for small (less than 3-cm) AVMs, surgery is indicated because the average rate for spontaneous bleeding is 2% to 3% per year. When an AVM is large or inaccessible, arterial embolization may be attempted as preliminary or, in some cases, definitive therapy.

II. ANESTHETIC MANAGEMENT

A. Goals

Because the operation on an AVM may be lengthy and tedious, the anesthesiologist must maintain optimal brain conditions for long periods of time and safeguard the patient from injury secondary to improper positioning as well as from hemodynamic instability attributable to large blood losses.

B. Preoperative Preparation

1. Each patient with an AVM must have a complete cerebral angiogram that clearly defines the feeding arteries and the draining vein(s).

2. In addition to noting signs of focal weakness or spasticity, the anesthesiologist should discuss the intraoperative use of blood products, as well as the anticipated length of the operation, with the patient and patient's family to allay anxiety.

3. As most surgery for AVMs is done on an elective basis, premedication with 5 to 10 mg diazepam orally as well as the maintenance of anticonvulsant medications is appropriate.

C. Monitors

Monitors are much the same as those for cerebral aneurysm operations, including an arterial catheter, one or two large-bore peripheral IVs, as well as a CVP pressure monitor. A Foley catheter is placed after induction.

D. Induction

1. Because as many as 7% of patients with AVMs have coexisting cerebral aneurysms, the induction sequence should avoid wide fluctuations in blood pressure.

2. Small doses (50–100 μg) of fentanyl while monitoring lines are being secured, followed by a thiopental induction (3–4 mg/kg) and the use of vecuronium or the combination of metocurine and pancuronium, result in hemodynamic stability during induction.

3. Additional increments of fentanyl and lidocaine, with or without a potent inhalational agent, will blunt the autonomic response to endotracheal intubation.

E. Maintenance Anesthesia

1. Fentanyl and N_2O supplemented by isoflurane maintain intraoperative hemodynamic stability. As these cases may extend for several hours, additional increments of fentanyl usually are required.

2. If the patient does not manifest signs of an intracerebral steal, hyperventilation to a $PaCO_2$ of 28 to 32 mmHg (which could further reduce flow to a poorly perfused brain), as well as diuresis with furosemide or mannitol, will promote brain relaxation.

F. Fluid Management

Maintenance fluids (normal saline solution) without glucose are administered during surgery. Blood loss, frequently considerable, is often replaced initially with 5% albumin. When blood loss exceeds 15% of the patient's estimated volume, replacement with blood products is initiated.

G. Induced Hypotension

1. Deliberate hypotension, induced to a MAP of approximately 50 to 70 mmHg, aids the surgical dissection and helps control bleeding. Isoflurane, nitroglycerin, and nitroprusside are suitable agents to induce and maintain deliberate hypotension, while the addition of beta-blockers attenuates the tachycardia that often accompanies the use of these agents. Labetalol and isoflurane is a useful combination.

2. Rarely, especially during surgery on large AVMs, cerebral circulatory "breakthrough" occurs. Shortly after dissection begins, the adjacent cortex begins to swell while the surface arteries dilate. Profound hypotension is required to facilitate hemostasis, and the patient may require prolonged ventilation and maneuvers to decrease the ICP for days postoperatively.

H. Intraoperative Angiography

1. Because postoperative hemorrhage from a residual AVM is the most feared surgical complication, occa-

sionally, an intraoperative arteriogram is performed. The anesthesiologist must be alert to the possibility of a reaction to contrast medium, as well as to the potent osmotic diuretic effect of these agents.

2. In cases where intraoperative arteriography is not performed to exclude residual AVM, induced hypertension (usually with a phenylephrine infusion) may demonstrate subtle hemorrhage to the surgical team.

I. Emergence from Anesthesia

1. After complete resection of the AVM, inhalation agents are gradually reduced to a low level. If hypertension develops, labetalol is administered in 5- to 10-mg increments per bolus.

2. Once the pin head holder has been removed, muscle relaxants are reversed, N_2O is removed, and the patient is extubated when responsive. All monitoring is continued during transportation to the PACU or ICU.

III. POSTOPERATIVE CARE

A. On occasion, removal of the AVM causes sudden transmission of high arterial pressures to the brain surrounding the resected lesion. This abrupt increase in perfusion may result in severe cerebral edema or hemorrhage secondary to the loss of autoregulation. Should this problem become apparent, it is best to leave the patient intubated and ventilated to control the $PaCO_2$ and to facilitate barbiturate loading.

B. Many centers maintain moderate hypotension in the initial postoperative period with head elevation, diuretics, or antihypertensive agents.

IV. SUMMARY OF ANESTHETIC CONSIDERATIONS

Maintaining tight control of perioperative blood pressure is important in the management of patients with AVM. The medications used for induction and maintenance anesthesia are similar to those used during cerebral aneurysm anesthesia. Profuse bleeding is associated with this surgical procedure, and hypotensive anesthesia is helpful in decreasing blood loss. Profound hypotensive anesthesia is needed to facilitate hemostasis if cerebral circulatory breakthrough occurs. Maintenance of mild hypotension postoperatively will help decrease bleeding. Hyperventilation, diuretics, and barbiturate loading may be necessary if severe cerebral edema or hemorrhage develops postoperatively.

Hypertensive Intracerebral Hematoma

I.   INCIDENCE AND PRESENTATION

   A.   Over the past decade in the US, the incidence of stroke secondary to occlusive cerebrovascular disease has declined, whereas the incidence of spontaneous hypertensive intracerebral hemorrhage has remained relatively stable. In those cases where the hemorrhage extends into the ventricular system, the mortality rate can approach 70%.

   B.   Seventy to ninety per cent of all spontaneous brain hemorrhages are associated with hypertension. Hypertensive brain hemorrhages tend to occur in specific sites: putamen, thalamus, cerebellum, and pons. Lobar hemorrhages may be related to hypertension but can also occur in association with normal blood pressure and without radiographic evidence of a specified etiologic factor. The most common sources of bleeding in hypertensive hemorrhages are the small penetrating arteries at the base of the brain and the paramedium branches of the basal arteries.

   C.   The advent of CT has markedly improved the management of these lesions by localizing the hemorrhage, providing clues to the etiology, and quantitating edema in adjacent brain tissue. However, the proper roles for both medical and surgical therapy for patients with these lesions are still being defined.

   D.   In general, surgical removal of the hematoma is indicated in lobar, putamen, and cerebellar hemorrhages when the patient is deteriorating in spite of vigorous medical therapy. Under experimental conditions, secondary brain-tissue edema, hemorrhage, and necrosis can be minimized by rapid hematoma evacuation.

II.   PERIOPERATIVE MANAGEMENT

   A.   Evaluation

   1.   A CT scan is indicated in any patient suspected of having a brain hemorrhage. Frequently, anesthesia personnel will be called on to sedate or monitor these patients so that the diagnostic study can be obtained. Anesthetic management should reflect concern for the potential of increased ICP.

   2.   Intubation may be necessary for the stuporous or comatose patient, utilizing a modified rapid-sequence technique with cricoid pressure, a large dose of a nondepolarizing muscle relaxant, thiopental, and intravenous lidocaine to control ICP.

3. Maintenance anesthesia for the study can be provided with low-dose isoflurane, and small doses of intravenous narcotics. Ventilation should be controlled to reduce $PaCO_2$ moderately (range 28–32 mmHg), and mannitol and furosemide may be necessary in attempts to decrease ICP. An ICP monitor is most helpful to guide therapy.

B. Maintenance of Cerebral Perfusion Pressure
Recalling that cerebral perfusion pressure (CPP) equals MAP minus ICP, vigorous attempts to lower MAP may, if ICP remains elevated, reduce CPP and produce secondary ischemic damage. To titrate blood pressure, trimethaphan may be preferable to sodium nitroprusside in the situation where ICP is increased, because, as a ganglionic blocking agent, it causes no direct cerebrovascular dilation or reflex tachycardia. The disadvantages to the use of this drug include prolonged pupillary dilation and gastrointestinal ileus. Sympathetic blocking agents, such as labetalol or esmolol, are very helpful in these situations and do not have the disadvantages of trimethaphan.

III. ANESTHETIC MANAGEMENT

A. Goals
In providing perioperative care to the patient with an intracerebral hematoma, the anesthesiologist should maintain or improve the patient's hemodynamic status while providing optimal operating conditions for the neurosurgeons. The adequacy of the CPP must be maintained and, if possible, monitored electrophysiologically to prevent secondary ischemic damage.

B. Preoperative Preparation

1. During review of the patient's chart, the anesthesiologist should note the range of preoperative blood pressure, the use of antihypertensive therapy, and the range of ICP if this has been monitored.

2. Adequate intraoperative hemostasis is a frequent problem. Coagulation studies and the availability of blood should therefore be noted.

3. Many of these patients are elderly and have concurrent medical problems, especially of the cardiovascular system, which will influence the selection of anesthetic agents.

    4. All patients are provided with prophylactic anticonvulsant coverage.

C. Monitors

    1. An arterial catheter is essential for this procedure, and CVP monitoring may be very helpful in managing fluid therapy. Concomitant cardiovascular disease may indicate pulmonary artery catheterization.

    2. If intraoperative EEG or SSEP monitoring is available, the adequacy of CPP can be better assessed.

D. Induction

    1. If a patient is to be transported from the ICU already intubated and hyperventilated, hyperventilation should be continued and adequate sedation provided to prevent any marked increases in blood pressure.

    2. If the patient is stuporous on arrival in the operating room but not intubated, a carefully orchestrated anesthesia induction following the placement of monitors is indicated.

        a. After preoxygenation, a dose of thiopental (2–4 mg/kg) is followed by a nondepolarizing muscle relaxant such as vecuronium or atracurium given in a dose of 1.5 to 2.0 times the usual intubating dose to decrease onset time.

        b. The patient is ventilated while cricoid pressure is applied to decrease the possibility of aspiration.

        c. Intravenous lidocaine or a bolus of narcotic is given before endotracheal intubation. A peripheral nerve stimulator should demonstrate profound muscle relaxation to help decrease the sympathetic response to intubation.

E. Maintenance Techniques

General anesthesia is maintained utilizing narcotics such as fentanyl with the addition of N_2O and isoflurane. Modest hyperventilation to a $PaCO_2$ of approximately 30 mmHg may help to improve disordered autoregulation.

F. Fluid Management

Glucose-free fluids (increased plasma glucose can potentiate cerebral injury during ischemia) are provided in volumes sufficient to ensure adequate renal perfusion. Blood transfusion may be required for anemia, or fresh frozen plasma or platelets may be necessary to reverse previous anticoagulant or antiplatelet therapy.

G. Emergence from Anesthesia
In general, it is prudent to continue mechanical hyperventilation into the postoperative period. Careful titration of blood pressure can be achieved more easily if the patient remains sedated and intubated. Postoperative cerebral swelling can be detected by ICP monitoring. Patients must be transferred from the operating room to the ICU with adequate monitoring and ventilation, and appropriate vasoactive drugs should be utilized as needed.

IV. POSTOPERATIVE CARE
Postoperatively, the ICP is frequently monitored. Patients should be observed carefully to detect the syndrome of inappropriate antidiuretic hormone secretion as well as hydrocephalus, both of which occasionally occur postoperatively.

V. SUMMARY OF ANESTHETIC CONSIDERATIONS
Patients with hypertensive intracerebral bleeding that requires drainage are usually stuporous and should not require any preoperative sedation. Many are already intubated and mildly hyperventilated to decrease the ICP. Hyperventilation should continue during transport and intraoperatively. Invasive blood pressure and CVP monitoring is important, as it is for all intracranial operations. Induction and maintenance anesthesia should be aimed at maintaining cerebral perfusion pressure and limiting fluctuations in blood pressure. Postoperative hyperventilation is often necessary. This is most easily achieved by leaving the patient intubated and sedated.

Carotid Artery Disease

I. INCIDENCE AND PRESENTATION
A. Despite declining stroke rates in recent years, symptomatic ischemic cerebrovascular disease continues to be a significant source of morbidity and death in the US. In 1982, 82,000 procedures on carotid arteries were performed in an effort to decrease the incidence of stroke in a large population at risk.
B. Currently, the least controversial indications for carotid endarterectomy are:
1. The presence of transient ischemic attacks (TIAs),

neurologic dysfunctions lasting only a few minutes or, rarely, a few hours.

2. Prolonged reversible ischemic neurologic deficits (PRINDs), neurologic dysfunctions generally persisting for more than 24 hours but resolving completely within a few days).

3. Angiographically demonstrated stenosis or ulceration in the compatible intracranial artery.

II. TREATMENT

A. Medical Therapy

1. In 1965, Millikan proposed that most TIAs were embolic in origin. Many neurologists believe that antiplatelet drugs or anticoagulants, when administered to carefully selected TIA patients under close supervision, reduce the incidence of stroke. The Canadian Cooperative Study Group (1978) demonstrated that aspirin alone and aspirin combined with sulfinpyrazone reduces the number of TIAs and strokes in men by almost one-half. Interestingly, the incidence of TIAs and strokes in women was not affected by these drugs.

2. Aspirin inhibits platelet cyclooxygenase, the enzyme that initiates the metabolism of arachidonic acid to thromboxane A_2 and other prostaglandins, whereas sulfinpyrazone appears to work through inhibition of many platelet functions and decreases the production of thromboxane A_2.

B. Indications for Operative Management

1. The goal of carotid endarterectomy is to increase blood flow through stenotic vessels and to reduce the risk of embolization from ulcerated plaques. This operation is usually offered to a patient who has had TIAs and who remains neurologically normal or has a mild, stable neurologic deficit.

2. Other indications, such as the presence of hemodynamically significant, asymptomatic carotid stenosis or asymptomatic atheromatous plaques, are less clear. The management of patients with asymptomatic carotid bruits is controversial. Approximately 5% of the population over age 50 has an asymptomatic carotid bruit, and two large studies have shown that there is an increased incidence of stroke in patients with bruits. However, there is no significant correlation between the stroke and the

location of the bruit, and there is no clear evidence that prophylactic carotid endarterectomy prevents strokes in these patients.

III. ANESTHETIC MANAGEMENT

    A. Goals

Freedom from pain for the patient, a quiet operative field for the surgeon, and maintenance of stable cardiovascular features are all important anesthetic goals during carotid endarterectomy. In addition, intraoperative monitoring of some measure of neurologic function may facilitate early detection and treatment of neurologic deterioration.

    B. Preoperative Preparation

        1. More than 50% of the patients entering the hospital for carotid endarterectomy will be hypertensive. Other frequent problems that may require special attention from the anesthesiologist are diabetes, generalized atherosclerosis, and coronary artery disease. Myocardial infarction is the leading single cause of early postoperative death. After the initial cardiovascular evaluation of the patient, cardiac catheterization and angiography may be indicated, as 30% to 50% of patients undergoing carotid endarterectomy have angiographic evidence of significant coronary disease.

        2. In addition to cardiovascular workup and treatment, preoperative assessment should emphasize neurologic assessment. Residual deficits from a previous cerebrovascular accident can influence the choice of muscle relaxant, and patients with prior cortical injury may be extremely sensitive to sedatives. The patient is at risk both during and after surgery for the appearance of new neurologic deficits, which may be recognizable only in comparison with the preoperative findings.

        3. Renal insufficiency is also an important finding, as the nephrotoxic effects of angiographic contrast medium may further compromise renal function.

        4. A reassuring preoperative interview, providing necessary information, can greatly allay patient anxiety. Generally, if the procedure is to be performed under regional anesthesia, no premedication is given, as these drugs might interfere with intraoperative neurologic assessment. Patients are reassured that they will be comfortable and monitored continually throughout the procedure.

C. Anesthetic Techniques

    1. Regional anesthesia

        a. Advantages to the utilization of regional anesthesia for carotid endarterectomy include the fact that higher integrative function can be assessed on a moment-to-moment basis just by speaking with the patient. Optimal provision of regional anesthesia requires careful cooperation of both the surgical and anesthetic teams. The patient must remain quietly supine for approximately 2 to 3 hours, and rapport is the best means of establishing patient cooperation. In experienced hands (on the part of both the anesthesia and surgical teams), regional anesthesia is remarkably effective.

        b. A superficial cervical plexus block is performed utilizing approximately 30 ml of 0.5% bupivacaine instilled primarily at the midpoint of the sternomastoid muscle. With this block, supplementation by the surgeon with additional local anesthetic is generally necessary when the carotid artery sheath is approached.

        c. Shortly before the carotid artery is cross-clamped, an infusion of 0.004% phenylephrine is initiated to increase the directly recorded blood pressure to approximately 20% above the mean blood pressure recorded on the patient's chart. While monitoring the patient's verbal responses, a V_5 lead on the EKG is scrutinized to detect ST depression. Heparin, 5000 units, is administered intravenously, and a test cross-clamping of the carotid artery is performed. The patient is instructed to go through a series of maneuvers designed to detect small differences in neurologic status. If no problems are discovered, the operation proceeds.

        d. Should the patient suffer acute neurologic deterioration with the test cross-clamping, the blood pressure is further elevated; if symptoms persist, the procedure is aborted. General anesthesia is then provided for surgery employing a prophylactic shunt.

    e. Monitoring of the patient's blood pressure via the arterial catheter is maintained throughout the postoperative period, including the transfer from operating room to PACU. Hypotension occurs commonly in patients who have undergone carotid endarterectomy under regional anesthesia; many patients require a phenylephrine infusion in the immediate postoperative period to maintain the systolic blood pressure at preoperative levels.

2. General anesthesia

    a. Ideally, when a carotid endarterectomy is performed under general anesthesia, an electrophysiologic monitor of cerebral function is employed to gauge the adequacy of cerebral blood flow.

    b. In addition to an ECG with V_5 and lead II and other standard monitors, an arterial line is utilized.

    c. In view of the large number of patients with coexistent coronary artery disease, the aim of a general anesthetic for carotid endarterectomy is to avoid myocardial ischemia while assuring adequate CPP.

    d. Doses of thiopental in the range of 2 to 3 mg/kg, followed by a short-acting nondepolarizing muscle relaxant such as vecuronium, are utilized for induction. Small doses (1–2 μg/kg) of fentanyl titrated to a total dose of 5 to 10 μg/kg and lidocaine given intravenously (1 mg/kg) shortly before intubation help prevent large fluctuations in blood pressure.

    e. Nitrous oxide may be added for the maintenance of anesthesia. Despite concerns about "coronary steal," isoflurane is the potent inhalational agent of choice for carotid surgery because, with this agent, the lowest values for regional cerebral blood flow (rCBF) are tolerated without EEG changes indicative of ischemia.

    f. The use of thiopental, via either continuous infusion or bolus at the time of cross-clamping, may be considered. The agent's theoretical value in terms of cerebral protection must be balanced against the loss of EEG as a monitor (at burst suppression doses), myocardial depression, and probable prolonged anesthetic emergence.

g. Because of the possibility that hypercarbia will generate intracerebral steals and hypocarbia will decrease CBF, normocarbia ($PaCO_2$ 35–40 mmHg) is maintained throughout the procedure. Systemic arterial blood pressure is raised, via the addition of a phenylephrine infusion, to approximately 20% over the patient's baseline during carotid cross-clamping. The V_5 lead on the EKG is monitored continuously for signs of myocardial ischemia. An infusion of nitroglycerin is begun if ST–T-wave depression is noted.

h. Smooth extubation is accomplished through adequate reversal of muscle relaxants, the occasional use of intravenous lidocaine to prevent coughing, and careful control of blood pressure. The patient's neurologic status is assessed rapidly in the operating room at the conclusion of surgery. Monitoring is maintained during transport to the PACU.

IV. POSTOPERATIVE CARE

Postoperatively, patients are monitored carefully for any deterioration of neurologic status. In addition, systemic hemodynamics are carefully controlled so that hypertension, a significant source of morbidity following general anesthesia, is treated quickly. Excessive bleeding within the surgical site can rapidly compromise the airway and necessitate reexploration of the wound. If so, fiberoptic intubation may be necessary. Hypotension, which may contribute to carotid thrombosis or to cerebral hypoperfusion, must likewise be avoided in the postoperative setting.

V. SUMMARY OF ANESTHETIC CONSIDERATIONS

Prior to carotid endarterectomy, all patients should have a thorough evaluation of their cardiovascular system, with therapy initiated if necessary. As many as 50% have significant coronary artery disease.

Regional anesthesia can be successful for carotid endarterectomies. Communicating with the patient and having simple maneuvers performed is the most sensitive method of detecting changes in neurologic status. More commonly, patients receive general anesthesia for this procedure. In addition to the usual monitors, including arterial catheterization, an electrophysiologic monitor is useful to gauge the adequacy of cerebral blood flow. Maintaining normal $PaCO_2$ is important, because hypercarbia or hypocarbia can decrease regional blood flow. Hemodynamic stability is very important in this case, as hypotension may decrease cerebral blood flow and cause myocardial ischemia. Anesthesia with the least myocardial-depressant and vasodilating effects should be used.

Postoperatively, wide swings in blood pressure are seen. Both extremes must be corrected immediately. Any significant deterioration in neurologic status may indicate carotid occlusion and need for immediate exploration of the surgical site. Close observation of the patient's respiratory status is necessary. Rapid bleeding within the surgical site can quickly compromise the airway.

Recommended Reading

Allen GS, Ahn HS, Preziosi TJ, et al. Cerebral arterial spasm: a controlled trial of nimodipine in patients with subarachnoid hemorrhage. N Engl J Med 1983;308:619.

Asiddao CB, Donegan JH, Whitesell RC, et al. Factors associated with perioperative complications during carotid endarterectomy. Anesth Analg 1982;61:631.

Day AL, Friedman WA, Sypert GW, et al. Successful treatment of the normal perfusion pressure breakthrough syndrome. Neurosurgery 1982;11:625.

Gamache FW, Patterson RH. Surgical management of cranial arteriovenous malformations. In: Schmidek HH, Sweet WH, eds. Operative neurosurgical techniques. 2nd ed. Orlando: Grune & Stratton, 1988;905.

Grundy BL, Heros R. Ischemic cerebrovascular disease. In: Matjasko J, Katz J, eds. Clinical controversies in neuroanesthesia and neurosurgery. Orlando: Grune & Stratton, 1986:1.

Hunt WE, Hess RM. Surgical risk as related to time of intervention in the repair of intracranial aneurysms. J Neurosurg 1968;28:14.

Kassell NF, Drake LG. Timing of aneurysm surgery. Neurosurgery 1982;10:514.

Kassell NF, Peerless SJ, Durward QJ, et al. Treatment of ischemic deficits from vasospasm with intravascular volume expansion and induced arterial hypertension. Neurosurgery 1982;11:337.

Messick TM, Casement B, Sharborough FW, Milde LN, Michenfelder

JD, Sundt TM. Correlation of regional cerebral blood flow (rCBF) with EEG changes during isoflurane anesthesia for carotid endarterectomy: critical rCBF. Anesthesiology 1987; 66:344.

Millikan CH. The pathogenesis of transient focal cerebral ischemia. Circulation 1965;32:438.

Newberg LA, Michenfelder TD. Cerebral protection by isoflurane during hypoxemia or ischemia. Anesthesiology 1983;59:29.

Ojemann RG, Heros RC. Spontaneous brain hemorrhage. Stroke 1983;14:468.

Peerless SJ. Pre- and postoperative management of cerebral aneurysms. Clin Neurosurg 1979;26:209.

Vermeulen M, Lindsay KW, Murray GD, et al. Anti-fibrinolytic treatment in subarachnoid hemorrhage. N Engl J Med 1984;311:432.

≡ Increased Intracranial Pressure and Space-Occupying Lesions

Patricia H. Petrozza
Donald S. Prough

Intracranial Pressure Control

I.   CEREBRAL PHYSIOLOGY AND METABOLISM
   A.   Anatomy
        The bony, rigid cranium contains three separate components: brain tissue and water (80%), blood (12%), and cerebrospinal fluid (CSF) (8%). Changes in cerebral blood volume can rapidly change the intracranial pressure (ICP).
   B.   Factors Affecting Cerebral Blood Flow
        1. $PaCO_2$
             For each 1 mmHg that the $PaCO_2$ increases or decreases, cerebral blood flow (CBF) increases or decreases by about 4%, respectively. The response of cerebral blood vessels to CO_2 is mediated by alterations in hydrogen ion concentration in CSF and brain extracellular fluid, as CO_2 diffuses freely across the blood–brain barrier.

2. PaO_2

As PaO_2 declines to less than 50 mmHg, the CBF increases rapidly. As PaO_2 increases within the clinical range from 50 to over 300 mmHg, the CBF declines slightly.

3. Cerebral metabolism

In general, an increase in cerebral oxygen metabolism ($CMRO_2$) is closely paralleled by an increase in CBF. The nature of this coupling mechanism is not well understood, but local release of adenosine or membrane fluxes of sodium, potassium, and calcium may be involved. Seizures, as well as pain, anxiety, and fever, cause large increases in $CMRO_2$ and CBF.

4. Autoregulation

The cerebral vasculature can alter its resistance to flow so that the CBF is maintained at a constant level (45–50 ml/100 g of brain per min) over a wide range of cerebral perfusion pressure (CPP). The autoregulatory response is not immediate, taking up to 2 minutes before the response of cerebrovascular resistance to a change in perfusion pressure is complete. Autoregulation may function through an intrinsic (myogenic) response of vascular smooth muscle to the distention or relaxation caused by differences in intraluminal pressure.

5. Temperature

Within a 5° to 7°C range of 37°C, $CMRO_2$ declines as body temperature is reduced. The $CMRO_2$ and CBF are reduced approximately 7% per degree Celsius of temperature change.

6. Blood rheology

Increases in cerebrovascular resistance secondary to increased blood viscosity reduce CBF. In polycythemia vera, the CBF can decline to half normal values. In contrast, in severe anemia, a decrease in blood viscosity may not be the sole factor responsible for an increase in CBF. Rather, this compensatory increase in CBF may be attributable to the reduced oxygen-carrying capacity of the blood. Isovolemic hemodilution elevates CBF in humans.

7. Anesthetic agents

   a. Anesthetic drugs alter $CMRO_2$ and cerebrovascular resistance. The inhalational anesthetics (halothane, enflurane, isoflurane, and N_2O) cause uncoupling of blood flow (increase) and metabolism (decrease).

    b.   Nitrous oxide and isoflurane cause the least increase in CBF, whereas halothane at 1 MAC concentration causes an increase of 190%. Hyperventilation initiated prior to the introduction of the volatile anesthetics may blunt increases in the CBF.

    c.   The effects of anesthetic agents on CSF production and reabsorption have been described recently. Enflurane increases the rate of production and increases the resistance to reabsorption. Isoflurane and fentanyl, in contrast, do not change the production of CSF but do lower the resistance to its absorption, factors that may be important in lengthy operations.

    d.   With the exception of ketamine, which increases both CBF and $CMRO_2$, intravenous agents, including the ultra-short-acting barbiturates, the narcotics, and the benzodiazepines, decrease CBF and $CMRO_2$. Thiopental, in high but clinically applicable doses, can eliminate brain electrical activity, reducing both $CMRO_2$ and CBF to approximately half of normal.

II.   INCREASED INTRACRANIAL PRESSURE

    A.   Pressure–Volume Response

        1.   The initial compensation for an intracranial mass (tumor, blood clot) involves the translocation of the CSF into the distensible spinal subarachnoid space. Increased CSF reabsorption may also occur. Decreasing cerebral blood flow further compensates for increasing ICP.

        2.   Eventually, however, these mechanisms are exhausted, and small increases in intracranial volume will produce large increases in intracranial pressure (Fig. 5-1).

    B.   ICP Monitors

        1.   Monitors have the greatest utility in the care of patients with head injuries in the ICU setting. Their value in the operating room has been less well documented, although large increases in ICP have been

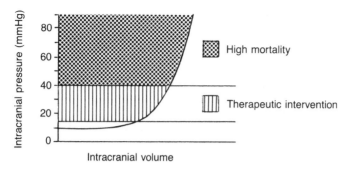

Figure 5-1 Intracranial pressure–volume curve.

detected during such maneuvers as endotracheal intubation and scalp incision.

2. The most commonly utilized monitors are an intraventricular catheter, a subarachnoid bolt, and an intraparenchymal fiberoptic pressure transducer. The ventriculostomy catheter permits the therapeutic withdrawal of CSF to control ICP, while the subarachnoid bolt and fiberoptic device reduce the danger of ventriculitis.

C. Causes of Increased ICP (IICP)

1. The ICP can be increased, not only by mass lesions such as traumatic intracranial hematomas or neoplasms, but by cerebral edema. Visible on CT scan as a decrease in brain density, cerebral edema is an accumulation of fluid within the brain parenchyma associated with the volumetric enlargement of brain tissue. It generally has been classified into three main types: interstitial (associated with hydrocephalus), vasogenic, and cytotoxic.

2. Vasogenic brain edema forms as a result of injury to the blood–brain barrier, permitting an increase in cerebrovascular permeability. This allows a protein-rich plasma filtrate to leak into the cerebral interstitial space. This type of edema surrounds neoplasms, hematomas, cerebral abscesses, and traumatized areas of the brain.

3. Cytotoxic edema, in contrast, is caused by an increase in water content, which is mainly intracellular, astrocytes being principally affected. This type of edema usually results from hypoxic injury. Fail-

ure of the intracellular ATP-dependent sodium pump, and consequent intracellular sodium accumulation accompanied by rapid increases in intracellular water, may account for the origin of this type of edema.

D. Control of IICP

    1. Mechanical measures

        a. Early endotracheal intubation with hyperventilation, as well as meticulous attention to oxygenation, are the easiest and most effective means of acutely controlling IICP. The ability of hyperventilation to effect cerebral vasoconstriction diminishes with time, but the avoidance of hypoxia and hypercapnia, as well as the careful control of blood pressure, remain important.

        b. Attention to the patient's head position (elevated 15 degrees and not rotated), preventing the endotracheal tube tape from constricting jugular venous drainage, and permitting sufficient expiratory time during mechanical ventilation are other important considerations in the care of the patient with IICP.

    2. Medications

    When adequate ventilation of the patient permits the reduction of $PaCO_2$ to approximately 25 mmHg and other simple mechanical maneuvers fail to reduce IICP to a normal range of about 15 mmHg, other therapy may be required.

        a. Diuretics

            1) Mannitol, in a 20% solution, is the generally preferred diuretic. As a hypertonic solution, it acts by the osmotic withdrawal of water from normal rather than edematous cerebral tissue. An initial intravenous dose of 0.5 g/kg of body weight administered over approximately 15 minutes is usually effective, although the large osmotic load may cause a transient increase in blood pressure and cerebral blood volume. Subsequent doses of approximately 0.25 g/kg may be employed to maintain the ICP at a lower level. When large doses of mannitol are necessary, serum osmolality should be followed closely. Enormous mannitol doses have caused acute renal failure.

2) The loop diuretics, furosemide and bumetanide acid, also reduce ICP. Furosemide decreases brain volume secondary to systemic diuresis and also decreases CSF production. It can be utilized either as the sole diuretic (1 mg/kg) or as an adjuvant to mannitol. Close attention must be paid to serum electrolytes, particularly potassium, when potent diuretics such as mannitol and furosemide are employed.

b. Corticosteroids

Although corticosteroids do not acutely reduce ICP, they exert a marked effect on vasogenic cerebral edema. Dexamethasone, in an initial dose of 8 to 10 mg followed by 4 mg every 6 hours, dramatically reduces edema around focal lesions such as glioblastomas and cerebral abscesses. Corticosteroids appear to provide little benefit in the management of closed head injury.

c. Barbiturates

In cases where IICP remains refractory to hyperventilation, diuretics, and steroids, barbiturate therapy is commonly employed. Barbiturates cause dose-dependent neuronal metabolic depression and reduced CBF and ICP. A commonly used regimen includes an initial IV dose of pentobarbital (3 to 5 mg/kg) followed by maintenance doses such that the serum level is maintained at approximately 30 to 40 μg/ml or such that burst suppression is produced on the EEG. Because barbiturate therapy causes considerable cardiovascular depression, a pulmonary artery catheter is frequently utilized to facilitate hemodynamic management.

3. Other measures

a. If medical management fails to control IICP, subtemporal decompression may increase the space available for the intracranial contents.

b. Careful nursing measures, such as the use of

small doses of thiopental (1.0–1.5 mg/kg) or lidocaine (1.5 mg/kg) prior to suctioning, as well as attention to the maintenance of muscle paralysis in a patient who might "buck" against the ventilator, help to control IICP.

Space-Occupying Lesions

I.   SUPRATENTORIAL TUMORS
    A. Etiology
       1. Metastatic tumors
          a. Metastatic tumors are the most common intracranial neoplasms; common primary sites are the lung, breast, kidney, and gastrointestinal tract.
          b. Surgical excision is offered to those patients with a relatively accessible solitary lesion. Metastatic lesions tend to be highly vascular and to cause extensive peritumoral edema.
       2. Primary intracranial tumors
          a. Common primary intracranial neoplasms arising from the cellular components of the brain are termed gliomas.
          b. Astrocytomas, a type of glioma, are the most common primary tumors found in the supratentorial compartment. They are generally well differentiated and slow growing, although they may undergo cystic degeneration. The malignant glioma is a rapidly growing tumor characterized by a brief clinical history with focal neurologic deficits and signs of IICP.
          c. Malignant gliomas, comprising almost 25% of all primary cerebral neoplasms, are frequently associated with a midline shift and CT evidence of cerebral edema.
          d. The benign, slowly growing meningioma arises from the dura mater. This tumor tends to compress but not invade cerebral tissue. Large abnormal feeding vessels arising from both intracranial and extracranial sources supply the tumors, which are often highly vascular. Meningiomas commonly arise in multiple sites, including the convexity of the cerebral hemi-

spheres, the falx tentorium, the base of the skull, and the sphenoid wing.

e. Several neoplasms arise in or around the ventricular system. Ependymomas are derived from cells lining the ventricular system, and papillomas arise from the choroid plexus. Frequently, these lesions present as obstructive hydrocephalus. Complete removal is often difficult because of the proximity to the hypothalamus or brainstem.

B. Perioperative Management

1. The preoperative visit to the patient scheduled for a supratentorial craniotomy should include an accurate assessment of the neurologic status. Particular attention should be paid to the presence of nausea, vomiting, focal neurologic deficits, decreased mental alertness, and faulty memory as clinical signs of IICP. A review of the CT scan is helpful in ascertaining the extent of the proposed resection, the presence of edema, and requirements for surgical positioning.

2. Because the use of preoperative corticosteroids reduces cerebral edema, many patients will be quite alert and may benefit from a conservative amount of preoperative sedation such as diazepam 0.1 mg/kg orally 1 hour before coming to the operating room to reduce anxiety and sympathetic stimulation without causing respiratory depression.

C. Anesthetic Management

1. Goals

Because the exact position of a particular patient on the pressure–volume compliance curve is unknown, it is wise to proceed with an anesthetic designed such that even small increases in intracranial volume are avoided.

2. Monitors

a. We recommended the judicious use of small amounts of narcotics to sedate patients while inserting monitoring devices such as arterial lines and CVP catheters.

b. A CVP line is particularly useful as a secure high-volume catheter and to measure intravascular volume for highly vascular tumors such as meningiomas.

    c.   Some centers use ICP monitors, placed while the patient is still awake, to monitor this important variable during induction and positioning.

    d.   A urinary catheter is inserted after induction, as is an esophageal stethoscope, temperature monitor, and oral gastric tube. A pulse oximeter, as well as a capnograph or mass spectrometer, is also utilized in each case.

3.   Induction

    a.   An effective induction sequence for patients with supratentorial tumors is oxygenation followed by thiopental, approximately 4 mg/kg IV. After the loss of the lid reflex and assurance that the patient can be ventilated manually with a face mask, a nondepolarizing muscle relaxant such as pancuronium or vecuronium (0.1 mg/kg) is administered.

    b.   As ventilation by mask is continued, incremental doses of thiopental and small amounts of fentanyl are administered. Intravenous lidocaine 1.5 mg/kg is administered approximately 1 minute before laryngoscopy, and any increases in blood pressure noted with laryngoscopy are treated promptly with additional thiopental.

4.   Maintenance techniques

Nitrous oxide, fentanyl, and isoflurane in a concentration less than 1 MAC usually provide satisfactory maintenance for a craniotomy. Depending on the anticipated length of the case, fentanyl in doses up to approximately 15 µg/kg may be utilized.

5.   Fluid management

Glucose-free fluids are administered, and the water deficit resulting from the previous night's fast is not replaced. Occasionally, furosemide, approximately 0.5 mg/kg, is added to promote diuresis. Normal saline solution is administered as maintenance fluid at the rate of 100 ml/hour once the dura has been opened, and blood loss of less than 15% of estimated volume is replaced with colloid solutions such as hetastarch or 5% albumin. Greater losses are replaced with blood.

6. Emergence from anesthesia

a. When dural closure begins, the concentration of inhalational agents is reduced. If hypertension occurs, labetalol, 5 to 10 mg IV, or other sympathetic blocking agent is effective in controlling blood pressure.

b. Once the patient is removed from the pin head holder, the muscle relaxants are reversed, but N_2O is maintained. When full muscle relaxant reversal has been demonstrated, the patient is placed on 100% oxygen, and spontaneous breathing is permitted to resume. Once spontaneous or prompted eye opening occurs with adequate spontaneous ventilation and oxygenation, the patient is extubated, given oxygen by face mask, connected to a portable arterial pressure monitor, and transported to the PACU or ICU.

D. Postoperative Care

Patients are monitored closely for changes in mental status that might reflect the accumulation of a subdural hematoma or bleeding into the tumor bed. Careful attention is paid to the maintenance of blood pressure within a normal range and to abnormalities in electrolytes or blood glucose that may have been precipitated by the intraoperative administration of diuretics and steroids.

II. INTRASELLAR TUMORS

A. Etiology

1. The pituitary gland is protected within the body of the sphenoid by the bony sella turcica. Although pituitary tumors are the most common abnormalities in the sellar region, many other processes may be found here as well. These include neoplasms such as craniopharyngiomas, meningiomas, and metastatic tumors and inflammatory lesions.

2. Abnormal endocrine function, visual loss, headache, or abnormal radiographic findings without apparent symptoms are all presentations of sellar lesions. Four endocrine syndromes relevant to pituitary tumors are well described.

a. The most common is prolactin hypersecretion, with a level of approximately 200 ng/ml generally accepted as indicating a prolactinoma. Galactorrhea/amenorrhea in women and a subtle loss of libido in men are the common presenting symptoms.

    b.   In adults, hypersecretion of growth hormone results in the syndrome of acromegaly. Cardiac disease, the most frequent cause of death in acromegaly, may be the result of hypertensive coronary artery disease or compensatory hypertrophy as a result of generalized somatomegaly.

    c.   Cushing's disease, the most serious of the pituitary–endocrine syndromes, has many clinical signs. Oversecretion of ACTH results in hypertension, diabetes, muscle weakness and atrophy, and changes in mental status.

    d.   Finally, patients with pituitary tumors may exhibit the syndrome of panhypopituitarism, where all pituitary hormones, as well as the hormones released secondary to stimulation by pituitary hormones, may be low.

B.   Perioperative Management

    1.   Most patients should have determinations of serum growth hormone, thyroid hormones, prolactin, and cortisol before surgery on the pituitary gland.

    2.   In addition, if a suprasellar mass is present on CT scan, the patient should undergo visual field testing.

    3.   An unusual presentation of a pituitary tumor is pituitary apoplexy, a condition in which hemorrhagic infarction of the gland stimulates the severe sudden headache and obtundation of a subarachnoid hemorrhage.

    4.   Severely hypothyroid patients should have several weeks of replacement therapy before surgery. Corticosteroid supplementation may be necessary in the perioperative period.

C.   Anesthetic Management

    1.   Goals

    Anesthetic management of a patient undergoing transsphenoidal removal of a pituitary lesion should include careful assessment of the patient's fluid and electrolyte status and an anesthetic plan that permits rapid recovery of consciousness to facilitate early postoperative evaluation of visual and motor function.

2. Preoperative preparation and monitors

    a. In the preoperative interview, it is important to assess the airway, particularly in those patients with Cushing's disease or acromegaly. Intubation is not a frequent problem in patients with acromegaly, although the anesthesiologist should be aware that certain patients may require fiberoptic intubation because of glottic stenosis resulting from soft-tissue overgrowth.

    b. An arterial catheter is useful for most transsphenoidal procedures. For those patients whose tumors extend into the cavernous sinus, appropriate monitoring for air embolism, such as the precordial Doppler, end-tidal CO_2 monitoring, and a central venous catheter placed at the superior vena cava–right atrial junction, are indicated.

3. Induction

The basic principles of neuroanesthesia described previously are employed for surgery involving the pituitary gland. Modest hyperventilation with the $PaCO_2$ approximately 28 to 32 mmHg generally is suitable. The anesthesiologist may be requested to perform a Valsalva maneuver or to increase the patient's $PaCO_2$ to permit visibility of the entire tumor within the sella.

4. Positioning

The anesthesiologist is usually positioned to the patient's left, necessitating added attention to the security of the inaccessible endotracheal tube and the use of extended breathing hoses. The patient is positioned on a padded head holder with the head mildly elevated and turned slightly.

In many centers, it is customary to pack the sella with fat taken from a separate abdominal incision after the removal of the tumor.

5. Maintenance technique

    a. An N_2O–narcotic technique is appropriate for this operation, as long as intracranial air studies have not been completed shortly before surgery. On occasion, a lumbar CSF drain is employed, and the anesthesiologist may be asked to inject air to outline the sella further. In this case, N_2O should be eliminated from the technique.

b.   Because the transsphenoidal approach to the sella is commonly employed, prophylactic antibiotics, usually penicillin, are administered. Hemostasis of the nasal mucosa is achieved through the use of cocaine and epinephrine. The neurosurgeon should notify the anesthesiologist when these vasoactive substances are employed.

6.   Fluid management
Diabetes insipidus sometimes develops intraoperatively after transsphenoidal resection of a pituitary tumor. Should it occur, hypotonic fluids should be administered and normovolemia maintained. If necessary, intravenous desmopressin will control diuresis without causing vasoconstriction.

7.   Emergence from anesthesia
After the resection of the pituitary tumor, the nose is carefully packed, and a large dressing is applied. Patients must be instructed to breathe only through the mouth; it is essential that patients be alert enough to maintain the airway and to allow a simple examination of the visual fields before extubation.

D.   Postoperative Care
Visual field examination should be performed shortly after surgery in order to detect hematoma formation early. Diabetes insipidus will usually appear during the first 12 to 24 hours after surgery but will gradually and spontaneously resolve. If the diagnosis is clear, desmopressin is commonly employed as a short-term agent.

III.   INFRATENTORIAL TUMORS
A.   Incidence and Presentation
1.   The structures in the posterior cranial fossa that lie below the tentorium are the pons, the medulla (brainstem), and the cerebellum. Primary tumors in this location occur more commonly in children, whereas adults frequently present with metastatic tumors and acoustic neuromas.

2.   Infratentorial tumors may obstruct the outflow of CSF; therefore, patients commonly present with headache and vomiting as well as other signs of IICP.

3.   Frequently, hydrocephalus develops, and pressure gradients may force the medulla and cerebellum

downward into the foramen magnum, causing compression and ischemia of the motor and sensory tracts. Rarely, upward herniation occurs when the vermis of the cerebellum is impacted in the posterior part of the tentorial notch.

B. Preoperative Management

Patients should be assessed preoperatively for the presence of cranial nerve dysfunction. Occasionally, a ventriculostomy or a ventriculoperitoneal shunt will be established to treat hydrocephalus and relieve IICP before general anesthesia is induced for tumor surgery.

C. Anesthetic Management

   1. Goal

The proximity of lesions and retractors to the brainstem in operations on the posterior fossa necessitates that anesthetic management be as precise as possible. Changes in blood pressure and pulse related to brainstem retraction or cranial nerve impingement can be detected if baseline hemodynamic status is extremely stable. In addition, the anesthesiologist should strive to provide an anesthetic that permits the rapid evaluation of patients postoperatively for the presence of adequate cranial nerve and brainstem function.

   2. Preoperative preparation

Anesthesiologists should be familiar with the CT findings and discuss intraoperative positioning with the surgeon. Basically, the infratentorium can be approached through three positions: prone, lateral, and sitting. Anesthesiologists should pay particular attention to the patient's cardiovascular and circulatory status when contemplating the sitting position.

   3. Monitors

      a. In addition to an arterial line, a central venous catheter is useful for operations on the posterior fossa, as the use of diuretics and hyperventilation make the patient's volume status difficult to quantitate.

      b. When the case is planned for the sitting position, an end-tidal CO_2 monitor (capnograph or mass spectrometer) and precordial Doppler, the most sensitive monitor of venous air embolism that is widely available, should be employed.

c. A central venous catheter with the tip positioned at the junction of the superior vena cava and right atrium, used to remove air embolism, is mandatory. Venous air embolism, reported most frequently during surgical procedures in the sitting position, may also occur in the prone and lateral positions.

4. Induction

The principles of neuroanesthesia previously discussed should be observed during the induction and careful attention paid to the patient's blood pressure, because hypovolemia from vomiting, a frequent problem in this group of patients, makes hypotension more likely with decreasing sympathetic tone.

5. Positioning

a. The sitting position offers many advantages to the surgeon in terms of operative exposure. The position is safe when carried out in centers familiar with its use, providing close attention is paid to the detection of air embolism and the avoidance of neurologic injury secondary to improper positioning.

b. The patient's head is placed in a pin head holder, and the patient is raised to the sitting position gradually while the blood pressure is monitored carefully. Excessive flexion of the neck on the sternum is avoided while care is taken that the tongue is protected within the mouth; otherwise, macroglossia may result from obstruction of the venous and lymphatic drainage. In addition, all extremities should be padded and elevated so that there is no stretch on the sciatic, ulnar, or brachial plexus nerves.

c. The lateral position offers wide exposure to the back of the head for resection of tumors in the cerebellopontine angle. A brachial plexus injury will be avoided if an axillary roll is utilized to prevent stretch on the dependent axilla. In addition, care must be taken to avoid an acute angle between the neck and dependent shoulder so that jugular compression does not produce cerebral venous distention.

d. The prone position is also utilized for surgery in the infratentorial area. The abdomen must be carefully supported so that diaphragmatic movement is not impeded and increased intra-abdominal pressure is not transmitted to the epidural veins.

6. Maintenance techniques

A technique combining narcotics, N_2O, and isoflurane is satisfactory for operations in the posterior fossa. An effort is made to establish a stable baseline with narcotics and isoflurane so that changes that occur because of surgical manipulation of the brainstem will be evident. The $PaCO_2$ should be maintained at approximately 28 to 32 mmHg using controlled ventilation.

7. Fluid management

Fluid management does not differ from that of surgery for supratentorial tumors, although the anesthesiologist must be aware of occult blood loss into the drapes, especially with operations performed in the sitting position.

8. Emergence from anesthesia

After posterior fossa procedures, it is imperative that the demonstration of a good gag reflex and adequate alertness by the patient be made before extubation. If there has been extensive manipulation of the brainstem, it may be wisest to ventilate the patient for a time postoperatively to avoid the consequences of cerebral edema or hemorrhage.

D. Postoperative Care

1. Pressure on the brainstem by edema or a hematoma may cause sudden deterioration a few hours postoperatively in patients who have apparently made a good recovery from anesthesia. Arterial hypertension, bradycardia, and respiratory irregularity necessitate immediate reintubation and re-exploration.

2. Staff should be alert to airway obstruction as well as obtunded laryngeal reflexes secondary to pressure on the 9th, 10th, or 12th nerves. On occasion, tension pneumocephalus has followed operations performed with the patient in the seated position.

IV. CHRONIC SUBDURAL HEMATOMA

A. Presentation

1. A subdural hematoma is an extracerebral collection of blood and serum, both clotted and liquid, that forms under the dura mater but does not extend into

the subarachnoid space or the basal cistern or other CSF systems. A chronic subdural hematoma is a collection of dark, liquified blood or serum of varying consistency that appears days or, more often, weeks after a head injury that is almost always minor and may not even be recollected.

2. Usually, chronic subdural hematomas occur at the extremes of life; in the aged and in the infant with cranial sutures that have not yet fused. Characteristically, there is fluctuating confusion, drowsiness, and mild hemiparesis; the ICP is usually only minimally elevated.

B. Intraoperative Management

1. Generally, hyperventilation is not employed during the anesthetic because shrinkage of the brain away from the bridging veins may cause tearing and so increase the accumulation of blood.

2. Large swings in blood pressure should be avoided, as the vasculature is fragile.

3. Attention must also be directed to the replacement of volume in patients who may be dehydrated because of poor intake over a long period of time.

4. After the hematoma has been evacuated through surgical bur holes, frequently the anesthesiologist will be asked to compress the jugular veins or to let the $PaCO_2$ rise to expand the brain parenchyma. If a large space is left when the dura is closed, bleeding may again occur and a clot reaccumulate.

C. Postoperative Management

1. Emergence from anesthesia should be smooth without coughing and bucking. Neurologic status should be evaluated as soon as possible after surgery.

2. Patients should be monitored carefully in the PACU for any change in mental status or increasing confusion, which might indicate reaccumulation of the hematoma.

V. BRAIN ABSCESS

A. Etiology

Brain abscesses arise most often from septic hematogenous emboli from distant infections, from adjacent sites of infection such as the paranasal sinuses and the middle ear, or as complications of intracranial surgery. In time, an abscess collection will become surrounded by a thick capsular wall, and the outer layer will begin to compress brain tissue. In addition, large amounts of edema often surround brain abscesses. A high index of suspicion is necessary for the presence of a brain abscess, for which the CT scan has become the single most valuable diagnostic tool.

B. Anesthetic Considerations

1. Preoperatively, because of the large amount of edema surrounding the abscess, steroids should be instituted as soon as possible after the initiation of antibiotics. In addition, prophylaxis with anticonvulsants is commonly employed.

2. Because of widespread use of antibiotics, brain abscesses occur infrequently. Excision remains the preferred method of therapy. Anesthetic considerations do not differ markedly from those for an intracranial tumor, with particular attention being paid to the possible origin of the infective foci.

3. Occasionally, after drainage of the abscess, patients demonstrate intractable cerebral edema, preventing the replacement of the bone flap. In these patients, postoperative ventilation and control of ICP will be necessary.

Summary of Anesthetic Considerations

Increased intracranial pressure may be associated with mass lesions and cerebral edema. Optimally, IICP should be controlled with hyperventilation, diuretics, barbiturates, or steroids prior to anesthesia. Patients with IICP usually have nausea, vomiting, lethargy, and focal neurologic deficits. Head CT will show decreased ventricular size, loss of cerebral sulci, and shift of midline structures. These patients must be hyperventilated before induction and given thiopental or other intravenous agents that will decrease cerebral blood and ICP for induction. Maintenance anesthesia with isoflurane will produce the least effect on cerebral blood flow. Halothane at 1 MAC can cause an increase in cerebral blood flow of 190%. Enflurane may increase ICP by increasing both cerebral blood flow and the rate of CSF production, as well as by inhibiting the absorption of CSF.

Treatment of IICP is facilitated by ICP monitoring. The intraventricular catheter is the only device that allows monitoring as well as therapeutic withdrawal of CSF.

All intracranial procedures must be monitored with an arterial catheter and a central venous catheter. These monitors are especially needed in patients who undergo tumor surgery in the sitting position. The CVP catheter can be used for assessing intravascular volume as well as for aspirating out air emboli. These patients should be monitored for air emboli with precordial Doppler and end-tidal CO_2.

It is especially important to maintain a very stable blood pressure and pulse rate during cerebellar and brainstem surgery to help differentiate the change in hemodynamics secondary to anesthesia or cardiovascular problems from that caused by brainstem manipulation.

The patient should be awake at the end of surgery. It is critical to be able to evaluate the patient's neurologic status postoperatively. Any deterioration in consciousness or development of focal neurologic deficit may indicate acute intracranial bleeding, increased cerebral edema, or ischemia, which would demand immediate treatment.

Recommended Reading

Artru AA. New concepts concerning anesthetic effects on intracranial dynamics: cerebrospinal fluid volume and cerebral blood volume. ASA Refresher Course Lecture 1987;133:1.

Hamill JF, Bedford RF, Weaver DC, et al. Lidocaine before endotracheal intubation: intravenous or laryngotracheal? Anesthesiology 1981;55:578.

Lanier WL, Stangland KJ, Scheithauer BW, et al. The effects of dextrose infusion and head position on neurologic outcome after complete cerebral ischemia in primates: examination of a model. Anesthesiology 1987;66:39.

Lassen NA. Cerebral and spinal cord blood flow. In: Cottrell JE, Turndorf H, eds. Anesthesia and neurosurgery. 2nd ed. St Louis: CV Mosby, 1986:1.

Oliver S, Cucchiara R. Comparison of outcome following posterior fossa craniectomy done in either a sitting or horizontal position. Anesthesiology 1986;65:A305.

Wright RL. Surgical management of intracranial and intraspinal infections. In: Schmidek HH, Sweet WH, eds. Operative neurosurgical techniques. 2nd ed. Orlando: Grune & Stratton, 1988:71.

≡ Head Trauma and Seizures

Patricia H. Petrozza
Donald S. Prough

Trauma

I. PRESENTATION

In a motor vehicle accident, head trauma is a common injury, either alone or in combination with other organ system trauma. Seventy-five per cent of the deaths following cranio-cerebral trauma related to car accidents occur within 48 hours. However, with rapid, intensive, and aggressive therapy, the mortality rate of patients with severe head injury (Glasgow coma score less than 8) has declined over the last 30 years.

II. ACUTE ASSESSMENT AND MANAGEMENT

   A. Airway Management

      Preoperative management of the patient with a head injury begins at the site of the accident, where emergency personnel must stabilize the neck and ensure that the patient's airway, ventilation, and oxygenation are maintained. Hypercarbia and hypoxemia have been associated with poor outcome of head injury, so adequate control of the airway by endotracheal intubation as soon as possible is recommended.

   B. Neurologic Assessment

      1. The Glasgow Coma Scale (GCS) has been adopted widely as a reproducible measure of neurologic status (Table 5-2). There is a close correlation with outcome, although brainstem abnormalities such as pupillary responses and extraocular movements are not included in the assessment.

      2. CT scanning is the diagnostic study of choice in assessing head injuries. In the majority of cases, a study without contrast enhancement suffices. If a patient is hemodynamically stable, a CT scan should have priority in the initial trauma assessment.

      3. The addition of CT data helps to predict outcome, as acute subdural hematomas with GCS scores of 3 to 5

Table 5–2. Glasgow Coma Scale

Observation	Points
Eye opening	
Spontaneous	4
To speech	3
To pain	2
None	1
Best verbal response	
Oriented	5
Confused	4
Inappropriate	3
Incomprehensible	2
None	1
Best motor response	
Obeys commands	6
Localizes pain	5
Withdraws from pain	4
Flexes to pain	3
Extends to pain	2
None	1

have the worst outcome (74% mortality rate and 8% good recovery), whereas coma of 6 to 24 hours' duration associated with diffuse injury and a GCS score of 6 to 8 has a 9% mortality rate and a 68% good recovery rate.

   C.   Associated Injuries

Thirty-five per cent of patients with severe head injuries have one other major system injury, and 25% have two other major system injuries.

III.   OPERATIVE MANAGEMENT

   A.   Anesthetic Management of Acute Subdural and Epidural Hematomas

      1.   Goals

The prevention of secondary injury caused by hypoxia, hypercarbia, cerebral edema, and ischemia are the main goals of the operative management of acute mass lesions.

      2.   Preoperative preparation

Optimally, the anesthesiologist is involved from the time the patient has presented to the emergency room. An assessment of peripheral injuries, as well as of volume status, level of consciousness, and pulmonary status, must be accomplished rapidly before the patient is transported to the operating room.

3. Monitors

Because of the imminent danger of transtentorial herniation from lesions such as acute epidural hematomas, some monitors (i.e., the intra-arterial line) may be placed after the induction of anesthesia.

4. Induction

   a. A rapid-sequence induction for the "tight head, full stomach" patient is a matter of some controversy. A generally safe technique in the patient who is not severely hypovolemic involves the use of thiopental 3 to 4 mg/kg following by a large dose of pancuronium bromide, 0.2 mg/kg, and lidocaine, 1.5 mg/kg, after the patient is oxygenated and cricoid pressure is applied.

   b. When necessary, hyperventilation with cricoid pressure may be accomplished while waiting 90 seconds for the muscle relaxants to become effective. In some patients, the use of succinylcholine following treatment with a small dose of a nonpolarizing agent may be the safest course of action despite a possible rise in the ICP.

5. Maintenance techniques

   a. Principles of neuroanesthesia such as hyperventilation, the use of narcotics, and thiopental with modest amounts of inhalational agents generally work well in a situation of acute head trauma.

   b. Acute cerebral edema may follow the evacuation of the hematoma and will necessitate the use of furosemide or mannitol. Large doses of steroids are not effective in limiting the morbidity of head injury.

6. Fluid management

   a. Volume resuscitation with isotonic fluids is important in maintaining the patient's blood pressure.

   b. In certain instances, the use of a pulmonary

artery catheter will be necessary to assess volume status and achieve optimal cardiac output, particularly in the presence of other major systemic injuries.

7. Emergence from anesthesia
Most often, the patient who has required evacuation of an acute subdural or epidural hematoma will remain intubated for a time postoperatively while the ICP is monitored.

IV. POSTOPERATIVE CONSIDERATIONS
  A. Concepts of Primary and Secondary Head Injury
    1. A brain contusion, shear injury, or laceration that occurs at the time of impact is a primary injury and cannot be reversed with treatment.
    2. Management of the head-injured patient currently focuses on the prevention of secondary injury, caused by insults such as intracranial hypertension, cerebral ischemia, systemic hypotension, hypoxia, sepsis, and mass lesions that arise after impact.
  B. Sequelae of Head Injury
    1. Cardiopulmonary
      a. Attention to the respiratory status of patients with closed head injury must be scrupulous. Comatose patients are subject to many pulmonary abnormalities, including aspiration, atelectasis, pneumonia, and neurogenic pulmonary edema.
      b. Neurogenic pulmonary edema, which occurs rarely, probably results from a diffuse and massive sympathetic discharge that both overloads the left ventricle and increases pulmonary capillary permeability.
      c. Atrial fibrillation following closed head injury not necessarily associated with IICP has been reported.
      d. Animal studies have demonstrated bradycardia, shortened QT interval, elevated ST segment, nodal rhythm, and increased T-wave amplitude after experimental concussion.
    2. Metabolic
A hypermetabolic state similar to that seen in burn and multitrauma victims follows closed head injury. The outcome may be improved if nutritional support is instituted early. However, excessive fluid and glucose loads must be avoided.

3. Hematologic
Coagulation abnormalities are very common in patients with closed head injury. Brain tissue thromboplastin causes accelerated fibrinolysis, the severity of which correlates with the severity of the injury. In addition, head trauma impairs platelet aggregation in vitro and in vivo.

4. Endocrinologic

a. Acute increases in ICP can stimulate antidiuretic hormone production and release. The syndrome of inappropriate antidiuretic hormone secretion (SIADH) features high renal sodium excretion, hyponatremia with corresponding hypo-osmolality of the serum and extracellular fluid, urine osmolality greater than serum osmolality, and normal renal and adrenal function. Fluid restriction is effective in establishing a negative fluid balance, but diuresis does not occur for 36 to 48 hours. SIADH must be distinguished from a natriuretic syndrome that is common with neurologic disease.

b. Diabetes insipidus is relatively common after craniofacial trauma. The signs of antidiuretic hormone deficiency include polyuria, polydipsia, hypernatremia, high serum osmolality, dilute urine, and a urine-to-serum osmolality ratio less than 1.0, implying a negative water balance. Post-traumatic diabetes insipidus is commonly transient, but occasionally, long-term therapy with desmopressin (DDAVP; 1-desamino-8-D-arginine vasopressin) is necessary. Daily weights, carefully recorded intake and output, serum BUN and electrolytes, urine specific gravity, and osmolality are keys to management. The patient's hourly urine output is replaced, plus the usual fluids for insensible loss, with solutions containing water and little or no electrolytes. In certain patients, the use of lysine vasopressin nasal spray or aqueous vasopressin or desmopressin will be necessary.

V. NEUROSURGICAL INTENSIVE CARE MANAGEMENT

A. Monitors
Most investigators have suggested that aggressive management of closed head injury, including ICP monitoring

and control, improves outcome from traumatic coma. Intracranial pressure monitoring is justified in a group of severely head injured patients (GCS ≤8), with either high- or low-density lesions on CT scan at the time of admission. ICP elevations occur in 63% and 53% of these patients, respectively. In addition, if an unstable patient requires immediate diagnostic studies, medical management, or surgical intervention, a means of continuously monitoring ICP allows for optimal care.

B. Therapeutic Modalities

1. In addition to long-term ventilatory support coupled with neuromuscular paralysis and sedation, IICP responds to other modalities previously discussed, such as mannitol and furosemide.

2. A recent prospective study of large doses of corticosteroids demonstrated that these agents do not improve outcome after traumatic coma, nor does prophylactic barbiturate administration.

C. Outcome

1. Elevated ICP (greater than 40 mmHg) usually implies a poor outcome. Almost uniform fatality is reported for those patients with hemispheric swelling and extracerebral masses.

2. The search continues for adequate clinical assessment scales and prognostic indicators that reliably predict the outcome in patients with head injuries. At present, accurate predictions are generally limited to those moribund or dying patients or those who recover very rapidly from coma.

D. Brain Death
Brain death is established if there is irreversible cessation of all function of the entire brain, including the brainstem. The criteria include deep coma, which may be confirmed by EEG or cerebral blood flow studies, and an absence of brainstem reflexes.

Seizures

I. ETIOLOGY
Recurrent seizure activity may follow head trauma, intracranial masses, CNS infection, or IICP. In 50% of the patients with recurrent seizures, no cause is found. Within the brain, a

sudden, excessive, and temporary electrical discharge from a few cells probably initiates a seizure; therefore, the successful management of epilepsy depends on the ability of treatment either to abolish these discharges or to prevent their spread throughout the nervous system.

II.   MEDICAL THERAPY

The history and EEG are used to determine the type of seizures. A variety of drugs are used as anticonvulsants, with phenytoin or phenobarbital being the most common for generalized seizures. Whereas most patients respond well to a single drug and have no further seizures, 20% to 30% of patients have seizures that are difficult to control with currently available drugs.

III.   SURGICAL THERAPY

   A.   The majority of patients considered for adjunctive surgical management of their epilepsy have intractable temporal lobe seizures. The goal of surgical resection is to reduce the critical mass of electrically unstable neurons that promote the abnormal activity.

   B.   Anesthetic management

   1.   Medical centers involved in epilepsy surgery use intraoperative electrocorticography to delineate areas of abnormal activity and to determine the extent of resection. For this reason, the preoperative use of drugs such as benzodiazepines, which can alter the electrocorticogram, are avoided. Corticosteroids are begun 24 hours preoperatively and continued postoperatively. In addition, most antiseizure medications are gradually reduced the week before surgery.

   2.   During the procedure with monitored anesthesia care, most patients are sedated with fentanyl and droperidol. Intraoperatively the patient will be asked to hyperventilate in an attempt to provoke abnormal activity. If a seizure occurs intraoperatively, methohexital 0.25 to 1.5 mg/kg is administered.

   3.   Although local anesthesia supplemented by analgesic drugs is considered optimal, on occasion, patients require general anesthesia. The use of N_2O, sodium methohexital, fentanyl, and a muscle relaxant is compatible with the goals of the procedure as long as the N_2O is discontinued before the electrocorticogram, as it obliterates epileptiform activity.

4. Postoperatively, phenytoin, phenobarbital, and hydrocortisone are continued. An antiseizure medication regimen is reinstituted for the first year after surgery; and, if the patient has been seizure free and has a nonepileptiform EEG, the medications are gradually reduced at 6- to 12-month intervals.

Summary of Anesthetic Considerations

After head trauma, the first priority is to establish airway control. Initiating hyperventilation and treating hypoxemia improves outcome. Establishing the baseline mental status before surgery is important for follow-up care. Injury to other major organ systems is present in 35% of patients with severe head injury. Unless these conditions are corrected, further brain damage may result.

Anesthetic management is aimed at preventing increases in ICP and maintaining hemodynamic stability. Rapid-sequence induction with small amounts of thiopental, large doses of pancuronium, and intravenous lidocaine has been successful. Maintenance anesthesia with narcotics and thiopental as a base and modest amounts of inhalational agents will work well. Intraoperative cerebral edema will respond well to mannitol or loop diuretics. To minimize fluid intake and maintain adequate cardiac output, a pulmonary artery catheter is helpful. Postoperatively, hyperventilation should be continued for 2 to 3 days until the danger of acute onset of cerebral edema and IICP from head trauma is low.

Recurrent seizures may develop after head trauma, brain metastasis, CNS infection, cerebral edema, and IICP. Most often, generalized recurrent seizures are well controlled with phenytoin or phenobarbital. Rarely, surgical resection of the epileptic focus is necessary. During anesthesia for such operations, drugs that can depress seizure activity must be avoided. Fentanyl and droperidol are often used in this situation. After surgical removal of the seizure focus, patients must be kept on antiseizure medication for at least 1 year before a trial off medication can be attempted.

Recommended Reading

Braakman R, Schouten HJA, Dishoeck MB, et al. Megadose steroids in severe head injury: results of a prospective double-blind clinical trial. J Neurosurg 1983;58:326.

Gennarelli TA, Spielman GM, Langfit TW, et al. Influence of the type of intracranial lesion on outcome from severe head injury. J Neurosurg 1982;36:26.

Jennett B, Bond M. Assessment of outcome after severe brain damage: a practical scale. Lancet 1975;1:480.

Manninen P, Contreras J. Anesthetic considerations for craniotomy in awake patients. Int Anesth Clin 1986;24(3):157.

Matjasko J, Pitts L. Controversies in severe head injury management. In: Matjasko J, Katz J, eds. Clinical controversies in neuroanesthesia. Orlando: Grune & Stratton, 1986:181.

Matjasko J. Multisystem sequelae of severe head injury. In: Cottrell JE, Turndorf H, eds. Anesthesia and neurosurgery. 2nd ed. St Louis: CV Mosby, 1986:188.

Sevitt S. Fatal road accidents in Birmingham: times to death and their cause. Injury 1973;4:281.

Ward JD, Becker DP, Miller DJ, et al. Failure of prophylactic barbiturate coma in the treatment of severe head trauma. J Neurosurg 1985;62:383.

≡ Neurologic Disorders and Spinal Cord Injuries

Lee Kearse

A broad spectrum of neurologic illnesses exists that present particular concerns and considerations for the anesthesiologist. Some of these illnesses represent abnormal neurologic function as a manifestation of systemic disease, such as the complications of diabetes mellitus. In other settings, the neurologic sequelae include the less well-understood consequences of degenerative processes specific to the central nervous system, such as the demyelinative disorders. Within each disease category, there is a range of patient disability and abnormality. For each patient, the anesthesiologist must understand the disease process itself, as well as how that process will be influenced by anesthetic techniques.

In this section, the perioperative management of patients with multiple sclerosis, Parkinsonism, myasthenia gravis, and spinal cord injuries will be described. The principal emphasis will be the interrelation between the abnormal nervous system and the potential complications from anesthetic management.

Multiple Sclerosis

I.   SIGNS AND SYMPTOMS
   A.   Generalized Multiple Sclerosis
        Multiple sclerosis (MS) is an autoimmune disorder in-
        volving the white matter of the central nervous system.
        The clinical expression of the disease is commonly of
        intermittent or remitting symptoms that may occur over
        several years. In rare cases, the symptoms are rapidly
        progressive or noticed over a matter of days or weeks.
        Potentially, disease in the cerebrum, brainstem, and spi-
        nal cord may transform a healthy adult into a comatose
        patient within 2 weeks. The symptoms may persist over a
        variable period, resolve either entirely or partially, and
        recur later with greater, more obvious involvement of the
        neuraxis. Symptoms often reflect disease in the optic
        nerves, spinal cord, cerebellum, brainstem, or cerebrum.
        This form of the disease represents a generalized or mixed
        type of MS.
   B.   Limited Forms of Multiple Sclerosis
        Often seen are the spinal form of MS, manifested as a
        spastic paraparesis or paraplegia, and the cerebellar or
        pontobulbar–cerebellar form. Optic neuritis and neuro-
        myelitis optica are other forms of the disease.
   C.   Principal Features
        The precise features of the illness vary considerably but
        implicate motor or sensory fibers, cerebellar and extra-
        pyramidal inputs, or both. Impairment of sensory func-
        tion is usually manifested as parasthesias or pain,
        whereas motor involvement produces weakness. Cerebel-
        lar damage may produce disturbances of gait and coor-
        dination. Visual disturbances, bladder dysfunction, and
        emotional lability may also be symptoms.

II.   ETIOLOGY
   A.   Current research strongly suggests that MS is an autoim-
        mune disorder. The typical pathologic "plaques" in the
        white matter tracts appear to represent an immunologic
        response of patients to their own myelin.
   B.   Despite speculation as to a causative agent, including
        various viruses and HLA type, neither an organism nor a
        specific genetic predisposition for the disease has been
        identified definitively.

III. MEDICAL TREATMENT AND ITS IMPACT ON ANESTHETIC MANAGEMENT

    A. Most medications used in multiple sclerosis treat the complications of the disease. The most common medications taken include propantheline (Pro-Banthine) for a spastic bladder and baclofen (Liorisal) for flexor spasms in patients with marked involvement of the spinal cord. Occasional use of dantrolene (Dantrium) and diazepam (Valium) has been reported for flexor spasms. These drugs, while reducing spasticity and spasms, may cause other significant side effects.

        1. Propantheline bromide

            a. Propantheline bromide is a synthetic quaternary ammonium compound with significant ganglion-blocking and antimuscarinic properties. In the customary doses of 15 to 45 mg/day, the patient may suffer from orthostatic hypotension as well as mild neuromuscular blockade.

            b. Propantheline at very high (>45 mg/day) doses blocks the neuromuscular junction.

            c. Gastric emptying is delayed, and gastric acid secretion is reduced.

            d. Although there are no published studies evaluating the interactions between muscle relaxants and volatile anesthetic agents in the MS patient taking propantheline, the anesthesiologist must anticipate the following:

                1) A potentially prolonged recovery of neuromuscular function;

                2) Increased patient difficulty in handling secretions;

                3) Significant hypotension after induction;

                4) An even greater propensity for gastric reflux.

        2. Baclofen

            a. Baclofen is derived from gamma-aminobutyric acid (GABA). Its mechanism for reducing flexor tone and spasm is thought to be inhibition at the presynaptic terminals of the motor neurons.

            b. At the customary dose of 20 mg four times a day, one of the side effects is muscle weakness.

      c. With toxic doses, marked respiratory depression and seizures have been reported.

      d. The patient should continue receiving this medication through the day of surgery, because abrupt withdrawal may cause central nervous system excitability, including hallucinations and pronounced anxiety.

      e. Short-acting nondepolarizing muscle relaxants are recommended to avoid slow recovery from muscle weakness.

   3. Dantrolene
Dantrolene reduces spasticity by inhibiting the excitation–contraction coupling of skeletal muscle through a reduction in calcium in the sarcoplasmic reticulum. Its principal side effect is generalized weakness.

   4. Diazepam

      a. Diazepam is a benzodiazepine with muscle-relaxant properties that is useful for managing spasticity in the MS patient. It appears to act at the spinal cord level by increasing the inhibitory influence of GABA-ergic transmission. In addition to producing sedation, it may cause generalized weakness.

      b. As a premedicant, diazepam may cause respiratory depression in the more debilitated patient because of sedation or generalized muscle weakness, even if diazepam has been taken long term.

  B. Experimental treatment protocols for the MS patient include trials using ACTH, azothiaprine, cyclophosphamide, cytosine arabinoside, and prednisone. Because of the side effects of these medications, the protocols lasted only a few weeks or months; the protocols themselves necessitated hospitalization. The anesthesiologist is not likely to manage the patient who receives these medications.

IV. ANESTHETIC MANAGEMENT

  A. Patients with Generalized MS

   1. For the patient with MS in whom the disease does not hamper lifestyle, no particular modifications of anesthetic technique are necessary.

   2. For patients who have become markedly dependent on others, the concerns of the anesthesiologist are similar to those in patients debilitated by any chronic illness.

3. In the advanced stages of MS, aspiration, atelectasis, and pneumonia often precipitate hospital admission.

   a. Respiratory failure may be secondary to demyelinative lesions of the cervical spinal cord or the respiratory centers of the medulla or to underlying parenchymal or pulmonary processes. Rarely, rapid demyelination of the respiratory centers causes acute loss of voluntary breathing.

   b. These two groups of patients must be intubated and mechanically ventilated in order to sustain life.

4. In less-compromised patients, the extent of respiratory disability must be determined through pulmonary function studies. Even if the patient appears comfortable while breathing, tells you he clears secretions well, and has an adequate cough, he may have marked respiratory compromise.

   a. The ambulatory MS patient may have normal or near-normal function, but the wheelchair-bound patient has markedly reduced pulmonary function.

   b. Values for forced vital capacity, maximal voluntary ventilation, and maximal expiratory pressure may be reduced by as much as two-thirds. Muscles involving expiration may be severely affected.

   c. Despite severe muscle weakness, patients may have excellent ventilation–perfusion matching and thus normal arterial blood gas values.

5. The patient with MS may be susceptible to changes in temperature, especially from cool to warm environments. Unmyelinated fibers conduct more slowly in warm temperatures; increases in ambient temperature and pyrexia caused by infections may exacerbate symptoms, perhaps increasing weakness and clouding the sensorium. In the operating room, such a response may influence both the ability to arouse the patient and the patient's ability to sustain breathing fully. The anesthesiologist should monitor the core temperature of all MS patients; the

temperature should not rise above the patient's baseline.

6. As with many patients who have chronic demyelination, MS patients may be at risk for excessive potassium release with the use of succinylcholine. This drug should not be used in the presence of pyramidal tract disease and demyelination unless absolutely necessary. Rapid-onset nondepolarizing muscle relaxants such as atracurium or vecuronium are better alternatives.

B. Patients with Pseudobulbar Palsy or Other Bulbar Impairment

1. The patient with severe brainstem and cerebellar findings will have difficulties with pharyngeal muscle control and may lack a gag reflex and coordination of the musculature of the mouth and pharynx as a result of abnormal cerebellar input.

2. Aspiration is a potential problem because the patient cannot swallow properly and has little control over secretions. The anesthesiologist should minimize the potential for aspiration in the perioperative period.

3. Judicious preoperative use of H_2 blockers such as cimetidine or ranitidine to lower gastric acidity and metaclopramide to facilitate stomach emptying is recommended for the patient who is to undergo a general anesthetic. These medications have central nervous system effects, including excitability and depression, which may need to be addressed.

4. The patient with little or no gag or cough reflex should have an awake or rapid-sequence intubation and be extubated only when adequately awake.

C. Patients with Weakness and Principal Spinal Cord Disease

1. Spontaneous tidal volumes may be adequate in the awake patient but completely inadequate under or upon emergence from general anesthesia. Sufficient respiratory efforts are especially important in the patient who has a transverse myelitis with a sensory or motor level in the thoracic or cervical region. Quadriplegia in this setting is rare. All patients with sensory or motor complaints involving the cervical cord are at risk of having some compromise in respiratory function.

2. Depending on the level of impairment, the individual may respond similarly to a patient with high traumatic spinal cord injury, such as autonomic hyperreflexia during urologic procedures.

    a. For urologic surgery, a high spinal anesthetic in a patient with respiratory compromise may precipitate an unwanted intubation and prolonged mechanical ventilation as a result of muscle relaxation. A lumbar epidural catheter with 2% lidocaine slowly titrated to the T8 sensory level may offer a satisfactory alternative.

    b. A combination of beta-blockers and venous and arterial dilators may be needed to control hypertension once the reflex has occurred. Deepening the general anesthetic before the surgery does not appear to alter the autonomic response.

V. POSTOPERATIVE EXACERBATION OF SYMPTOMS
Although emotional and physical stresses are associated with exacerbations of MS symptoms, there appears to be no intrinsic risk of exacerbation with anesthesia and surgery.

VI. SUMMARY OF ANESTHETIC CONSIDERATIONS
Breathing is significantly affected by multiple sclerosis secondary to demyelinative lesions in the respiratory centers of the medulla and the cervical and thoracic spinal cord. A full pulmonary evaluation is necessary. A patient wth generalized MS may not complain of shortness of breath but may have minimal respiratory reserve. Pharyngeal muscle control is often affected in patients with brainstem and cerebellar disease. Swallowing, gag, and cough reflexes are adversely affected.

Most patients will benefit from perioperative administration of H_2 antagonists to increase gastric pH and metaclopramide to increase gastric emptying. Patients with extensive spinal cord involvement may respond similarly to those with a high traumatic cord injury. Use of succinylcholine should be avoided because of the potential of excessive potassium release. Autonomic hyperreflexia had been recorded with inadequate anesthesia. Spinal or epidural anesthesia can be used in these patients after careful documentation of their neurologic problems. Intraoperative use of muscle relaxants must be carefully monitored. Many of the drugs taken to relieve symptoms of MS, such as propantheline and baclofen, can prolong the recovery of neuromuscular function. Excessive intraoperative warming must be prevented, as hyperthermia can exacerbate most symptoms. Postoperatively, patients should not be extubated until they demonstrate the ability to protect the airway.

Parkinson's Disease (Paralysis Agitans)

I.   CLINICAL FEATURES
   A.   Parkinson's disease reflects degeneration of the dopaminergic connections between the substantia nigra and the striatum. There is a strong correlation between the clinical symptoms and the loss of pigmented cells in the substantia nigra, locus ceruleus, and dorsal motor nucleus of the vagus.
   B.   There is a triad of symptoms.
      1.   A rhythmic, four per second, "pill-rolling" tremor noted at rest;
      2.   A paucity of voluntary movement marked by a slowness and deliberateness in the initiation (akinesia) as well as in the execution (bradykinesia);
      3.   An increase in muscle tone that has a peculiar "cogwheel" characteristic.
   C.   The typical Parkinson's patient is middle-aged to elderly with a "masked" facies, chronic stare, festinating gait, prominent tremor, monotonous soft voice, and micrographic writing.
II.   ANTI-PARKINSON MEDICATIONS
   A.   Medical Treatment
      Most evidence suggests that the symptoms are related to a deficiency of the neurotransmitter dopamine in the brain. Therapy thus has been directed toward providing more brain dopamine. The drugs used do not retard or prevent the further degeneration of neuronal cells in the substantia nigra but have been helpful in treating the symptoms. Surgical treatment by implanting adrenal medullary cells into the hypothalamus is still experimental.
   B.   Commonly Used Medications
      1.   L-Dopa
         L-dopa (L-dihydroxyphenylalanine) has until recently been the most successful drug in reversing some of the symptoms of Parkinsonism. The medica-

tion is usually administered as a combination of a decarboxylase inhibitor and L-dopa (Sinemet). The decarboxylase inhibitor prevents the aromatic L-amino decarboxylase from converting L-dopa into dopamine peripherally and so makes more of the drug available for conversion within the striatum.

2. Amantidine hydrochloride
   Amantadine hydrochloride (Symmetrel), an antiviral agent, is thought to act by causing a release of dopamine from dopaminergic neurons in the striatum.

3. Diphenhydramine hydrochloride
   Diphenhydramine hydrochloride (Benadryl) is an H₁ blocker with central anticholinergic action. This antimuscarinic property appears to alleviate some of the central excitatory effects of the cholinergic system in the Parkinson patient.

4. Anticholinergics
   Anticholinergic agents such as benztropine mesylate (Cogentin) and trihexphenidyl (Artane) are often used as an adjunct to levodopa and have their greatest effect on reducing the tremor.

5. Bromocriptine mesylate
   Bromocriptine mesylate (Parlodel) is an ergot derivative with dopaminergic agonist properties. It stimulates dopaminergic terminals to secrete dopamine.

III. PERIOPERATIVE MANAGEMENT
   A. Preoperative Medications and Assessment
   1. Medication review
      a. A thorough review of the medical regimen is necessary to make certain the patient is not given medication that will contribute adversely to the disease.
      b. Dopamine-blocking agents such as phenothiazines and butyrophenones, as well as drugs that deplete dopamine stores, such as reserpine, may precipitate or worsen symptoms.
      c. Monoamine oxidase inhibitors interfere with the catabolism of catecholamines, risking marked increases in blood pressure and body temperature if used in combination with L-dopa.
      d. Pyridoxine may accelerate the breakdown of

L-dopa through the pyridoxine-dependent L-amino acid decarboxylase.

2. Airway and respiratory status

   a. The patient has limited abilities to protect himself or herself from aspiration and may not have enough pulmonary reserve to compensate for the loss of accessory muscles.

   b. A full evaluation of pulmonary function in advance of surgery helps to determine the impact of the anesthetic on the respiratory reserve and to anticipate any need for intubation and ventilation into the postoperative period.

   c. Tremor, bradykinesia, akinesia, and muscle rigidity in the extremities also involve the oropharyngeal and chest wall muscles. The anesthesiologist must pay particular attention to findings of bulbar function. Drooling may reflect bradykinesia of the swallowing apparatus.

   d. Rigidity is prominent in both the primary and accessory muscles of breathing. The ability to generate a forceful gag or cough may be dramatically diminished in the moderately to severely affected patient.

   e. Notice should be made of unusual movements such as titubation of the head, orobuccolingual dyskinesias, or abnormal breathing patterns. Depending on the site of the surgery, these movements may complicate the postoperative plans.

3. CNS status

   a. Parkinson's disease is associated with dementing illnesses. Also, L-dopa may cause behavioral changes that include hypomania, depression, psychotic delusions, and delirium.

   b. The patient's disturbed sensorium must be noted before the anesthetic is administered in order to avoid expensive, time-consuming, and unnecessary neurologic tests postoperatively seeking to explain a "new" mental status.

4. Fluid and nutritional status

   a. Because of inability to swallow and eat, some patients become dehydrated and protein deficient. An evaluation of volume status may be accomplished by examination of tissue turgor and mucous membrane moisture.

b. The tilt test may not be useful, because many Parkinson's patients have some degree of orthostatic hypotension secondary to a postural reflex impairment.

c. In the very debilitated and cachectic patient, increased serum sodium, hematocrit, and blood urea nitrogen indicate hypovolemia.

5. Anti-Parkinson medications and cardiac status

a. L-dopa may cause cardiac dysrhythmias and either hypotension or hypertension, all of which may be attributable to dopamine's effects on the cardiovascular system. Vasodilating effects on dopaminergic receptors in the renal and splanchnic beds may be the cause of hypotension. Beta stimulation of the myocardium and indirect release of catecholamines from sympathetic nerves may cause dysrhythmias such as ventricular extrasystoles and tachycardia, atrial flutter and fibrillation, and sinus tachycardia. In higher doses, stimulation of alpha-receptors in the peripheral vasculature may produce vasoconstriction and hypertension.

b. Currently, discontinuing L-dopa prior to surgery is not recommended, as withdrawal from the medication may render some patients entirely immobile with rigidity and may trigger hemodynamic instability and cardiac dysrhythmias, particularly in the patient with coronary artery disease.

c. The recommended approach to the preoperative use of L-dopa is to continue the customary regimen until the day of surgery. Dysrhythmias that occur during L-dopa administration can be controlled with beta-adrenergic blocking agents, which can be given intraoperatively.

d. Little is known regarding the withdrawal of other anti-Parkinson medications.

B. Intraoperative Management

1. Patients with few symptoms who are taking no medication require no special procedures. No studies

conclude that any one anesthetic technique is superior.

2. In most situations, the severely affected patient with bulbar involvement and extreme rigidity should be intubated using cricoid pressure and a rapid-onset nondepolarizing agent or succinylcholine. Muscle rigidity and tremor respond to either depolarizing or nondepolarizing agents. Under general anesthesia with volatile agents, patients have some muscle relaxation, and the movement disorder is suppressed. Supplemental muscle relaxants may be indicated for certain abdominal or musculoskeletal operations.

3. Extubation should be performed only after the patient is fully awake and demonstrates at least a baseline ability to protect the airway. Recovery of motor function should be supported by information from a nerve stimulator. Before extubation, evacuation of the stomach contents with an oral gastric tube and suction aspiration of the oral cavity may help prevent aspiration.

4. Regional techniques may be employed safely. However, the patient's head, neck, and trunk may move as one, making these techniques somewhat difficult to implement. Epidural and spinal techniques may cause respiratory complications secondary to relatively high spinal levels.

IV. POSTOPERATIVE ASSESSMENT

Postoperative assessment of the patient's return of baseline motor and mental function is complicated, especially in patients with communicative and movement disorders.

V. SUMMARY OF ANESTHETIC CONSIDERATIONS

The patient with Parkinson's disease is at increased risk for perioperative complications because of dysfunction of the gag, swallowing, and cough reflexes. The patient is further compromised because of the lack of ability to respond to hypotension secondary to blunting of the baroreflex mechanism.

The usual treatment medication, L-dopa, can cause cardiac dysrhythmias and hemodynamic instability. This medication should not be discontinued before surgery, however, as its withdrawal also can cause cardiac dysrhythmias as well as render the patient completely rigid, compromising the gag reflex and the ability to expand the chest wall on inspiration.

Regional anesthesia can be used safely. However, high

levels of motor block from spinal or epidural anesthesia can markedly worsen the patient's already compromised accessory muscles of breathing.

Rapid-sequence induction or awake intubation should be used for airway protection. Use of muscle relaxants will decrease the rigidity of Parkinson's disease and increase the ease of intubation and ventilation. All inhaled anesthetics will decrease muscle rigidity and suppress involuntary muscle movement. Extubation should be attempted only when the patient is alert and appears to be able to protect the airway. Multiple adjustments in the medication regimen may be needed before movement disorder and rigidity can be brought back to preoperative levels.

Myasthenia Gravis

I. ETIOLOGY
Myasthenia gravis is an autoimmune-mediated disease causing muscle weakness. The clinical manifestations are thought to be secondary to a reduced number of acetylcholine receptor sites in the neuromuscular junction caused by immune destruction. The clinical expression is fatigability of contraction with repetitive muscle activity.

II. INCIDENCE
The incidence of the disease is between 1 in 10,000 and 1 in 50,000 and has different forms. It can occur in any age group, but the peak incidence is in the 20 to 30 age group, with women two to three times more likely to be affected. This group also has more involvement of the musculature, with weakness in the extremities as well as in muscles innervated by the motor nuclei of the brainstem. In 50- to 60-year-olds, men and women are affected equally.

III. PRESENTATION
    A. The illness varies considerably, but in most situations, the patient becomes aware of the disease gradually. It is not until activities that were performed easily, such as talking, swallowing, and breathing, become difficult that the patient seeks medical advice.
    B. The diagnosis may become evident quickly during pregnancy in young women or after a patient has undergone a general anesthetic, when spontaneous breathing does not resume within an expected period.

    C. In the elderly, the most common findings are weakness in the bulbar, facial, masticatory, lingual, and ocular muscles. Rarely, truncal muscles, the diaphragm, and the abdominal wall, intercostal, bladder, and bowel muscles are involved.

IV. PREANESTHETIC MANAGEMENT

    A. Important Physical Findings

        1. Myasthenia gravis should be regarded as a systemic disorder in which all muscles are involved. Although formal pulmonary function studies need not be performed on all patients, preoperative knowledge of the patient's tidal volume, vital capacity, and forced expiratory volume enables the anesthesiologist to determine an appropriate anesthetic technique and to anticipate problems during and after surgery.

        2. In order to make airway management decisions, the anesthesiologist must assess the patient's ability to gag, cough, handle secretions, and protect the airway. A comprehensive neurologic assessment is important because it enables change to be documented.

    B. Medication History

        1. Understanding cycles of patient fatigue and the patient's medication will guide the anesthesiologist in altering medication dosage. Most patients take pyridostigmine (Mestinon) regularly, depending on the duration of the patient's strength between doses. More frequent doses thus reflect a greater extent of disease.

        2. Patients on steroids are often markedly debilitated and are subject to the complications of steroid use.

        3. There is an association between myasthenia gravis and hyperthyroidism, systemic lupus erythematosus, rheumatoid arthritis, and polymyositis. If thyroid disease is suspected, thyroid studies should be performed before surgery. The other diseases usually do not pose a threat if they are asymptomatic.

        4. Three cardinal features of the disease are:

            a. Easy fatigability of voluntary muscle with repetitive activity;

            b. Restoration of power generally occurring with rest;

            c. Anticholinesterase treatment improves performance but may cause a cholinergic crisis.

V. PREOPERATIVE MEDICATIONS

   A. Intravenous Anesthetics

      Sedatives and narcotics should be reduced or eliminated in patients with tenuous respiratory reserve. Drugs that may inhibit respiratory drive or adversely influence neuromuscular transmission should be avoided. Although benzodiazepines and opiates affect neuromuscular transmission, they may be used safely with attention to respiratory effects.

   B. Anticholinergics

      Patients with specific bulbar involvement should be evaluated to determine whether antisialologues and H_2 blockers are indicated and can be given safely. Anticholinergics may increase physiological "dead space," contribute to the difficulty of clearing secretions, depress central control of muscle tone, or increase gastroesophageal sphincter tone. The anesthesiologist may have to use cricoid pressure during induction and intubation.

   C. Anticholinesterase

      1. An edrophonium test is often recommended to assess the adequacy of pyridostigmine or neostigmine. With a specific marker for strength (ptosis improvement, hand grip, vital capacity), the patient is tested before the intravenous administration of 2 mg of edrophonium and 30 to 90 seconds after. An improvement indicates the patient may need more of his or her customary medication before the operation. No change or worsening indicates the patient is adequately medicated and may be at risk for a cholinergic crisis if medication is increased.

      2. Anticholinesterase medications increase gastric volume. Airway protection measures are therefore warranted.

      3. Withdrawing anticholinesterase medications 24 to 48 hours before surgery could precipitate a respiratory crisis and does not reduce postoperative complications. Preoperatively, the patient can be given his or her customary medications as scheduled, as they do not affect the postoperative time to return to baseline neurological status.

VI. ANESTHETIC MANAGEMENT

   A. Muscle Relaxants and Reversal Agents

      1. Use of muscle relaxants to facilitate intubation and muscle relaxation is controversial. The myasthenic patient may be resistant to depolarizing muscle relaxants such as succinylcholine and may develop a Phase II block with that drug. The mechanism may be secondary to the fewer acetylcholine receptors available for binding. Therefore, succinylcholine should be used only for emergencies. Also, because succinylcholine hydrolysis is mediated by pseudocholinesterase, patients taking anticholinesterases and given succinylcholine may develop an extraordinarily prolonged muscle blockade necessitating extended postoperative mechanical ventilation.

2.   Myasthenic patients may have variable responses to nondepolarizing muscle relaxants because of the variability in the stages of the disease and the medications taken for preoperative control. Dosages may be titrated as necessary to achieve muscle relaxation without causing a significant delay in the return of muscle strength as measured with a peripheral nerve stimulator. Latency between administration of the relaxant and the onset of the block, duration and depth of block, and the dose required for achieving 90% twitch suppression all differ significantly.

3.   Neuromuscular blockade reversal may be equally problematic because an overdose of anticholinesterase may increase weakness and precipitate a cholinergic crisis. Titration of the reversal doses is also indicated. Pyridostigmine given intravenously in 1-mg increments over 5 minutes or neostigmine at a dose of 2.5 mg every 5 minutes have been recommended. Edrophonium has also been given in incremental doses. The evoked twitch response may be used as a guide.

B.   Maintenance Anesthesia

1.   No anesthetic technique is problem free for the myasthenic patient. Even when no supplemental muscle relaxation has been utilized, weakness and other symptoms have occurred. There appears to be no specific benefit enjoyed by one inhalational or intravenous agent over another.

2.   Regional anesthesia may be employed, but there is risk of respiratory compromise secondary to an unanticipated high spinal level or effects on accessory muscles. Systemic absorption of local anesthetics may also cause generalized weakness.

VII. POSTOPERATIVE MANAGEMENT

    A. Postoperatively, the anesthesiologist must be prepared for long-term management of all myasthenic patients. Mechanical ventilation must be made available preoperatively. Because the outcome is unpredictable, the patient should be told before surgery of the possibility of a long hospital stay.

    B. The interplay between the disease, the surgical procedure, and the anesthesia offers much potential for complications. Procedures involving either primary or accessory muscles of breathing, such as major abdominal and chest procedures, are particularly troublesome. Weaning the patient from the ventilator may be a challenge with any procedure. The minimal extubation criteria are a vital capacity greater than 15 ml/kg, a tidal volume of greater than 10 ml/kg, and a negative inspiratory force of greater than -25 mmHg. These values may need to be reassessed in a patient with an inadequate cough or with bulbar involvement and a limited gag reflex for possible reintubation.

    C. Other issues may become important, such as making certain that no other drug is being given that has neuromuscular blocking properties, including antibiotics such as aminoglycosides, magnesium for pre-eclamptic pregnant patients, or sedatives such as benzodiazepines.

VIII. SUMMARY OF ANESTHETIC CONSIDERATIONS

Myasthenia gravis is associated with easy fatiguability of the voluntary muscles with repetitive activity. Maintaining normal vital capacity, expiratory force, and gag and cough reflexes is difficult without medication. Pyridostigmine (Mestinon), an anticholinesterase and the drug most commonly used to treat myasthenia gravis, must be constantly adjusted to maintain patient strength. This drug can increase gastric emptying and gastric sphincter tone.

    Preoperatively, pyridostigmine should be given to the time of surgery. If there is any question about the adequacy of the medication regimen, an edrophonium test can be performed. Prophylaxis against aspiration is recommended, as well as intubation techniques that reduce the risk of aspiration.

    Succinylcholine should be avoided. The short-acting nondepolarizing muscle relaxants are most appropriate if paralysis is necessary. For optimal management, using a nerve stimulator to titrate muscle relaxants is necessary. Reversal of neuromuscular blockade is equally problematic because the additional anticholinesterase may increase weakness and precipitate a cholinergic crisis.

No specific inhaled or intravenous anesthetic has proved to be best for these patients. Regional anesthesia may be used, but in spinal or epidural blocks, unexpected high levels can cause respiratory failure.

Before extubation, these patients must have objective assessment of their respiratory strength in addition to the evaluation of respiratory rate, hand grip strength, and head lift time. Other criteria for extubation include a vital capacity of at least 15 ml/kg and an inspiratory force of no less than −25 mmHg.

Spinal Cord Injury

I. INCIDENCE
In the United States and Canada, the incidence of spinal cord injuries is approximately 40 per 1,000,000. Approximately 40% of these injuries are sustained in automobile accidents, 28% in recreational or sports activities, and 18% in work-related accidents. Those who survive the initial period have a very good prognosis for long-term survival even if the cervical spine is involved. The challenge in managing these patients is in handling individuals whose physiological responses are constantly changing. Because most anesthetic management problems arise in the patient with cervical or thoracic cord damage, those areas of concern will be addressed. Patients with lumbar injuries with cauda equina abnormalities usually do not have the life-threatening array of complications seen in those with upper cord lesions.

II. PREOPERATIVE EVALUATION
A. Cervical Stability
Every precaution should be implemented during any movement of the patient, including proper immobilization of the head and neck and limited or no flexion of the neck during intubation for a surgical procedure. Even if the patient has normal cervical spine films, he or she may suffer from cervical cord injury. This approach will help prevent further cord compromise.
B. Respiratory Status
1. Inspiration
a. The respiratory status assessment should cover rate, rhythm, tidal volume, and pattern of breathing.

b. One should look particularly for paralysis of specific muscle groups to confirm suspicion of the level of spinal cord injury. The primary muscles of inspiration include the diaphragm and the external intercostals. Because the diaphragm is innervated by the phrenic nerve, which originates from C3 through C5, and the external intercostals from T1–T12, the anesthesiologist may determine the functional debility by observing the pattern of breathing. For example, the paradoxical rise of the abdomen and concomitant contraction of the chest wall during inspiration indicate that the phrenic nerve is the principal source for the patient's breathing and that there is impairment of the intercostals. Thus, the lesion probably exists below C5 and above T6. This lack of chest wall mobility suggests a severe compromise of inspiratory capability.

2. Expiration

a. To determine the patient's ability to protect the airway, the anesthesiologist must evaluate the primary muscles necessary to generate a forceful cough. The principal muscles for expiration include the internal intercostals and the abdominals. The former are innervated at the level of T1 through T11, the latter from T7 through T11.

b. In the awake patient, a chest wall that expands symmetrically and fully with each breath strongly suggests an injury below the mid-thoracic level. Even without using the abdominal muscles, these patients may have adequate ventilatory capacity and may generate an adequate cough despite a decrease in tidal volume and vital capacity.

3. Patient position and respiratory capability

a. In the patient with abdominal muscle paralysis, position has direct bearing on tidal volume and vital capacity. The ability to wean a patient from a ventilator may therefore be determined on the basis of the patient's position.

b. In the upright position, the visceral contents and gravity limit the excursion capability of the diaphragm. In the supine position, the diaphragm has a higher resting level, and more diaphragmatic excursion is possible.

    c.   The ability to generate an adequate cough may be limited by the upright position.

4.   Other potential respiratory complications

    a.   With extreme respiratory compromise, many accessory muscles are recruited, especially during inspiration. These muscles, primarily elevators of the ribs, include the sternocleidomastoid, trapezii, serratus anterior, pectoralis minor, and scaleni. Careful evaluation may reveal significant bronchoconstriction, pulmonary infection, pneumothorax, and aspiration. Rib fractures, pulmonary contusions, hemothorax, as well as underlying pulmonary disease such as chronic obstructive or restrictive diseases, will further complicate respiratory mechanics.

    b.   In the more cephalad-injured patient, there is a diminished respiratory drive sensitivity to arterial pCO_2. Abnormal breathing patterns may intervene, including Cheyne-Stokes and apnea. The greatest danger for sleep apnea occurs between 3 and 18 days after injury.

5.   Generally, the anesthesiologist should evaluate the spinal cord-injured patient according to the vital capacity and tidal volume in both the erect and supine positions, the breathing pattern, ability to generate an adequate cough and to clear secretions, respiratory rate and rhythm, the ability of the chest wall to expand, the use and strength of the accessory muscles, the fatigability of the patient in various positions, and arterial blood gases. This information is helpful in developing a plan to handle anticipated intraoperative problems, and it facilitates postoperative management.

C.   Cardiovascular Considerations

    1.   Patients with a spinal cord injury often have markedly altered hemodynamic status and cardiovascular responses. Those with more cephalad involvement tend to be hypotensive and bradycardic. Depression in blood pressure has been attributed to diminished activity in the sympathetic vasomotor fibers, thus reducing vasomotor tone. Sympathetic

discharges in muscle nerves are related temporally to the cardiac cycle, and in the spinal cord-injured patient, this regulatory mechanism is altered.

2. Low levels of plasma norepinephrine in the quadriplegic patient may be another mechanism contributing to hypotension. The heart rate tends to be slow because of normal vagal innervation to the heart and diminished sympathetic innervation. Cardiac output is also reduced. Vagal input from tracheal suctioning or other painful stimuli may cause severe bradycardia and cardiac arrest, particularly in patients with high cervical or thoracic cord injuries.

3. Because of low spontaneous sympathetic activity to the skin, thermoregulation becomes deficient, as there is no automatic adjustment mechanism for heat conservation or loss. Sweating is impaired below the level of injury.

4. An exaggerated vasoconstrictor response to cutaneous stimulation may account for hypertension in some situations. There may also be increased sensitivity to norepinephrine.

D. Other Considerations

1. Gastrointestinal and urinary complications are common after spinal injury. Immediately after injury, there is marked bowel and bladder atony. Gastrointestinal atony may continue for many days, in part because of a reflex ileus, but also because these patients tend to swallow much air. There may be further compromise of the patient's breathing, and bowel rupture may result. Intermittent mild suction through a nasogastric tube during this period is clearly indicated.

2. An indwelling catheter may be necessary after the injury to prevent further bladder injury. After 10 days, the return of sacral innervation to the bladder may be evaluated and a regimen for bladder control established. A distended bladder may cause either a significant combination of bradycardia and hypotension or a hypertensive response, especially when the patient undergoes surgery.

E. Neurologic Injury

1. Spinal shock

Spinal shock is that condition in which there is no motor or sensory function below an identifiable level of injury. Spinal neuron reflexes that normally have supraspinal controls are affected. The two most significant reflexes for the anesthesiologist are the stretch reflex and the blood pressure reflex.

2.   Spinal recovery
Spinal shock may have a duration of 24 hours to a few months, with an average of 3 to 10 days. After the shock period, there is a general increase in spinal reflexes and all phasic muscle reflexes. Often, the reflexes spread to include large groups of muscles, and the excitability or hyperactivity of these reflexes increases. For example, a mild tap on the right patellar tendon may cause an exaggerated response on the right with some spread to the left. Reflex systems begin to show some activity within 3 to 6 weeks after injury. Commonly, the bulbocavernosus reflex and the Babinski sign are the first to return. By the third month, all of the reflex systems have achieved a higher level of excitability, and spasticity is generally complete.

III.   ANESTHETIC MANAGEMENT
A.   Prevention of Autonomic Hyperreflexia
1.   Autonomic dysreflexia may be precipitated by any surgical stimulus below the level of the spinal lesion, especially in the bladder region. Manifestations of this response are muscular contractions of the abdominal wall, hip, and extremities; evacuation of the bowel and bladder; sweating; hypertension; and reflex erythema. This reflex is most likely to occur when the spinal lesion is above T6. Less-noxious stimuli, such as lightly stroking the skin below the lesion, may cause marked increases in blood pressure, heart rate, and temperature. Infections, pressure sores, renal calculi, and mental distress may also cause autonomic dysreflexia.
2.   General anesthetics do not appear to diminish autonomic hyperreflexia.
3.   When appropriate, spinal or epidural techniques may blunt abnormal autonomic responses.
4.   Antihypertensive medications such as beta-blockers, ganglionic blocking agents, and venous and arterial vasodilators may block or treat those responses.
5.   Combinations of regional and general anesthesia have shown some promise.

      6. With any approach, the primary concern should be the ability to anticipate and control the response with medications.

B. Preventing Hyperkalemia

      1. There is particular sensitivity to the depolarizing effects of acetylcholine on denervated muscle membranes, especially 7 or more days after a spinal cord injury. After denervation, the muscle fibers, rather than just the motor endplate, become sensitive to acetylcholine.

      2. Succinylcholine has a similar effect. A rapid rise in the extracellular potassium concentration occurs with the use of succinylcholine 7 or more days after spinal cord injury. There is very little risk of a hyperkalemic response within 72 hours of the injury, but after 3 days, succinylcholine should not be used.

C. Respiratory Concerns

Within 6 months to a year, physiological changes in the patient become less volatile, residual deficits from the injury remain relatively stable, and no further significant improvements occur. Derangements exist, however, even if they are not readily apparent.

      1. Respiratory compromise may not appear imminent because the patient has learned to recruit more of the accessory muscles. After surgery and anesthesia, relearning often is necessary. Apnea may occur postoperatively.

      2. Administration of any anesthetic exacerbates all the abnormal tendencies observed in the few weeks after the injury. The anesthesiologist must be prepared for abnormal physiological behavior.

IV. SUMMARY OF ANESTHETIC CONSIDERATIONS

Most anesthetic management problems arise in patients with thoracic or cervical spinal cord injuries. Respiratory function is compromised, especially the ability to clear secretions, because of the loss of accessory muscles. Autonomic dysfunction is also present, and large fluctuations in blood pressure and pulse rate can be seen with stimulation below the spinal injury. Gastrointestinal ileus and bladder atony are common problems.

    Preoperative medication should include an H_2 blocker and metaclopramide as aspiration prophylaxis. Autonomic hyperreflexia can occur with painful stimuli or bladder distention under light general anesthesia. Deepening the anesthesia usually is not helpful. Intravenous vasodilators or beta-blockers are effective in treating the severe hypertension and cardiac dysrhythmias associated with autonomic hyperreflexia.

The incidence of autonomic hyperreflexia with spinal or epidural anesthesia is low. High levels of block must be guarded against because of the risk of compromising the accessory muscles of breathing.

For muscle relaxation, nondepolarizing agents are preferable. Three days after an acute spinal injury, the muscle fibers may become sensitized to acetylcholine. Administration of succinylcholine can then cause extensive depolarization and hyperkalemia.

Recommended Reading

Adams RD, Victor M. Principles of neurology. 3rd ed. New York: McGraw-Hill, 1985.

Bloom FE. Neurohumoral transmission and the central nervous system. In: Gilman AG, Goodman LS, Rall TW, Murad F, eds. Goodman and Gilman's the pharmacological basis of therapeutics. 7th ed. New York: Macmillan, 1985:236.

Brevan DR, Monks PS, Calne DB. Cardiovascular reactions to anaesthesia during treatment with levodopa. Anaesthesia 1973; 28:29.

Buzello W, Noeldge G, Krieg N, Brobmann GF. Vecuronium for muscle relaxation in patients with myasthenia gravis. Anesthesiology 1986;64:507.

Claus–Walker J, Halstead LS. Metabolic and endocrine changes in spinal cord injury II section 1: Consequences of partial decentralization of the autonomic nervous system. Arch Phys Med Rehabil 1982;63:569.

Davis R. Spasticity following spinal cord injury. Clin Orthop Rel Res 1975;112:66.

Defalque RJ, Musunuru VS. Diseases of the nervous system. In: Stoelting RK, Dierdorf SF, eds. Anesthesia and co-existing disease. New York: Churchill Livingstone, 1983;239.

Ellis FR. Neuromuscular disease and anaesthesia. Br J Anaesth 1974;46:603.

Gibbs PS, Kim KC. Skin and musculoskeletal diseases. In: Stoelting RK, Dierdorf SF, eds. Anesthesia and co-existing disease. New York: Churchill Livingstone, 1983;573.

Gimovsky ML, Ojeda A, Ozaki R, Zerne S. Management of autonomic hyperreflexia associated with a low thoracic spinal cord lesion. Am J Obstet Gynecol 1985;153:223.

Glynn CJ, Teddy PJ, Jamous MA, Moore RA, Lloyd JW. Preliminary communication: role of spinal noradrenergic system in transmission of pain in patients with spinal cord injury. Lancet 1986;2:1249.

Graham DH. Monitoring neuromuscular block may be unreliable in patients with upper-motor-neuron lesions. Anesthesiology 1980;52:74.

Greene LF, Ghosh MK, Howard FM. Transurethral prostatic resection in patients with myasthenia gravis. J Urol 1974;112:226.

Miller RD, ed. Anesthesia. 2nd ed. New York: Churchill Livingstone, 1986.

Plunkett PK, Wilkins RG, Edwards JD. Early management of spinal cord injury [letter]. Br Med J 1986;292:485.

Rolbin SH, Levinson G, Shnider SM, Wright RG. Anesthetic considerations for myasthenia gravis and pregnancy. Anesth Analg 1978;57:441.

Rothermel JE, Garcia A. Treatment of hip fractures in patients with Parkinson's syndrome on levodopa therapy. J Bone Joint Surg 1972;54[A]:1251.

Siemkowicz E. Multiple sclerosis and surgery. Anaesthesia 1976;31:1211.

Smeltzer SC, Utell MJ, Rudick RA, Herndon RM. Pulmonary function and dysfunction in multiple sclerosis. Arch Neurol 1988;-45:1245.

Stjernberg L, Blumberg H, Wallin BG. Sympathetic activity in man after spinal cord injury. Brain 1986;109:695.

Stjernberg L. Cutaneous vasomotor sensitivity to noradrenalin in spinal and intact man. Scand J Rehab Med 1986;18:127.

Stone WA, Beach TP, Hamelberg W. Succinylcholine: danger in the spinal cord injured patient. Anesthesiology 1970;32:168.

Taylor P. Anticholinesterase agents. In: Gilman AG, Goodman LS, Rall TW, Murad F, eds. Goodman and Gilman's the pharmacological basis of therapeutics. 7th ed. New York: Macmillan, 1985:110.

Taylor P. Neuromuscular blocking agents. In: Gilman AG, Goodman LS, Rall TW, Murad F, eds. Goodman and Gilman's the pharmacological basis of therapeutics. 7th ed. New York: Macmillan, 1985:222.

Vacanti CA, Ali HH, Schweiss JF, Scott RP. The response of myasthenia gravis to atracurium. Anesthesiology 1985;62:692.

Ward S, Wright DJ. Neuromuscular blockade in myasthenia gravis with atracurium besylate. Anaesthesia 1984;39:51.

Weiner N. Atropine, scopolamine, and related antimuscarine drugs. In: Gilman AG, Goodman LS, Rall TW, Murad F, eds. Goodman and Gilman's the pharmacological basis of therapeutics. 7th ed. New York: Macmillan, 1985:130.

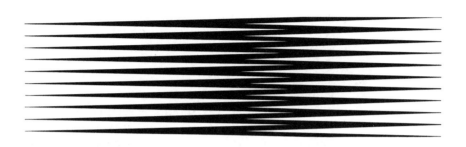

Gastrointestinal System Disorders

Eugene Y. Cheng
Jonathan Kay

Gastrointestinal and Pancreatic Disease

I. GASTROINTESTINAL DISEASE
    A. Anesthetic Concerns
        1. Hypovolemia
        Hypovolemia may result from ileus or bowel obstruction from poor oral intake, intraluminal collection of fluid, or gastrointestinal (GI) bleeding. Dangerous hypotension may occur on induction unless volume is restored and induction medication dosage decreased.
        2. Aspiration
        Pulmonary aspiration is a threat with any of these disorders. The airway should be secured by awake intubation if there is any uncertainty as to the patient's ability to tolerate a rapid-sequence induction or if intubation appears problematic. The presence of an endotracheal tube is incomplete protection against aspiration: several studies have documented the leak of gastric contents past inflated endotracheal and tracheostomy tube cuffs into the lungs. It is therefore prudent to keep the stomach well drained by nasogastric suction during intubation and to suction the pharynx periodically.
        3. Metabolic acidosis
        Metabolic acidosis from elevated lactate may be severe in the case of bowel infarction. A non–anion-gap (hyperchloremic) acidosis may be caused by nasogastric suction in the duodenum or by protracted diarrhea (bicarbonate loss from the pancreas or colon, respectively). Acidosis should be corrected as soon as possible, certainly prior to any surgical procedure, and the underlying problem eliminated.
        4. Splanchnic hypoperfusion
        Decreased splanchnic blood flow may result from beta-blocking drugs or alpha-agonist medications used to decrease GI bleeding, especially that from esophageal and gastric varices. Splanchnic blood flow can be enhanced by optimizing preload and with low-dose (2–4 µg/kg per min) dopamine infusion.
    B. Anesthetic Recommendations
        1. There is no specific preferred anesthetic technique. The most important factor in providing a safe anesthetic is good preoperative preparation.

2. Hypovolemia, if corrected before induction, will minimize problems with hypotension. Also, low intraoperative urine output will not be as troublesome with a full intravascular volume. A central venous catheter will provide a secure access for multiple fluid challenges and a port for vasoactive drugs if necessary. In older patients, especially those with underlying pulmonary and cardiovascular problems, a pulmonary artery catheter is indicated to help titrate fluid and vasoactive drug therapy.

3. These patients must all be considered as having full stomachs and at high risk for aspiration. Many patients will have a nasogastric (NG) tube already in place. Placing the tube to suction prior to induction will help decrease gastric volume and distention. Using H_2 antagonists will increase gastric pH. Metaclopramide is not recommended in patients with ileus or GI obstruction.

4. Postoperative fluid shifts from the intravascular space to the extravascular space are common. Careful attention to the intravascular volume status is important for hemodynamic stability and renal perfusion. Patients should be extubated only when fully awake and with recovered airway protective reflexes.

II. PANCREATITIS

Pancreatitis is an autolytic process, typically induced by trauma or alcoholism. Although it mandates no specific anesthetic technique, there are specific concerns for anesthesiologists.

A. Hypovolemia can be the consequence of the ascites and peritonitis that typically accompany severe pancreatitis.

B. Hypocalcemia may be multifactorial in etiology. One cause is the sequestration of Ca^{++} during the saponification of peripancreatic fat. Measurement of ionized calcium levels is required for diagnosis and to follow therapy. Restoration of normal levels is likely to improve myocontractility and coagulation.

C. Hypoglycemia or hyperglycemia can result from disordered insulin and glucagon synthesis and release.

D. Noncardiogenic pulmonary edema and disseminated intravascular coagulopathy (DIC) may accompany acute pancreatitis and probably result from circulating products of pancreatic cell lysis and circulating lytic enzymes.

Arterial blood gases and coagulation panels should be obtained early if any clinical suspicion of these disorders arises.

E. The "full stomach" states of these patients makes rapid-sequence induction and airway protection important anesthetic considerations.

Liver Disease

Hepatic dysfunction presents a special set of considerations in the anesthetic care of the critically ill patient. A number of studies performed since the 1960s have documented the variable, but generally high, mortality rate (5% to 70%) of patients with severe hepatic disease undergoing major surgical procedures. Recently, many anesthesiologists have developed expertise in the perioperative management of liver failure, in large part because of knowledge and skill gained from caring for liver transplant patients.

The key to successful anesthetic management of the patient with liver disease is preoperative assessment and preparation for likely complications. The three principal problems are altered drug metabolism, impaired energy substrate utilization, and abnormal coagulation.

I.   ALTERED METABOLIC ACTIVITIES
A. Protein Metabolism
1. The liver synthesizes coagulation enzyme precursors as well as fibrinolytic enzymes and inhibitors. Hemostasis is commonly impaired in hepatic disease, and the degree of impairment is an indication of the degree of liver dysfunction.
2. Diminished albumin production will affect protein binding, which may alter drug potency and duration (see below).
3. Pseudocholinesterase is produced by the liver; severe hepatic dysfunction may, rarely, prolong the action of succinylcholine.
B. Bilirubin Metabolism
1. Normally, most bilirubin in the body is eliminated by hepatic conjugation and subsequent excretion of the conjugates in the bile. In patients with hepatic dysfunction, large quantities of unconjugated bilirubin may appear.

2. Complications of increased bilirubin
   a. Cerebral O_2 consumption is increased by hyperbilirubinemia, which may render the central nervous system more susceptible to ischemic and hypoxic insults.
   b. Hyperbilirubinemia is a risk factor for the perioperative development of acute tubular necrosis.
   c. Hyperbilirubinemia may alter drug pharmacokinetics and pharmacodynamics by displacing drugs from albumin binding sites.

C. Glucose and Lactate Metabolism
   1. Hepatocytes are the primary site of gluconeogenesis. Hypoglycemia is associated with fulminant hepatitis because of the lack of glycogen stores and impaired gluconeogenesis.
   2. Anion-gap metabolic acidosis is a frequent complication of severe hepatic insufficiency because of the liver's impaired ability to metabolize lactate.

D. Drug Pharmacokinetics and Pharmacodynamics
   1. Decreased albumin enhances the immediate potency of numerous drugs (morphine, diazepam, etomidate, phenytoin, thiopental, quinidine) by leaving a higher fraction in the active, nonprotein-bound state. This effect may be further enhanced by hyperbilirubinemia, as bilirubin competes with these drugs for albumin binding sites.
   2. An increase in the effective volume of distribution is common in hepatic disease. A lower concentration of drug may actually be presented to the liver for metabolism. This, in addition to the decrease in metabolism by the impaired hepatocytes, will prolong drug effect.
   3. Duration of action is not prolonged for single-bolus injections of most opiates, sedatives, or hypnotics because of rapid distribution. Prolonged action might be expected with multiple doses of barbiturates or other long-acting intravenous drugs.
   4. The nondepolarizing muscle relaxants *d*-tubocurarine and pancuronium demonstrate an increased volume of distribution in hepatic failure, which decreases their apparent potency. Vecuronium, pancuronium and *d*-tubocurarine all exhibit decreased

clearance in hepatic insufficiency, which will prolong their duration of action between 50% and 100%. Rarely, the duration of action of succinylcholine is prolonged because of a deficiency in pseudocholinesterase. The prolongation is not as profound as that seen with genetically defective pseudocholinesterase. Atracurium undergoes metabolism by Hoffman's elimination; therefore, its effect is not prolonged in patients with liver failure.

5. Meperidine, morphine, and alfentanil exhibit increased potency secondary to decreased protein binding. Meperidine and alfentanil clearance is decreased, prolonging the duration of action (100% increase); morphine kinetics are unchanged. Fentanyl pharmacodynamics and pharmacokinetics do not appear to be altered in cirrhosis. Normally, sufentanil is highly protein bound. Its protein binding can be expected to decrease during acute hepatic disease. Its duration of action would be expected to be prolonged secondary both to the increased volume of distribution and to impaired hepatic metabolism, although confirming data are not available.

6. Intravenous benzodiazepines (diazepam, chlordiazepoxide, and midazolam) exhibit decreased clearance and prolonged duration of action in liver disease. Lorazepam, another benzodiazepine given intravenously, is not metabolized by the liver oxidative system; rather, it is renally excreted after glucuronidation. Clearance of this drug is minimally affected by liver failure. In general, benzodiazepines exhibit an apparent increase in potency and duration in hepatic disease because of decreased protein binding and potentiation of hepatic encephalopathy.

7. Inhalation anesthetics' pharmacodynamics and pharmacokinetics are not discernibly altered.

II. COMPLICATIONS
A. Hypoxemia
Intrapulmonary shunting, with resultant hypoxemia, is an occasional feature of long-standing hepatic insufficiency. The mechanism is not well understood, and the phenomenon does not reverse rapidly after liver transplantation. The hypoxemia may not be responsive

to supplemental oxygen and positive end expiratory pressure.

B. High-Output Failure

Cirrhotics often have a high cardiac output and low systemic blood pressure secondary to systemic vasodilation and increased arterial–venous shunting. Severe hepatic dysfunction can induce a high-output shock state that may be attributable to endotoxemia without other signs of infection.

C. Hepatic Encephalopathy

1. Progressive stupor leading to coma is a grave complication of severe hepatic dysfunction.

2. The pathophysiology of hepatic encephalopathy is not well understood; a high blood ammonia concentration is typically associated with depressed mental status, although ammonia may not be the primary etiologic agent. False neurotransmitters such as octopamine and increased concentrations of inhibitory neurotransmitters such as gamma-aminobutyric acid may also have a role.

3. A high percentage (>30%) of patients with hepatic coma have cerebral edema, which may cause cerebral ischemia, herniation, and death. Cerebral edema from liver failure responds well to osmotic diuresis. Steroids are ineffective.

4. Patients with Reye's syndrome present with encephalopathy, intracranial hypertension, and hepatocellular injury. This condition is rare and usually (although not invariably) limited to the pediatric population following a characteristic viral prodrome. Prompt diagnosis is important because intracranial hypertension is particularly severe in Reye's syndrome, and the key to successful outcome is the aggressive reduction of intracranial pressure.

D. Portal Hypertension and Ascites

1. Hepatic venous obstruction (portal and intrahepatic hypertension) is a prerequisite for the development of ascites in most cases of liver disease. Increases in hydrostatic pressure along the length of the hepatic sinusoids causes a transudation of plasma, which eventually overcomes the ability of the lymphatics to return lymph to the systemic circulation. Excess lymphatic fluid then accumulates in the peritoneal cavity.

2. Expansion of the splanchnic circulation, the development of extensive portosystemic collateral channels, and the loss of lymphatic fluid leads to a decreased effective intravascular volume. The reduction in circulating volume causes the release of antidiuretic hormone and activation of the renin–angiotensin–aldosterone system, which will lead to more fluid retention.

3. Ascites may cause a restrictive pulmonary defect by limiting diaphragmatic and chest wall motion. In addition, ascites may displace the diaphragm upward against the lungs, causing atelectasis and hypoxemia.

4. The presence of esophageal varices should be assumed in patients with ascites unless specifically excluded. The potential for esophageal varices, combined with thrombocytopenia from associated hypersplenism and coagulopathy, make GI bleeding a common problem for these patients. This increases the risks of occult hypovolemia and blood aspiration.

E. Metabolic Acidosis

1. Lactic acid is often responsible for the metabolic acidosis in patients with liver failure. This results from increased production because of high-output failure and decreased liver metabolism.

2. Management of lactic acidosis is initially with sodium bicarbonate to keep the pH above 7.2. If the patient is intubated, hyperventilation may be used. The underlying cause of lactic acidosis must be sought and aggressively treated. The buffer tris-hydroxymethylaminomethane (THAM) is an alternative to sodium bicarbonate, especially if CO_2 production from sodium bicarbonate is of significant concern.

3. Alternatives to bicarbonate administration currently under investigation include dichloroacetate, which stimulates pyruvate dehydrogenase (the rate-limiting enzyme for aerobic metabolism of pyruvate), and "carbicarb," an equimolar solution of sodium carbonate and sodium bicarbonate, which buffers without changing CO_2 levels. Neither is available for clinical use at this time.

III. PREOPERATIVE ASSESSMENT
    A. History
        Frequently, the patient will be encephalopathic or intubated and thus a "nonhistorian." A good physical examination, including a thorough neurologic evaluation, is often the basis of diagnosis and treatment. The ICU nurse is often helpful in providing insight into the patient's baseline neurologic function.
    B. Physical Examination
        1. The diagnosis of hepatic encephalopathy depends on documentation of mental obtundation, asterixis, and fetor hepaticus. Early symptoms are fatigue, lassitude, and drowsiness.
        2. Characteristic cutaneous manifestations include palmar erythema over the hypothenar region, spider angiomata, and a bronze discoloration. Large bruises or bleeding from vascular access sites is common if the patient has a coagulopathy. Petechiae indicate platelet dysfunction.
        3. Other typical findings include gynecomastia, testicular atrophy, and evidence of portal hypertension (splenomegaly, ascites, periumbilical varicosities).
        4. Acutely injured livers will usually be boggy and enlarged. The cirrhotic liver will be small and firm, and occasionally, large regenerative nodules will be felt on the surface.
        5. Portal hypertension increases the likelihood of esophageal varices and the risk of GI hemorrhage. With active bleeding, there is a characteristic odor, difficult to describe but unmistakable once experienced, that should alert the practitioner to the risk of aspiration on induction or to the presence of occult hypovolemia.
    C. Laboratory Evaluation
        1. Coagulation tests
            a. In patients who have biliary obstruction or cholestasis (and in patients who are malnourished or who have been on broad-spectrum antibiotics), there may be a deficiency of vitamin K-dependent factors (II, VII, IX, and X) resulting in a prolonged prothrombin time. Patients with such a coagulopathy should re-

ceive vitamin K (10 mg IV slowly or IM daily for 3 days) or fresh frozen plasma.

b. Partial thromboplastin time

The partial thromboplastin time is frequently prolonged, because the liver is responsible for producing many other coagulation factors (V, XI, XII, XIII, fibrinogen). Fresh frozen plasma is used to correct the problem.

c. Bleeding time

Platelets should be administered prior to surgery to correct a count less than 50,000. Hypersplenism may be the cause of thrombocytopenia, in which case platelet transfusion may be ineffective. In patients who are uremic or hyperbilirubinemic, platelet function should be assessed with a template bleeding time. If the bleeding time is prolonged, DDAVP (desmopressin) will promote platelet aggregation. Its clinical efficacy is documented in postcardiopulmonary bypass and in uremia.

2. Glucose

a. The liver is the primary site of lactate metabolism and gluconeogenesis and the main glycogen store in the body. With severe hepatocellular disease, hypoglycemia can occur secondary to impaired gluconeogenesis and low glycogen stores. If the patient is hypoglycemic, dextrose solutions should be titrated to maintain adequate blood glucose. In general, fluids containing dextrose should not be used for fluid challenges or as drug flushes because of the risk of causing hyperglycemia.

b. Hyperglycemia is the more common problem in critically ill patients with or without hepatic dysfunction and is caused by stress (elevated cortisol and catecholamines) and overfeeding.

c. Hyperalimentation can be continued during anesthesia. If for some reason hyperalimentation must be discontinued, the patient should be maintained on a 5% dextrose solution, and serum glucose determinations should be made to avoid rebound hypoglycemia.

3.   Arterial blood gases
Arterial blood gases should be checked prior to anesthesia to identify hypoxemia and pH alterations. Hypoxemia is usually multifactorial and may include an element of intrapulmonary shunting from hepatic failure. Patients with hepatic disease are more likely to hyperventilate spontaneously (respiratory alkalosis). Metabolic acidosis, if present, should be explored, and the serum anion gap ($[Na^+] - \{[Cl^-] + [HCO_3{}^-]\}$) should be calculated. If the anion gap is greater than 12, the presence of an occult anion (typically lactate) should be suspected, and serum lactate should be measured. Marked lactate elevation suggests either global hypoperfusion (cardiogenic or hypovolemic shock), specific tissue infarction (bowel or renal), sepsis, or severe hepatic dysfunction.

4.   Albumin, bilirubin, and ammonia
   a.   Hepatic dysfunction reduces the levels of albumin and total protein because of decreased production. The reduction in intravascular protein diminishes drug binding and enhances drug potency.
   b.   Hyperbilirubinemia may be secondary to biliary obstruction, hemolysis, or cholestasis. Cholestasis may result from sepsis, drugs, or hepatocellular injury. Hyperbilirubinemia increases cerebral metabolism. Bilirubin also occupies albumin binding sites for drugs, which increases free (nonprotein-bound) drug concentrations and hence potency.
   c.   Elevated ammonia is caused by the liver's inability to metabolize nitrogenous products, primarily amines and aromatic amino acids. Ideally, serum ammonia should be tested from an arterial sample to avoid the increased variability caused by muscle uptake. Ammonia is a marker for hepatic encephalopathy, and its level is increased by the inability of the liver to handle oral protein intake or the protein that results from GI bleeding. Lactulose, employed primarily as an acidifier and purgative in the

GI tract, helps reduce ammonia levels when given as an enema or by mouth.

5. Blood urea nitrogen and creatinine

a. Elevated BUN with normal creatinine (azotemia) usually marks diminished renal blood flow (prerenal state), whether secondary to maldistribution of cardiac output or to reduced intravascular volume.

b. The hepatorenal syndrome differs from acute tubular necrosis in that the kidneys are sodium avid (urine sodium <10 mEq/L) and there is no apparent renal parenchymal pathology. Nonetheless, it is associated with elevated BUN and creatinine and is usually unresponsive to maneuvers to improve renal blood flow (i.e., volume administration, low-dose dopamine).

c. Elevated creatinine is common in patients with severe hepatic disease and does not automatically imply the hepatorenal syndrome. Drug metabolism and excretion may be problematic in patients with combined hepatic and renal insufficiency.

6. Liver function tests

a. Hepatic enzymes are not always helpful in the assessment of hepatic dysfunction; these assays (AST [SGOT], ALT [SGPT], GGT) measure the enzymes released into the bloodstream by hepatocyte necrosis. Normal levels of enzymes may merely reflect an overall paucity of hepatocytes, as in end-stage cirrhosis, or may result from a liver that has undergone acute necrosis and is now "burned out." Nonetheless, it is prudent to assay these enzymes. An elevated level prior to anesthesia may reveal unsuspected hepatic dysfunction and can establish the existence of hepatocellular injury prior to exposure to anesthetic agents.

b. In obstructive or cholestatic liver disease, alkaline phosphatase and bilirubin will both be elevated. In hyperbilirubinemia secondary to hemolysis, lactate dehydrogenase (LDH) will be elevated, and the hematocrit will drop. Widespread hemolysis may cause a direct (conjugated) hyperbilirubinemia, because excretion appears to be the rate-limiting step in hemoglobin metabolism.

7. Hepatitis screen

    a. Any patient with acute hepatocellular injury (elevated AST, ALT, GGT) should be screened for viral hepatitis.

    b. Acute hepatitis A is diagnosed by the presence of specific IgM antibodies. Prior infection can be diagnosed with specific IgG antibodies. Although the infection is usually benign and self-limited, occasional cases of hepatitis A-induced fulminant hepatic failure are known.

    c. Active hepatitis B infection is diagnosed by the presence of hepatitis B surface antigen (HBsAg) in the blood. Hepatitis B surface antibody (HBsAb or anti-HBs) indicates either resolved infection or immunization. The hepatitis B antigen (HBeAg) is a marker of infectivity. The anti-hepatitis core antibody (anti-HBc) serves to identify those patients with hepatitis B whose HBsAg has decreased below detectable levels but who are still infected.

    d. Non-A, non-B hepatitis is a common cause of acute hepatitis. Diagnosis is suggested by elevation of serum AST and the presence of anti-HCV. Assay for anti-HCV is specific for non-A, non-B hepatitis.

    e. Delta-agent hepatitis is a diagnosis of exclusion. Delta agent superinfects patients with hepatitis B, increases the severity of the acute hepatitis, and increases the likelihood of the development of chronic active hepatitis, cirrhosis, and hepatoma.

    f. Screening high-risk groups (drug addicts, institutionalized patients, extensively transfused patients, hemophiliacs, and health workers with blood product exposure) and patients with obvious symptoms or signs of hepatic disease is reasonable. Although the results of such screening may not directly influence anesthetic management, appropriate protection for caregivers can be instituted, and the results may identify the cause of the hepatic dysfunction.

g.   A vaccine for hepatitis B is available. The series of three injections poses minimal cost and little risk and confers a high degree of protection against the virus and its complications (chronic active hepatitis, fulminant hepatic failure, death).

8.   Imaging studies
Specific diagnostic studies such as liver ultrasound, iminodiacetic acid scan, and technetium-labeled sulfur colloid scan can differentiate obstructive jaundice from the hyperbilirubinemia of cholestasis, hemolysis, or fulminant hepatic dysfunction.

IV.   ANESTHETIC CARE

A.   Preanesthetic Preparation
Cerebral edema, hypoglycemia, coagulopathy, and electrolyte and fluid imbalances should be treated prior to surgery rather than trying to correct the abnormalities in the early anesthetic period.

1.   Decreased intravascular volume is frequent in patients with severe liver disease. Use of lactulose for high ammonia levels, treatment of ascites or cerebral edema with diuretics, and poor nutritional states may all contribute to the problem. Preoperative hydration is frequently necessary to optimize preload. Excessive fluid administration must be guarded against, as it can worsen ascites and edema. A pulmonary artery catheter is helpful in this situation by virtue of its ability to estimate left ventricular preload and cardiac output.

2.   Coagulopathies from liver disease should be corrected preoperatively to help minimize bleeding during placement of invasive monitors and the surgical procedure.

3.   Anemia should be corrected to a hematocrit of approximately 30% to provide a buffer against the frequent occurrence of intraoperative bleeding.

4.   Electrolyte, metabolic, and glucose imbalance should be corrected preoperatively.

B.   Intraoperative Monitoring

1.   Routine monitors (ECG, esophageal stethoscope, temperature probe, noninvasive blood pressure, and pulse oximetry) should be utilized.

2. A Foley catheter should be employed to follow urine output.

3. Patients with hepatic failure usually are hemodynamically unstable and need arterial catheterization for continuous blood pressure and arterial blood gas analysis.

4. A pulmonary artery catheter will provide a more reliable indication of intravascular volume than a central venous catheter. Also, many hepatic failure patients have a limited cardiac reserve from high-output failure, and determination of cardiac output is helpful in titrating inotropic or vasopressive agents.

5. Serial arterial blood gases should be followed. Development of metabolic acidosis is a marker of tissue hypoperfusion.

6. Prothrombin and partial thromboplastin times, platelet count, and occasionally thromboelastography or sonoclot are used to identify causes of coagulopathies and guide replacement therapy.

C. Intraoperative Management

1. Induction of anesthesia

   a. Because of the unpredictable potency and duration of many drugs administered intravenously to patients with hepatic disease, caution should dictate therapy. An awake intubation with minimal intravenous medication may be preferable to a rapid-sequence induction. After awake intubation, titration of narcotics and benzodiazepines can be undertaken prior to paralysis to assess the patient's susceptibility to these drugs.

   b. Monitoring the effect on the neuromuscular junction of small incremental doses of relaxant will quickly alert the anesthesiologist to changes in potency and duration of these agents in individual patients.

2. Maintenance anesthesia

   a. Hepatic perfusion is a function of arterial blood pressure, splanchnic vascular resistance, and metabolic rate. The maintenance anesthetic will influence hepatic perfusion.

   b. Inhalational anesthesia tends to decrease splanchnic perfusion despite stable blood pressure. If an inhalational agent is to be used, isoflurane may be preferable because it has the least effect on splanchnic perfusion of the three currently used agents. Drug-induced hepatitis has been associated with halothane and, very rarely, with enflurane or isoflurane.

c. Nitrous oxide is an inhibitor of methionine synthetase in the liver, and after long use, patients may exhibit signs of vitamin B_{12} deficiency postoperatively. Chronic exposure studies in animals suggest that N_2O may be hepatotoxic. There is no supporting evidence in human studies.

d. Carefully titrated doses of intravenous narcotics and benzodiazepines are frequently sufficient to provide surgical planes of anesthesia, especially if augmented by supplemental N_2O (if pulmonary status allows) or "light" inhalation anesthesia. Splanchnic perfusion may, however, be decreased with this technique despite stable blood pressure because of different regional responses to catecholamines. Large doses of intravenous anesthetics should be avoided unless a period of postoperative mechanical ventilation is anticipated and acceptable.

e. Reversal of neuromuscular blockade requires special diligence in patients with severe hepatic dysfunction. Unforeseen alterations in the kinetics of neuromuscular blockers and reversal drugs makes blockade monitoring desirable.

f. Spinal and epidural anesthesia effectively blocks sympathetically induced decreases in splanchnic blood flow. However, if blood pressure is not maintained, there will be a parallel drop in hepatic perfusion. The maintenance of systemic pressure with vasopressors may not restore regional hepatic blood flow.

V. POSTOPERATIVE CARE

Patients with severe liver dysfunction often have dysfunction or failure of other organ systems. These patients are most prudently left on mechanical ventilator support until consciousness and respiratory adequacy are clearly established.

VI. Invasive monitors should be observed carefully to help ensure adequate intravascular volume and cardiac output. Any significant change from the patient's normal state can cause the hepatorenal syndrome.

SUMMARY OF ANESTHETIC CONSIDERATIONS

Liver failure patients are at high risk for perianesthetic complications from alteration of drug distribution and elimination, coagulopathies, fluid and electrolyte imbalance, tenuous cardiovascular reserve, and compromised pulmonary status. Preoperatively, coagulopathy should be corrected with vitamin K, fresh frozen plasma, or cryoprecipitate. Decreasing ascites with a good diuretic regimen will help improve pulmonary and cardiovascular function. Correcting a poor nutrition state will improve liver metabolism, protein production, and fluid–electrolyte balance. Lactulose should be used to reduce ammonia levels and improve mental status before surgery.

Intraoperative monitoring should include arterial catheterization and central venous catheters in patients with liver disease significant enough to cause ascites, pulmonary dysfunction, and a high cardiac output state. In these patients, serum protein is low and the volume of distribution is increased. This can produce an initial increase in the potency of intravenous drugs and a longer duration of action. All inhaled anesthetics decrease hepatic perfusion, but isoflurane causes the smallest decrease and thus may be the best inhaled agent for maintenance anesthesia. Spinal and epidural anesthesia can be used in patients with liver failure if coagulopathy is not a problem. Splanchnic blood flow is preserved in these patients because of the block of sympathetically induced vasoconstriction. However, if cardiac output and blood pressure are not maintained, there will be a parallel drop in hepatic perfusion.

Postoperative ventilatory support and invasive monitoring should be continued in patients with severe liver disease until consciousness and cardiorespiratory adequacy are established.

Recommended Reading

Bihari DJ, Gimson AES, Williams R. Cardiovascular, pulmonary and renal complications of fulminant hepatic failure. Semin Liver Dis 1986; 6:119.

Bihari D, Gimson AES, Lindridge J, et al. Lactic acidosis in fulminant hepatic failure: some aspects of pathogenesis and prognosis. J Hepatol 1985; 1:405.

Brown BR Jr, ed. Anesthesia and the patient with liver disease. Philadelphia: FA Davis, 1981.

Browne RA, Chernesky MA. Viral hepatitis and the anaesthetist. Can Anaesth Soc J 1984; 31:279.

Cameron AG. Acute respiratory failure in acute pancreatitis. Anaesth Intens Care 1975; 3:244.

Flute PT. Clotting abnormalities in liver disease. In: Progress in liver disease, vol VI. New York: Grune & Stratton, 1979:301.

Fraser CL, Arieff AL. Hepatic encephalopathy. N Engl J Med 1985; 313:865.

Friedman LS, Maddrey WC. Surgery in the patient with liver disease. Med Clin North Am 1987; 71:453.

Kaplowitz N, Aw TY, Simon FR, Stolz A. Drug induced hepatotoxicity [review]. Ann Intern Med 1986; 104:826.

Kreisberg RA. Pathogenesis and management of lactic acidosis. Annu Rev Med 1984; 35:181.

Krowka MJ, Cortese DA. Pulmonary aspects of chronic liver disease and liver transplantation. Mayo Clin Proc 1985; 60:407.

McCammon RL. Diseases of the liver and biliary tract. In: Stoelting RK, Dierdorf SF, eds. Anesthesia and co-existing diseases. New York: Churchill Livingstone, 1983:327.

McCammon RL. The gastrointestinal system. In: Stoelting RK, Dierdorf SF, eds. Anesthesia and co-existing diseases. New York: Churchill Livingstone, 1983:363.

McCloy RF. Metabolic problems associated with gastrointestinal and pancreatic disease. Br J Anaesth 1984; 56:83.

Russell GJ, Fitzgerald JF, Clark JH. Fulminant hepatic failure. J Pediatr 1987; 111:313.

Saik RP, Chadwick C, Katz J. Gastrointestinal disorders. In: Katz J, Benumof J, Kadis LB, eds. Anesthesia and uncommon diseases. Philadelphia: WB Saunders, 1981:384.

Secor JW, Schenker S. Drug metabolism in patients with liver disease. Adv Intern Med 1987; 32:379.

Williams RL, Mamelok RD. Hepatic disease and drug pharmacokinetics. Clin Pharmacokinet 1980; 5:528.

Wood M. Plasma drug binding: Implications for anesthesiologists. Anesth Analg 1986; 65:786.

CHAPTER
7

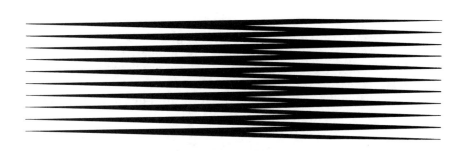

Endocrine Disorders

Jonathan Kay

≡ Diabetes Mellitus

Diabetes mellitus is chronic systemic disease caused by a relative or absolute lack of insulin. Its primary manifestations are hyperglycemia, glycosuria, and degeneration of the small vessels.

I.   DIAGNOSIS AND CLASSIFICATION
  A. Diagnosis
      Serum glucose is measured every 30 minutes after a standard oral glucose load. Serum glucose levels that remain inappropriately elevated are indicative of a diabetic state. Specific diagnostic criteria are listed in Table 7-1.
  B. Classification
      1. Type 1: juvenile-onset, insulin-dependent, or keto-acidosis-prone (IDDM).
      2. Type 2: maturity-onset, non-ketosis-prone, non-insulin-dependent (NIDDM).
  C. Etiology
      1. A possible mechanism for Type 1 diabetes involves attack by the immune system on the pancreas brought on by a viral illness. There is a genetic component, as indicated by the common association with certain HLA types.
      2. Type 2 diabetes may be inherited in either an autosomal dominant or a recessive pattern. Obesity causes endogenous insulin resistance and contributes to the development of the disorder.

II. INSULIN PHYSIOLOGY
  A. Insulin is a polypeptide anabolic hormone secreted by pancreatic beta cells. The normal daily output is 50 units (approximately 2U/hour).

Table 7–1.   Interpretation of Glucose Tolerance Test Results

Timing of Sampling after Glucose Load (minutes)	Blood glucose concentrations (mg/dl)	
	Nondiabetic	*Diabetic*
Control	<100	>110
30	<160	>160
60	<160	>160
90	<140	>140
120	100–110	>120

(Stoelting RK, Dierdorf SF, eds. Anesthesia and co-existing disease. 2nd ed. New York: Churchill Livingstone, 1988.)

B. The effects of insulin include facilitation of glucose transfer across cell membranes into cells. Insulin enhances glycogen formation while inhibiting lipolysis and gluconeogenesis and promotes the transport of glucose into adipose tissue for conversion to and storage as fatty acids. It also enhances the passage of potassium into cells along with glucose.

C. Fasting causes a decline in insulin levels, which, in turn, forces catabolic hormones to maintain blood glucose concentrations at the expense of tissue breakdown. During surgery, the release of cortisol and catecholamines results in insulin resistance. This effect is most dramatic during hypothermic cardiopulmonary bypass.

III. TREATMENT

A. Oral Hypoglycemics (NIDDM)

1. Oral hypoglycemic agents (Tables 7-2 and 7-3) are usually given when diet alone does not control glucose in NIDDM. They stimulate insulin release from pancreatic beta cells.

2. Side effects

   a. The drugs enhance the effects of thiazide diuretics, barbiturates, and anticoagulants.

   b. They may cause prolonged hypoglycemia and lactic acidosis (phenformin) and possibly are associated with an increased risk of sudden death.

B. Insulin

1. There are several insulin preparations (Table 7-4). The most frequently used regimen combines NPH or lente insulin, the intermediate-acting form, with

Table 7–2. Oral Hypoglycemic Drugs

Category	Generic Name	Trade Name
Sulfonylureas	Tolbutamide	Orinase
	Acetohexamide	Dymelor
	Tolazamide	Tolinase
	Chlorpropamide	Diabinese
	Glipizide	Glucotrol
	Glyburide	DiaBeta, Micronase
Biguanides	Phenformin	DBI, Metrol

(Stoelting RK, Dierdorf SF, eds. Anesthesia and co-existing disease. 2nd ed. New York: Churchill Livingstone, 1988.)

Table 7–3. Comparison of Sulfonylureas

	Tolbutamide	Acetohexamide	Tolazamide	Chlorpropamide	Glipizide	Glyburide
Relative potency	1	25	5	5	100	150
Duration (hr)	6–8	8–12	12–18	24–72	12–18	16–24
Daily dose	0.5–3 g	0.25–1.5 g	0.1–1 g	0.1–0.5 g	2.5–30 mg	1.25–20 mg
Doses per day	2 or 3	1 or 2	1 or 2	1	1 or 2	1 or 2
Inactivation	Hepatic	Renal	Hepatic	Hepatic/renal	Hepatic	Hepatic
Diuretic	Yes?	Yes	Yes	No	No	Yes
Antidiuretic	Yes?	No	No	Yes	No	No
Antabuse effect	No	No	No	Yes	No	No
Frequency of hypoglycemia	Rare	<1%	<1%	2%–3%	3%–5%	4%–6%

(Oh MS, Carroll HJ. Electrolyte and acid–base disorders. In: Chernow B, ed. The pharmacologic approach to the critically ill patient. Baltimore, Williams & Wilkins, 1988.)

Table 7–4. Insulin Preparations

Type of Insulin	Action	Protein	Peak Action (hr)*	Duration (hr)*	Route	Dose (U/ml)
Regular (crystalline)[†]	Rapid	None	1–3	5–7	IV, SC, IM	100, 500
Semilente	Rapid	None	2–4	10–16	SC	100
NPH[†‡]	Intermediate	Protamine	6–14	18–28	SC	100
Lente[†]	Intermediate	None	6–14	18–28	SC	100
Ultralente	Prolonged	None	18–24	30–40	SC	100
PZI[‡]	Prolonged	Protamine	18–24	30–40	SC	100

* After subcutaneous injection. [†] Available as human insulin. [‡] NPH = neutral protamine; PZI = protamine zinc.
(Oh MS, Carroll HJ. Electrolyte and acid–base disorders. In: Chernow B, ed. The pharmacologic approach to the critically ill patient. Baltimore: Williams & Wilkins, 1988.)

regular insulin before breakfast and again before the evening meal.

2. Side effects

   a. The Somogi effect is the morning glycosuria associated with rebound hyperglycemia from insulin-induced hypoglycemia at night. Its discovery should call for reduction of the evening dose of long-acting insulin.

   b. Patients who have been treated with protamine-containing insulin preparations are 50 times more likely to have life-threatening allergic reactions to intravenous protamine used to reverse the effects of heparin.

IV. COMPLICATIONS WITH ANESTHETIC IMPLICATIONS

   A. Atherosclerosis

   Accelerated atherosclerosis accounts for the high incidence in diabetics of myocardial infarction, cerebrovascular accident, and peripheral vascular disease at an early age. A 20-year-old patient with 10 years of IDDM is similar to a much older person in the likelihood of coronary disease.

   B. Microangiopathy

   Thickened and leaky capillary walls most commonly affect the kidneys and eyes, with consequent proteinuria, azotemia, and blindness. The proteinuria reduces the serum albumin level, which, in turn, reduces the gradient between the colloid osmotic pressure and pulmonary artery occlusion pressure, making pulmonary edema more likely in this group of patients.

   C. Neuropathy

   Segmental demyelination from microangiopathy of the vasa nervorum results in significant neurologic deficits of importance to the anesthesiologist. Orthostatic hypotension may occur secondary to lack of vasoconstriction as a result of sympathetic dysfunction. Resting tachycardia is common, as is loss of the normal beat-to-beat variability. These last two phenomena may represent parasympathetic excess, and diabetics may be resistant to atropine as a result. Gastroparesis (delayed gastric emptying) makes airway management more hazardous because of the likelihood of the stomach being full even many hours after a meal. Painless myocardial infarction is more common, and autonomic nervous system dysfunction is a predisposing factor in cardiac arrest in diabetics.

IV.   MANAGEMENT OF ANESTHESIA
The goals are to avoid hypoglycemia and ketoacidosis and to maintain blood glucose in a reasonable range perioperatively.

A.   Preoperative Evaluation

1.   It is necessary to know whether the patient is insulin dependent and the current regimen and quality of blood sugar control. A high glycosylated hemoglobin level implies long-term poor control. It is essential to confirm the absence of ketoacidosis, as this condition is an absolute contraindication to elective surgery.

2.   A search must be made for end-organ dysfunction, the patient being examined for signs of coronary and cerebrovascular disease, hypertension, renal dysfunction, peripheral neuropathy, and autonomic nervous system dysfunction. The examiner should ask specifically about early satiety, lack of sweating, lack of pulse rate change with orthostatic maneuvers, impotence, and paroxysmal nausea or vomiting.

B.   Management of Glucose Perioperatively

1.   If the patient can be scheduled for surgery early in the day, there is less need for repeatedly altering intravenous glucose and hypoglycemic agents when the patient is not under direct observation.

2.   Oral hypoglycemics are best withheld the evening before surgery because of their ability to produce hypoglycemia 24 to 36 hours after their administration. If glucose control is needed, human insulin is recommended. Insulin derived from animal sources is associated with rapid development of resistance to insulin effect with intermittent dosing.

3.   For insulin-dependent diabetics having minor surgery, two regimens are popular.

a.   "No insulin—no glucose." The fasting diabetic is given no insulin or glucose before surgery. Glucose is monitored with one of the readily available glucometers, analyzing blood obtained from a finger stick for rapid bedside results. Values are adjusted with a sliding scale of intravenous regular human insulin. With this method, high glucose values may occur perioperatively, but no adverse sequelae have been noted clinically despite higher levels of cortisol and glucagon and a more negative nitrogen balance.

b. On call to surgery, an intravenous infusion of 5% glucose in water is begun at 100 to 150 ml/hour. One half to $1/3$ of the usual NPH or lente insulin dose is given subcutaneously. Glucose is measured before the fluid infusion is started, and the value recorded on the front of the chart. Glucose is measured 15 minutes after surgery starts, approximately 1 hour after each insulin bolus, and again in the postanesthetic care unit by a glucometer. Subsequent regular insulin doses are given intravenously based on a sliding scale (10 U for more than 400 mg/dl down to 2 U for 200–250 mg/dl).

4. Insulin-dependent diabetics having major surgery

a. Plasma glucose and potassium are determined the morning of surgery, with the results posted to the front of the chart before the patient arrives in the operating room. An infusion of 5% glucose in water is begun at 100 ml/hour. "Piggybacked" to this infusion, an insulin drip of 25 U in 250 ml of normal saline is begun according to the equation:

$$\text{Insulin (U/hour)} = \frac{\text{plasma glucose (mg/dl)}}{150}$$

(A bolus of 25 ml of this solution is flushed through the tubing before starting the insulin drip to saturate the insulin binding sites of the polyvinylchloride).

b. If the patient is receiving corticosteroids, is markedly obese, or has an infection, the equation is modified to:

$$\text{Insulin (U/hour)} = \frac{\text{plasma glucose (mg/dl)}}{100}$$

c. Serum glucose is measured every hour by either a glucometer or the hospital laboratory, and the infusion is adjusted accordingly using the insulin infusion formula to maintain serum glucose at 120 to 200 mg/dl.

d.   See the sample orders in the display below for insulin management of patients undergoing myocardial revascularization.

Preoperative and Postoperative Orders for Diabetic Patients Undergoing Myocardial Revascularization

PRE- AND POSTOPERATIVE ORDERS

Before surgery, measure glycohemoglobin.

On the day of surgery, do AccuChek on call to operating room. If greater than 180 mg/dl, give 6 U of Humulin regular insulin subcutaneously.

Measure glucose on arrival in cardiovascular ICU.

Start infusion of 100 U of Humulin regular insulin in 250 ml of 5% glucose in water at appropriate rate (No. 1 below). Run first 50 ml of infusion through tubing and discard.

AccuChek glucose every 2 hours and record findings on diabetic record sheet.

Adjust insulin infusion per hour as follows using Accu-Chek:

AccuChek (mg/dl)	Insulin Infusion (No. 1)	Restart Insulin Infusion (No. 2)
<110	None	None
110–150	5 ml (2 U)	3 ml (1.2 U)
151–200	10 ml (4 U)	5 ml (2 U)
201–250	20 ml (8 U)	15 ml (6 U)
>250	30 ml (12 U)	25 ml (10 U)

If insulin infusion is interrupted because glucose is below 110 mg/dl, do AccuChek hourly until glucose exceeds 110 mg/dl. Then restart modified infusion per No. 2 above.

If glucose is consistently less than 150 mg/dl, AccuChek can be performed every 2 to 4 hours as needed.

If AccuChek result is not below 200 mg/dl within 6 hours after patient arrives in cardiovascular ICU, increase rate of infusion to 40 ml (16 U per hour) until AccuChek is below 200 mg/dl.

For signs of hypoglycemia, do immediate AccuChek. If result is below 100 mg/dl, stop infusion and give half an ampule of 5% glucose in water IV.

Immediately before transfer of patient from cardiovascular ICU, stop insulin infusion and give 15 U of human NPH Insulin and 4 units of human Regular Insulin subcutaneously.

Subsequent insulin orders by: _____

_____ M.D.
(Signature)

(Courtesy of Dr. James Findling and Dr. Joseph Shaker, St. Luke's Medical Center, Milwaukee, Wisconsin.)

≡ Adrenal Disorders

I. PHYSIOLOGY OF ADRENAL HORMONES
   A. Glucocorticoids (Cortisol)
      1. Cortisol regulates carbohydrate, protein, lipid, and nucleic acid metabolism. The hormone works by binding to stereospecific intracellular cytoplasmic receptors, which stimulate specific mRNA that modulates the production of regulatory proteins.
      2. The serum half-life of cortisol is 80 to 110 minutes, but because its effects are exerted via intracellular receptors, the serum values vastly underestimate the duration of the effects. The effects of a single dose on glucose and pulmonary function can last as long as 24 hours. Treatment schedules are based on

twice-daily dosing to simulate the normal diurnal variation in cortisol level.

3. The normal output of cortisol is 30 mg/day, with maximal output thought to be between 150 to 300 mg. More than 30 mg is considered supraphysiologic and will cause mineralocorticoid effects, including salt and water retention, loss of potassium and hydrogen, and increase in serum bicarbonate.

4. Cortisol secretion is under the control of both the hypothalamus and the pituitary, with closed feedback loops to each.

B. Mineralocorticoids (Aldosterone)

1. Aldosterone is produced by the zona glomerulosa of the adrenal cortex. It causes reabsorption of sodium and secretion of potassium and hydrogen, predominantly in the distal renal tubule.

2. Aldosterone is regulated by the renin–angiotensin system. Decreases in renal perfusion pressure or intravascular volume trigger the release of renin from the juxtaglomerular cells in the macula densa located by renal afferent arterioles. Renin, in turn, converts angiotensinogen to angiotensin I, which is converted to angiotensin II in the lung. Angiotensin II stimulates the secretion of aldosterone.

II. EXCESS ADRENOCORTICAL HORMONE

A. The most common cause of glucocorticoid excess (Cushing's syndrome) is iatrogenic. Other causes are adrenal hyperplasia, adenoma, and carcinoma.

B. Symptoms and signs include moon facies, plethora, centripetal fat distribution, easy bruising, striae, hypertension (85%), diabetes mellitus (60%), mental status changes (46%), pathologic fractures secondary to osteopenia (38%), and renal calculi (20%).

C. Anesthetic Considerations

1. Common problems such as hypertension, diabetes mellitus, and intravascular volume depletion should be anticipated and treated before surgery.

2. Potassium should be restored in these patients, who have a tendency to hypokalemic metabolic alkalosis.

3. Gentle patient positioning is important because of the higher incidence of pathologic fractures.

4. If bilateral adrenal resection or manipulation is performed, replacement with 100 mg hydrocortisone

intravenously is begun before the incision. Hydrocortisone (100 mg) is then given every 12 hours as a continuous infusion, with gradual reduction to 20 to 30 mg/day over about 1 week.

5. Neuromuscular blocking agents may have enhanced potency because of the skeletal weakness common in these patients. A nerve stimulator should be used to monitor neuromuscular blockade.

III. HYPERALDOSTERONISM (CONN'S SYNDROME)

A. Primary aldosteronism results from excess secretion of aldosterone by a functional tumor independent of a physiologic stimulus. Secondary hyperaldosteronism is present when increased renin secretion is responsible for the excess aldosterone levels.

B. Signs and Symptoms
The signs and symptoms of hyperaldosteronism include those of increased sodium retention, which leads to volume-dependent blood pressure elevation. Aldosterone excess promotes renal excretion of potassium, resulting in hypokalemic metabolic alkalosis. Glucose tolerance is impaired in 50% of patients. The persistent hypokalemia may result in polyuric nephropathy.

C. Diagnostic Criteria
An increase in plasma aldosterone associated with increased urinary potassium (>30 mEq/dl) with hypokalemia is diagnostic. Selective adrenal venography and radionuclide scanning are helpful to distinguish hyperaldosteronism from functional tumors or adrenal hyperplasia.

D. Treatment and Anesthetic Management

1. Hyperaldosteronism is initially treated with potassium supplementation and a competitive aldosterone antagonist (e.g., spironolactone). If adrenal cortical hyperplasia is the cause, spironolactone may suffice.

2. Definitive therapy for aldosterone-secreting tumors is surgical excision.

3. Scrupulous volume assessment and potassium replacement are the cornerstones of anesthetic management.

4. Supplementation of cortisol will be necessary for bilateral mobilization of the adrenal glands even if resection is not performed (see section on adrenal insufficiency for dose regimens).

IV.   PHEOCHROMOCYTOMA

    A.   Pathophysiology

        1.   Pheochromocytoma is a catecholamine-secreting tumor originating in the adrenal medulla or in chromaffin tissue along the paravertebral sympathetic chain. Ninety-five per cent of these tumors are found in the abdominal cavity, 90% in the adrenal gland. Ten per cent of the time, both adrenal glands are involved.

        2.   Familial pheochromocytoma occurs in association with medullary carcinoma of the thyroid and parathyroid adenoma and is designated Sipple's syndrome or multiple endocrine neoplasia Type IIa. If, in addition, the syndrome involves mucosal neuromas and Marfanoid habitus, then it is called multiple endocrine neoplasia Type IIb.

        3.   A higher incidence of pheochromocytoma is also found in neurofibromatosis, von Hippel–Lindau disease, tuberous sclerosis, and Sturge–Weber syndrome.

    B.   Signs and Symptoms

        1.   Paroxysmal hypertension, diaphoresis, headache, tremulousness or weakness, and palpitations are common. Fatigue, weight loss, and orthostatic hypotension (the latter resulting from the characteristic chronic volume depletion) also occur.

        2.   Hyperglycemia reflects the predominance of alpha-receptor agonist effects, which inhibit insulin release.

        3.   Of critical importance to the anesthesiologist is the frequent finding of catecholamine-induced cardiomyopathy, which is associated with arrhythmias and high-output heart failure. Fifty per cent of the deaths in patients with unsuspected pheochromocytoma occur during anesthesia, surgery, or parturition.

    C.   Diagnosis

        1.   Measurement of plasma catecholamines is the standard test. A value of 1000 pg/ml or less rules out the diagnosis. Catecholamine values between 1000 to 2000 pg/ml are equivocal, and those above 2000 pg/ml are almost diagnostic.

        2.   In equivocal cases, a clonidine suppression test may be helpful. Clonidine (0.3 mg orally) will suppress the catecholamine output to less than 500 pg/ml in hypertensive patients who do not have a pheochromocytoma, whereas patients with a pheochromocytoma usually will not have suppression of catecholamines because the excess catecholamines are not under adrenergic control. The test should be performed by those knowledgeable in antihypertension drug interactions and in the treatment of pheochromocytoma. Appropriate monitoring should be available during the test.

3. The use of CT scanning is an important adjunct in the localization and diagnosis of pheochromocytoma. When suspicion of the disease is very strong and CT scanning is negative, ^{131}I-m-iodobenzylguanidine localization or T-2 weighted MR imaging may be helpful.

D. Treatment

1. Preparation with alpha-adrenergic receptor blockade is mandatory. Prazosin or phenoxybenzamine are titrated to control blood pressure while intravascular volume is gradually normalized. Prazosin may be preferable, as it is a selective alpha-1-receptor antagonist. By sparing alpha-2 receptors, prazosin allows released norepinephrine to exert negative feedback on continued catecholamine release.

2. Decreases in hematocrit associated with volume expansion are expected in the preparatory stage as an indication that euvolumia is being reached.

3. Persistence of tachycardia or cardiac arrhythmias despite alpha-adrenergic blockade is an indication for the addition of beta-blockade. Beta-blockade should never be instituted in the absence of alpha-blockade, because unopposed alpha effects may cause a paradoxical increase in blood pressure in these patients.

4. Alpha-methyltyrosine blocks the hydroxylation of tyrosine and thereby reduces catecholamine synthesis. Its use in the preparation for pheochromocytoma surgery is gaining popularity, although studies comparing its efficacy with that of current regimens is lacking.

5. A patient is considered ready for surgery when the following have been achieved:

   a. Volume expansion over 10 to 14 days

      b. No in-hospital blood pressure higher than 160/90 mmHg in the 24-hour period before surgery

      c. Orthostatic blood pressure above 89/45 mmHg

      d. ECG free of ST-T changes

      e. The number of premature ventricular contractions not exceeding 5 per minute.

E. Anesthetic Management

    1. Communication with the surgeon and endocrinologist is important for ensuring a smooth perioperative course. A preoperative visit with the patient is useful to establish rapport, which may offset some of the anxiety-provoked hypertensive paroxysms when the patient is prepared for surgery.

    2. Continuation of adrenergic blockade but at a reduced dose on the day of surgery has been most effective. Dose titration is based on amount of premedication, the blood pressure, and the volume status the day of surgery.

    3. Heavy premedication with nonhistamine-releasing compounds is desirable. Titration of midazolam and fentanyl for insertion of invasive monitors the night before surgery has proved useful and permits final volume and medication adjustments.

    4. Monitoring should include an arterial line, and strong consideration should be given to pulmonary artery catheterization or transesophageal echocardiography. The cardiomyopathy associated with the lesion has the potential for producing remarkable hemodynamic lability, which makes careful assessment of left-sided cardiac function desirable.

    5. Induction of anesthesia may be associated with marked lability of blood pressure. No study has demonstrated the superiority of any specific anesthetic agent. The author favors a combination of epidural and general anesthesia, with the invasive monitoring and the epidural block performed well in advance to allow for volume adjustments. Combinations of short-acting benzodiazepines and barbiturates in carefully titrated doses with the addition of nonsensitizing inhalational agents (isoflurane, enflurane to an adequate depth of anesthesia before intubation) is one approach. Maintenance of anesthesia with an inhalational agent allows for rapid titration of the anesthesia-to-blood pressure changes.

6. Lidocaine 1 to 2 mg/kg or the addition of a small dose of a short-acting opiate 1 to 2 minutes before intubation is useful in blunting the sympathetic response.

7. Drugs that release histamine or that stimulate the sympathetic nervous system (succinylcholine, ketamine, pancuronium, large amounts of atracurium) should be avoided.

8. Ready availability of drugs to control hypertension unresponsive to increasing the depth of anesthesia (nitroprusside, nitroglycerin, phentolamine) is crucial.

9. Care should be taken to prepare the abdomen gently and to be gentle in positioning the patient in order to avoid paroxysmal sympathetic discharge.

10. Innovar (the combination of fentanyl and droperidol) has been reported to provoke hypertension. The suggested mechanism is the interference with the uptake of norepinephrine into the postganglionic nerve endings by droperidol. However, others have used Innovar successfully.

11. Reductions in blood pressure may be precipitous when the venous drainage of the tumor is ligated. Volume infusion, reduction of the inhalational agent, and administration of catecholamines (norepinephrine or dopamine) may be necessary. Hypotension has not been a particular problem in combined regional–general techniques if the block has been performed well in advance of surgery with adequate volume replacement.

F. Postoperative Care

1. In patients who have had a combined regional (epidural with indwelling catheter)–general anesthetic technique, postoperative analgesia can be provided with epidural opiates.

2. It should be remembered that 50% of the patients will remain hypertensive for several days postoperatively and that the catecholamine levels are usually elevated for 10 days after surgery. Continued antihypertensive therapy may be needed for this time.

    3. Screening of family members may be advisable, given the hereditary tendency of this tumor.

V. ADRENAL INSUFFICIENCY

    A. Causes

    Causes of adrenal insufficiency include destruction of the adrenal cortex by granulomatous disease, cancer, or hemorrhage. Other, less common, causes include ACTH deficiency and long-term administration of exogenous corticosteroids, which depress the pituitary–adrenal axis.

    B. Signs and Symptoms

    The clinical manifestation of adrenal insufficiency differ according to the origin of the syndrome, either primary (adrenal cortical destruction) or secondary (anterior pituitary dysfunction).

        1. Primary adrenal insufficiency is associated with skeletal muscle weakness, weight loss, hypotension, hyperpigmentation (from excess secretion of melanocyte-stimulating hormone from the anterior pituitary), and circulatory collapse during stress. Laboratory findings include hyponatremia, hyperkalemia, hypoglycemia, and hemoconcentration.

        2. Secondary adrenal insufficiency is less likely to cause electrolyte derangements because aldosterone is still produced. The panhypopituitarism frequently associated with the secondary form results in a deficit of ACTH as well as of other important hormones (growth hormone, thyroid-stimulating hormone, gonadotropins).

    C. Diagnosis

        1. The diagnosis of adrenal insufficiency is made using the ACTH stimulation test. After obtaining a baseline plasma cortisol, 250 μg of synthetic ACTH is given intravenously, and the plasma cortisol is measured 30 and 60 minutes later. An increase of 7 to 30 μg/dl is normal. A rise of less than 7 μg/dl indicates a likelihood of adrenal insufficiency, and perioperative steroid coverage is indicated.

        2. If the administration of steroids cannot be delayed even the hour necessary to perform an ACTH stimulation test, the immediate use of dexamethasone is suggested. Dexamethasone is unique in that it will not invalidate the ACTH stimulation test. The practice of "covering" the patient with steroids without establishing a diagnosis should be resisted, as it may condemn the patient to a longer steroid exposure than necessary.

D. Treatment and Anesthetic Management

    1. Intravenous volume replacement with glucose-containing salt solutions and the monitoring of intravascular volume are important. The patient with circulatory collapse from suspected adrenal insufficiency requires emergency steroid replacement with 100 mg of intravenous cortisol (or steroid equivalent) followed by 50 mg every 4 to 6 hours for the first 48 hours of the crisis.

    2. The patient taking steroids for other medical indications who presents for elective surgery is a totally different and more common situation. Perioperative stress in such patients is related directly to the magnitude of the surgery and inversely to the depth of the anesthesia. The postoperative stress may be greater than the intraoperative stress. Although hypotension has occurred perioperatively in such patients, little documentation implicates steroid deficiency as the cause.

    3. Bearing in mind that there is little risk in short-term administration of high-dose steroids and that acute adrenal insufficiency may be life-threatening, the following is a rational approach to steroid replacement for patients already on steroids and undergoing elective surgery:

        a. Supplementation perioperatively for any patient who has received steroids in the last year.

        b. Never supplement with a lower dose than the patient has been receiving.

        c. For major surgery (a maximum-stress situation), approximately 200 mg hydrocortisone or steroid equivalent, which is $2/3$ of the maximum daily steroid output. One-quarter of the total dose is given as a bolus when the IV is started and the remainder by continuous infusion over the next 24 hours.

        d. For minor procedures, 100 mg of hydrocortisone equivalent per day, with $1/4$ of the dose given when the IV is started and the remainder by continuous infusion over 24 hours.

    4. Short-term steroid supplementation can (although seldom does) cause any of the side effects of chronic steroid use, including a delay in wound healing (partially offset by vitamin A therapy), aggravation of hypertension, hyperglycemia, fluid retention, psychosis, and stress ulceration.

5. Anesthetic considerations include the need to follow glucose, electrolyte, and volume status of the patient carefully. With the exception of the avoidance of etomidate because of its adrenal suppression, no specific anesthetic regimen is superior.

≡ Thyroid Disorders

I. PHYSIOLOGY

A. The synthesis and secretion of the two active thyroid hormones, triiodothyronine (T3) and thyroxine (T4), occurs in four phases:

1. Iodide trapping
Iodine absorbed by the gastrointestinal tract is concentrated by the epithelial cells of the thyroid, a process that is accelerated by thyroid-stimulating hormone (TSH). This process is slowed by increasing the circulating levels of iodide, thiocyanate, or perchlorate.

2. Oxidation and iodination
Inorganic iodide is incorporated into tyrosine residues (monoiodotyrosine, diiodotyrosine), which are nondiffusible forms. This process is accelerated by TSH and inhibited by propylthiouracil and methimazole.

3. Hormone storage
The two compounds above are coupled to form T3 and T4. These are then coupled to a protein carrier, thyroglobulin, and stored as colloid in the gland. This step is also TSH dependent and inhibited by propylthiouracil and methimazole.

4. Proteolysis and release
Thyroxine accounts for 95% of the hormone released, but T3 is the more potent and the less protein-bound entity and modulates almost all of the effects that we recognize as thyroid related. Triiodothyronine is produced mainly by the deiodina-

tion of T4 in the liver and kidney. The proteolytic effect responsible for the release of active hormone is stimulated by TSH and inhibited by elevated intra-thyroidal concentrations of iodide and lithium.

B. Basic Function of Thyroid Hormones
1. The active form of thyroid hormone (T3) is moved across the target-cell membrane by energy-dependent transport systems.
2. In the cytoplasm, T3 diffuses to receptors in the nucleus, where it alters the production of specific mRNA sequences.
3. Thyroid hormones have anabolic effects, promote growth, and advance normal brain and organ development.
4. Triiodothyronine also causes upregulation of adrenergic receptors, which may account for its cardiovascular effects.

II. THYROID FUNCTION TESTS

A. Total Plasma Thyroxine (T4)
Ninety per cent of patients with hyperthyroidism have high T4 levels, and 85% of those with hypothyroidism have low levels. Interpretation of the results will be affected by thyroid-binding globulin (TBG) levels, a low TBG causing falsely low T4 values in the absence of thyroid disease.

B. Resin Triiodothyronine Uptake (T3RU)
The T3RU test clarifies whether abnormalities in total T4 are secondary to dysfunction of the thyroid gland or to altered TBG levels. Resin uptake is greater if the number of TBG binding sites is lower.

C. Free T4 Index
Although T3 has greater biologic activity than T4, the diagnosis of thyroid disorders is most often based on a "free T4" index. A free T4 index is needed because total T4 values may be affected by the plasma concentration of TBG. The TBG values are increased in pregnancy, with oral contraceptives, and in infectious hepatitis and decreased in nephrosis, malnutrition (with hypoproteinemia), and acromegaly. By multiplying the T3RU by the total T4, one obtains the free T4 index.

D. Free Thyroxine
The free T4 test is useful when malnutrition in a hyperthyroid patient results in low levels of TBG. In such a

situation, the total T4 may be normal or low, but free T4 will be elevated.

E. Plasma T3

Plasma T3 is used primarily to detect hyperthyroidism in patients in whom the T3 elevation precedes thyroxine elevation or is the only hormone to be elevated. This is not a very good test for hypothyroidism, as it may be normal in half of such patients. Furthermore, T3 can be low in euthyroid patients with renal failure, malnutrition, and hepatic cirrhosis.

F. Radioactive Iodine Uptake

Uptake of ^{123}I or ^{131}I is used to quantitate total gland activity. It is not reliable in assessing overactivity.

G. Thyroid-Stimulating Hormone

Assay for TSH is the most sensitive test for hypothyroidism, as TSH may be elevated before symptoms are obvious or total plasma T4 is decreased. Secondary hypothyroidism (from hypothalamic or pituitary failure) will be suggested by a reduced TSH while total plasma T4 is low. Thyrotropin-releasing hormone (TRH) from the hypothalamus is responsible for augmenting the pituitary formation of TSH, and both hormones are inhibited by serum T4 elevations. Hyperthyroidism is suggested by a small or absent response of the TSH level to stimulation by TRH (a sensitive test for hyperthyroidism).

H. Thyroid Scan

The radionuclide scan is useful in differentiating benign from malignant disease of the thyroid. Functioning tissue is rarely malignant; nonfunctioning tissue may be either malignant or benign.

I. Antibodies to Thyroid Tissue

Immunologic testing is helpful in determining the cause of inflammation of the thyroid or, occasionally, the cause of hyperthyroidism. Hashimoto's thyroiditis typically causes elevated antibodies. This entity is associated with other autoimmune disorders such as diabetes mellitus and adrenal insufficiency.

III. HYPERTHYROIDISM

A. Causes

The most common cause of hyperthyroidism is multinodular diffuse toxic goiter (Graves' disease). Other causes are thyroiditis (Hashimoto's disease), thyroid adenoma, choriocarcinoma, and a TSH-secreting pituitary tumor (rare). Hyperthyroidism can be associated with pregnancy.

B. Clinical Manifestations

    1. Signs and symptoms include weight loss, diarrhea, warm moist skin, weakness of large muscle groups, menstrual abnormalities, nervousness, heat intolerance, tachycardia, cardiac dysrhythmias, mitral valve prolapse, heart failure, mild anemia, thrombocytopenia, increased serum alkaline phosphatase, hypercalcemia, muscle wasting, bone loss, exophthalmos, and retrobulbar edema with conjunctival erythema.

    2. The "apathetic" form of hyperthyroidism is seen frequently after the age of 60, and cardiac abnormalities are the dominant feature, with atrial fibrillation, heart failure, and papillary muscle dysfunction the usual findings.

C. Treatment

    1. Elective surgery should be postponed until the patient is clinically and chemically euthyroid, as the metabolic demands of the hyperthyroid state coupled with major surgery and anesthesia may take a staggering toll on end-organ function, especially postoperatively.

    2. Antithyroid drugs generally take at least 2 weeks to render the patient euthyroid. The patient should be reevaluated by competent endocrine consultation.

        a. Oral iodide (Lugol's solution or tablets) is effective in reducing the vascularity of the hyperplastic gland and inhibiting the release of T4 and T3. Potassium iodide orally or sodium iodide intravenously may accomplish the same goal.

        b. Propylthiouracil and methimazole inhibit the oxidation of inorganic iodide. They take several weeks to work. Both drugs may (rarely) cause agranulocytosis. Propylthiouracil is also associated with thrombocytopenia and hypoprothrombinemia.

        c. Beta-adrenergic blockers attenuate the manifestations of sympathetic overactivity characteristic of hyperthyroidism. Part of their efficacy comes from their interference with the deiodination of T4 to T3.

3. Subtotal thyroidectomy is an alternative to long-term drug therapy. Patients should be rendered euthyroid before surgery with either 6 to 8 weeks of specific antithyroid drugs (propylthiouracil or methimazole) and the vascularity of the gland reduced with 10 days of oral iodide therapy.

4. Radioactive iodine therapy carries a finite risk per year of inducing hypothyroidism.

D. Anesthetic Management

1. Elective surgery should be delayed in a clinically hyperthyroid patient, as the hyperkinetic circulation in untreated individuals may predispose patients with marginal cardiac reserve to heart failure. Patients whose hyperthyroidism is under good control generally have heart rates under 100/minute.

2. Heavy premedication without the addition of an anticholinergic drug is suggested.

3. Induction with a combination of barbiturates, benzodiazepines, and narcotics is ideal. Ketamine and pancuronium are usually avoided because of their sympathetic stimulatory effects.

4. Maintenance of anesthesia

   a. The hyperthyroid patient frequently has an elevated body temperature, which raises the inhalational agent requirement by 5% for each degree Celsius. Accelerated drug metabolism may predispose the patient to toxicity from halothane or enflurane.

   b. The use of isoflurane may be associated with reflex tachycardia from baroreceptor stimulation. Changing maintenance anesthesia or using beta-blockers may be needed to reduce heart rate. The concurrent use of beta-blockade is almost always required.

   c. The use of short-acting potent narcotic agents, with their tendency to depress the cardiovascular system slightly, combined with nitrous oxide is another attractive alternative for maintenance.

   d. Neuromuscular blocking drugs that neither stimulate the cardiovascular system nor release histamine are logical choices. Atracurium, given slowly, and vecuronium are good. The tendency to skeletal muscle weakness makes monitoring of neuromuscular blockade desirable. There is an increased incidence of myasthenia gravis in hyperthyroid patients as well.

e. Regional anesthesia should be accompanied by adequate sedation, as exaggerated responses to vasopressors may occur in these patients.

5. Hypotension should be treated with carefully titrated doses of vasopressors, because there will be a tendency toward exaggerated response. Directly acting agents are advised.

6. Monitoring should be tailored to detect thyroid storm as early as possible and should include at least two forms of temperature assessment. A cooling mattress, cold intravenous solutions, and ice packs should be readily available.

7. The cornea will require liberal amounts of ointment to prevent the drying and ulceration to which exophthalmic hyperthyroid patients are predisposed.

E. Treatment of Thyroid Storm

1. Storm is most likely 6 to 18 hours after surgery and is usually abrupt in onset. There is no predictive test for thyroid storm. Successful outcome is related to control of the underlying disease and to support of the threatened circulation.

2. Treatment of thyroid storm includes infusion of cold crystalloid solutions, sodium iodide (500–1000 mg IV q8h), hydrocortisone (100–200 mg IV q8h), propylthiouracil (200–400 mg q8h), and propranolol. Propranolol should be titrated to control the heart rate while monitoring left ventricular function. Corticosteroids are necessary because of the possibility of acute precipitation of adrenal insufficiency by the increased metabolism of thyroid storm. Aspirin should be avoided because it displaces T4 from carrier proteins.

IV. HYPOTHYROIDISM

A. Causes

The causes of hypothyroidism are divided into primary (the thyroid gland itself is deficient) or the more rare secondary (anterior pituitary failure to produce TSH or hypothalamic failure to produce TRH).

1. The primary disorders most commonly responsible

for hypothyroidism include thyroid gland destruction from previous subtotal thyroidectomy, ^{131}I therapy, neck irradiation, or Hashimoto's (autoimmune) thyroiditis.

2. Less common primary causes of hypothyroidism are iodine deficiency, excess iodine (which inhibits hormone release), and excess antithyroid drug.

B. Clinical Manifestations

1. Signs and symptoms vary greatly according to the patient's age and may be subtle. They include dry skin, husky voice, delayed reflexes, lethargy, weakness, and intolerance to cold and can be elucidated with careful examination and questioning.

2. Also found are decreased cardiac output, increased systemic vascular resistance, decreased blood volume, prolonged circulation time, pleural effusion, cardiomegaly, peripheral edema, and ascites.

3. Myxedema coma is the end-stage form of hypothyroidism, characterized by congestive heart failure, hypoventilation, spontaneous hypothermia, and depressed consciousness.

4. Associated adrenal insufficiency, with adrenal atrophy and the impaired ability to excrete water resulting in the characteristic hyponatremia of hypothyroidism, should be sought.

5. Two other syndrome complexes associated with hypothyroidism are commonly recognized.

   a. Subacute thyroiditis is a viral-like illness with a diffusely enlarged, tender gland. Twenty-five per cent of these patients will be hypothyroid for several months after the attack.

   b. Chronic (Hashimoto's) thyroiditis is an autoimmune disorder with associated pernicious anemia, myasthenia gravis, and adrenal insufficiency found with increased frequency. This disorder is the most common cause of hypothyroidism in adults.

C. Treatment

1. In general, thyroid replacement therapy should be instituted gradually to avoid precipitation of angina pectoris, cardiac dysrhythmias, or congestive heart failure brought on by sharply increased metabolism. Thyroxine takes 10 days to exert its physiologic effects.

2. Exogenous administration of cortisol will be necessary if adrenal insufficiency is discovered (testing for adrenal insufficiency should be done on all hypothyroid patients).

3. Digitalis for congestive heart failure may adversely affect the hypothyroid heart; thyroid replacement usually, but not always, reverses thyroid cardiomyopathy.

4. In the face of severe coronary artery disease, myocardial revascularization may have to be performed before the patient is subjected to the stress of thyroid replacement.

5. The adequacy of thyroid replacement should be confirmed by the normalization of serum TSH.

D. Management of Anesthesia

1. Elective surgery should be delayed until the patient is euthyroid. If surgery cannot be delayed, then the following items that affect anesthetic management should be noted and corrected:

a. Hypothyroid patients exhibit marked sensitivity to depressant drugs.

b. The cardiovascular system is characterized by a low cardiac output, high systemic vascular resistance, and low heart rate state.

c. Drug metabolism is slowed, especially for opioids.

d. Baroreceptors tend to be unresponsive and beta receptors downregulated.

e. Intravascular volume is decreased.

f. The ventilatory responses to hypoxemia and hypercarbia are blunted.

g. Free water clearance is impaired.

h. Gastric emptying is delayed.

i. Baseline hypothermia is common.

j. Normocytic anemia is common.

k. Primary adrenal insufficiency and consequent hypoglycemia are common.

2. Preoperative medication might include cortisol support. Little else beyond attempting to establish rapport is indicated.

3. Preinduction monitoring should include pulse oximetry and invasive blood pressure monitoring. Serious consideration should be given to monitoring of left ventricular function (e.g., pulmonary artery

catheterization or transesophageal echocardiography).

4. Induction in hypothyroid patients might include intravenous ketamine. The need to avoid cardiovascular depression implies avoidance of sodium thiopental. Short-acting muscle relaxants should be considered, because of both the ventilatory compromise and the underlying muscle weakness.

5. Maintenance of anesthesia should be designed to use the minimum amount of fixed, long-acting drugs or myocardial depressants.

   a. Small, carefully titrated amounts of short-acting agents such as opiates (alfentanil) and benzodiazepines (midazolam), ketamine, or nitrous oxide are reasonable.

   b. When volatile agents are used, the sensitivity of these patients to myocardial depression should be borne in mind. The actual dose of volatile agent necessary to prevent skeletal muscle responses to a noxious stimulus is not reduced. This may reflect the maintenance of cerebral metabolic activity for oxygen in the face of hypothyroidism. The reduction in cardiac output with the consequent rapid achievement of maintenance levels of anesthesia may account for the clinical impression that anesthetic requirements are reduced.

   c. Pancuronium is a good choice for muscle relaxation for longer cases in the setting of bradycardia and myocardial depression, but underlying muscle weakness makes titration to carefully monitored end points of the reduced dosage requirements desirable.

   d. The treatment of hypotension with sympathomimetic drugs may precipitate heart failure, because the hypothyroid heart may not be able to increase its output. The possibility of acute adrenal insufficiency should be part of the differential diagnosis of hypotension in hypothyroid patients. Hypothermia and hyponatremia commonly occur and must be promptly treated.

   e. Prolonged emergence is common, and prolonged respiratory depression may be a clue to previously undiagnosed hypothyroidism.

≡ **Pituitary Disorders**

Anterior (Adenohypophyseal) Pituitary

I. PHYSIOLOGY
   A. The hypothalamus controls anterior pituitary function. Thyrotropin-releasing hormone and corticotropin-releasing factor (CRF) are produced in the hypothalamus and transported via the hypophyseal portal system to the anterior pituitary, where they stimulate production and release of TSH and ACTH, respectively. Thyroid-stimulating hormone regulates the synthesis and release of active thyroid hormones. Adrenocorticotropic hormone regulates the release of cortisol and androgens from the adrenal cortex.
   B. Dopamine secreted by the hypothalamus inhibits prolactin secretion by the pituitary.
   C. Luteinizing hormone-releasing factor (hypothalamic origin) is responsible for stimulating the release of luteinizing hormone (LH) and follicle-stimulating hormone (FSH) from the pituitary. The former induces ovulation and stimulates the testes to produce androgens. The latter stimulates ovarian and testicular development.
   D. Somatostatin is the (hypothalamic) growth hormone-release inhibiting factor.
   E. Growth hormone (GH) stimulates skeletal development and increases protein synthesis and the rate of carbohydrate metabolism.
   F. Prolactin is necessary for lactation.
   G. Melanin-stimulating hormone (MSH) is necessary for the formation of melanin pigments.

II. HYPERSECRETION OF HORMONES
   A. Although the most common cause of anterior pituitary hormone excess is an adenoma producing prolactin, a basophilic adenoma is the most common cause of Cushing's disease.
   B. The condition of greatest importance for the anesthesiologist is the excess of GH. Hypersecretion of GH is called gigantism if it begins before epiphyseal closure and acromegaly if the onset is after closure of the epiphyses. In either case, it is caused by excess secretion of GH from an eosinophilic adenoma of the pituitary. The diagnosis is made by documenting an elevation of GH that does not

fall in response to glucose infusion. An enlarged sella turcica usually is also found.

C.   Clinical Manifestations

1.   Signs and symptoms of an eosinophilic adenoma include the effects of local invasion of adjacent structures or the far-reaching effects of excess GH.

2.   The pressure effects from local tumor invasion include headache, visual field abnormalities, rhinorrhea, and erosion of the bony sella turcica.

3.   The most important effects of GH for the anesthesiologist involve the airway. Prognathism; soft tissue overgrowth affecting the tongue, lips, epiglottis, and vocal cords; and recurrent laryngeal nerve paralysis from connective tissue overgrowth are all common. The airway in acromegaly may present a heroic challenge because of the increased thickness and length of the mandible, the massively enlarged tongue and epiglottis, polypoid masses in the pharynx, abnormal vocal cord movement (from recurrent laryngeal nerve paralysis), and decreased subglottic tracheal diameter.

4.   Other significant signs and symptoms of GH excess are peripheral neuropathy (most commonly carpal tunnel syndrome), visceromegaly, glucose intolerance, hypertension, congestive heart failure, muscle weakness, and osteoporosis.

D.   Anesthetic management of the acromegalic patient is directed primarily at securing the difficult airway.

1.   Distorted facial anatomy may necessitate a larger than normal face mask. A drying agent should be considered in the premedication. Enlarged nasal turbinates and pharyngeal polyps make the use of a nasal airway somewhat more risky than usual. The large tongue, reduced vocal cord mobility, and reduced tracheal diameter make fiberoptic intubation appealing. Reduced collateral circulation at the wrist makes radial artery cannulation more hazardous.

2.   Glucose should be monitored because of the increased incidence of glucose intolerance.

3.   Cortisol replacement is necessary and should include the equivalent of 200 to 300 mg of hydrocortisone divided into three doses. The first dose should be given before induction.

III. HYPOSECRETION OF HORMONES
  A. Causes
  1. The most common cause of anterior pituitary hyposecretion is a chromophobe adenoma (in the adult) or a craniopharyngioma (in a child).
  2. Necrosis of the anterior pituitary can follow postpartum hemorrhagic shock (Sheehan's syndrome).
  3. Less common causes include head injury, radiation therapy to adjacent structures, surgical hypophysectomy, or management of severe exophthalmus.
  B. The signs and symptoms of hyposecretion typically are slow in onset.
  1. Usually, the deficiency of LH and FSH presents as impotence or secondary amenorrhea.
  2. Hypoadrenocorticism may take 2 weeks to manifest symptoms after surgical hypophysectomy. Therapeutic replacement should, of course, begin earlier (see below).
  3. Posthypophysectomy, hypothyroidism may take up to a month to become evident.
  C. Anesthetic management must include corticosteroid support. The equivalent of 200 to 300 mg of hydrocortisone should be provided, divided into three doses intravenously. The first dose should be given before induction. Mineralocorticoid therapy is usually not required, because aldosterone release is sustained in the absence of ACTH.

Posterior Pituitary

I. PHYSIOLOGY
  A. Neurons from the hypothalamus terminate in the posterior pituitary and control the secretion of its two hormones, antidiuretic hormone (ADH or vasopressin) and oxytocin.
  B. ADH activates osmoreceptors in the hypothalamus in response to increased osmolarity. It also facilitates reabsorption of water by the renal tubules, which causes reduction in plasma osmolarity and increases in urine osmolarity. Free water clearance decreases, as does urine volume. Many other factors stimulate ADH secretion, in-

cluding pain, nausea, positive pressure ventilation, reduction in intravascular volume, and narcotics. Surgery is a much more intense stimulant than any of the anesthetic agents.

C. Oxytocin stimulates the contraction of the pregnant uterus and promotes milk secretion and ejection of milk by the mammary glands.

II.   DISORDERS

    A.   Diabetes Insipidus

        1.   Failure to produce adequate ADH results in diabetes insipidus (DI). The common causes are intracranial tumor, head trauma, and hypophysectomy.

            a.   DI from head trauma may be delayed for several days.

            b.   DI from pituitary surgery is generally reversible and transient.

            c.   Another form of DI occurs if the renal tubules are incapable of responding to ADH (nephrogenic DI).

        2.   The signs and symptoms include polydipsia (if the patient is awake and has access to water), low urinary specific gravity, high serum osmolarity, hypernatremia, and hypovolemia.

        3.   The treatment and anesthetic management is directed at close monitoring of urine output, intravascular volume, and electrolytes while administering appropriate amounts of vasopressin.

            a.   Nasal vasopressin (5–10 units every 4–6 hours) or intramuscular vasopressin in oil (beware of the prolonged effect, which may lead to water intoxication) have been used.

            b.   The use of desmopressin (a structural analog of arginine vasopressin), 5 to 100 μg in carefully titrated intravenous doses, carries less pressor effect and more antidiuretic effect.

    B.   Syndrome of Inappropriate ADH Secretion (SIADH)

        1.   The diagnostic criteria for SIADH are an elevated urinary sodium, elevated urinary osmolarity, hyponatremia, and decreased plasma osmolarity (also discussed in Chapter 3). Renal and adrenal insufficiency must be ruled out as well.

        2.   The common causes of SIADH include intracranial tumor and chest pathology of almost any variety.

Less commonly, hypothyroidism and porphyria are responsible.

3. Signs and symptoms of most concern involve the central nervous system. Disorientation, obtundation, and seizures may occur.

4. Treatment includes fluid restriction in the case of chronic SIADH with mild symptoms.

   a. If seizures and acute hyponatremia are present, administration of hypertonic saline is appropriate at a rate sufficient to increase sodium by 0.5 to 2.0 mEq/L per hour.

   b. A fatal disorder called *central pontine myelinolysis* has been associated with too-rapid correction of hyponatremia.

≡ Porphyria

I. PATHOGENESIS

The formation of heme and the pathogenesis of porphyria is illustrated in Figure 7-1. The basic defects are stimulation of aminolevulinic acid synthetase and decreased uroporphyrinogen synthetase, which lead to increased amounts of aminolevulinic acid and porphobilinogen.

II. ACUTE INTERMITTENT PORPHYRIA

A. Acute intermittent porphyria (AIP) is the most common and serious variety. It is inherited as an autosomal dominant condition.

B. The diagnosis is made by documenting increased urinary aminolevulinic acid. Aminolevulinic acid and porphobilinogen may be normal between attacks, but a decreased level of red cell uroporphyrinogen synthetase may help make the diagnosis even when the disease is quiescent.

C. The signs and symptoms include abdominal pain (sufficient to result in multiple scars from negative exploratory laparotomies), motor weakness, decreased peripheral reflexes, bulbar paralysis, cerebellar dysfunction, and autonomic nervous system dysfunction. The latter manifests as labile hypertension, orthostatic hypotension, and diaphoresis.

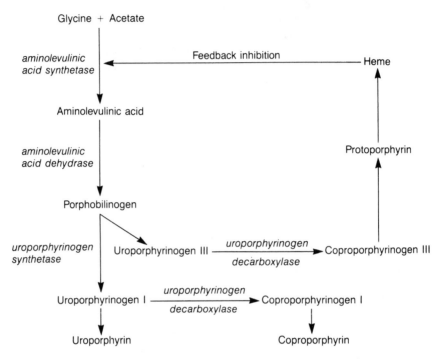

Figure 7-1 Heme synthesis. The first step in the synthesis of heme is the formation of aminolevulinic acid from glycine and acetate. The first step is catalyzed by aminolevulinic acid synthetase and inhibited by heme. The formation of porphobilinogen is catalyzed by aminolevulinic acid dehydrase. Excess amounts of both aminolevulinic acid and porphobilinogen, as seen in acute intermittent porphyria, occur as a result of stimulation of aminolevulinic acid synthetase activity, and decreased uroporphyrinogen synthetase activity. Decreased activity of uroporphyrinogen decarboxylase can lead to an accumulation of uroporphyrin, which is believed to cause porphyria cutanea tarda. (Stoelting RK, Dierdorf SF, eds. Anesthesia and co-existing disease. 2nd ed. New York: Churchill Livingstone, 1988.)

    D.   Careful preoperative evaluation should include a search for excessive R-R variability on ECG, orthostatic hypotension, and a failure of the pulse to increase with assumption of the upright position.

    E.   Treatment and Anesthetic Management

        1.   Provocative factors such as dehydration and starvation and provocative drugs such as barbiturates, benzodiazepines, ketamine, pentazocine, and etomidate must be avoided.

2. Therapy is summarized by the "four H's": hydration, hematin (3–4 mg/kg per day), hexose sugars (glucose), and "happy" patient (adequate pain medication).
3. Safe drugs to use for the anesthetic include opioids (except pentazocine), droperidol, nitrous oxide, volatile agents, chlorpromazine, promethazine, anticholinergics, anticholinesterases, and depolarizing and nondepolarizing neuromuscular blocking agents.

≡ Hyperparathyroidism

I. PATHOPHYSIOLOGY
Hyperparathyroidism involves the interaction of calcium, parathyroid hormone (PTH), and vitamin D. The hormone activates the enzyme necessary for vitamin D synthesis. Increased vitamin D, in turn, leads to increased tubular reabsorption of calcium and enhanced renal phosphorus clearance. PTH also stimulates osteoclastic activity, thereby releasing calcium from bone. In the gastrointestinal tract, PTH enhances the absorption of calcium and increases vitamin D synthesis.

II. CAUSES
A. Ninety per cent of the time, hyperparathyroidism is caused by a benign parathyroid adenoma.
B. Carcinoma is responsible for less than 5% of cases.
C. The remainder are attributable to hyperplasia, with all four glands usually involved.
D. Hyperparathyroidism may coexist with other endocrine disorders.
1. The syndrome of multiple endocrine neoplasia (MEN) type I includes adenomata of the parathyroid, pituitary, and pancreas.
2. MEN IIa is defined as an adenoma of the parathyroid coupled with medullary carcinoma of the thyroid and a pheochromocytoma.
3. MEN IIb includes mucosal neuromas, skeletal deformities, medullary carcinoma of the thyroid, a high (50%) incidence of pheochromocytoma, and a low incidence of parathyroid disease.

III. SIGNS AND SYMPTOMS

Clinical manifestations are arranged by organ systems in Table 7-5. Of particular note are hypertension with contracted intravascular volume, peptic ulcer disease (with the implications for "full stomach" precautions), and skeletal muscle weakness (with the implication of carefully titrated use of muscle relaxants and blockade monitoring).

IV. DIAGNOSIS

The diagnosis of hyperparathyroidism is made by documenting an elevated PTH despite an elevated ionized calcium level. However, the results of the PTH radioimmunoassay may take several weeks. Additional clues to the diagnosis include an elevated plasma chloride (usually greater than 102 mEq/L), reflecting the increased bicarbonate excretion, which causes

Table 7–5. Manifestations of Hypercalcemia Secondary to Hyperparathyroidism

Organ System	Manifestation
Renal	Polydipsia and polyuria
	Renal stones
	Decreased glomerular filtration rate
Cardiac	Hypertension
	Short Q-T interval
	Prolonged P-R interval
Gastrointestinal	Abdominal pain
	Vomiting
	Weight loss
	Peptic ulcer
	Pancreatitis
Skeletal	Bone pain and tenderness
	Skeletal demineralization
	Pathologic fractures
	Collapse of vertebral bodies
Nervous system	Somnolence
	Psychosis
	Decreased pain sensation
Neuromuscular	Skeletal muscle weakness
Articular	Periarticular calcifications
	Gout
Ocular	Calcifications (band keratopathy)
	Conjunctivitis
Hematopoietic	Anemia

(Stoelting RK, Dierdorf SF, eds. Anesthesia and co-existing disease. 2nd ed. New York: Churchill Livingstone, 1988.)

the typical mild metabolic acidosis; decreased plasma phosphorus; and increased excretion of cAMP.

V. TREATMENT

Treatment and anesthetic management are directed at reducing serum calcium through hydration with normal saline.

A. Because furosemide often is used to promote calcium excretion and because severe hypercalcemia causes an obligate diuresis, these patients may be severely volume contracted.

B. Frequently, hypertension coexists with intravascular volume depletion. This combination markedly increases the risk of hypotension during induction if preinduction hydration is not done.

C. Coexisting renal dysfunction from stones or prerenal azotemia should be suspected and anesthetic techniques adjusted accordingly (see Chap. 4).

D. Altered central nervous system (CNS) status makes the carefully titrated use of rapidly excreted agents desirable. Ketamine's lingering CNS effects may make it relatively contraindicated for this reason.

E. Muscle relaxants must be carefully titrated, as sensitivity to succinylcholine and resistance to atracurium have both been reported.

F. Restoration of magnesium and potassium may be required because both are frequently reduced by diuretic therapy.

G. Patients must be positioned gently to avoid the pathologic fractures to which they are prone.

H. For cases in which hydration and loop diuretics prove inadequate, several other treatment modalities are available.

   1. Glucocorticoids are effective in the hypercalcemia of sarcoidosis, multiple myeloma, vitamin D intoxication, and some malignancies. They are not effective in primary hyperparathyroidism.

   2. Mithramycin (25 μg/kg intravenously) works by inhibiting PTH-induced osteoclastic activity. It takes up to 24 hours to produce an effect, which lasts 3 to 5 days. The toxic effects include thrombocytopenia, hepatic dysfunction, azotemia, proteinuria, hypokalemia, and sodium retention.

   3. Calcitonin may be used (0.004 units/kg every 6 hours subcutaneously). Calcium decreases within 1 to 2 hours. Side effects are less serious than with mithramycin and include nausea, facial flushing, and diarrhea. Calcitonin works by inhibiting bone resorption.

Summary of Anesthetic Considerations

The preanesthetic diagnosis and the establishment of a stable management regimen of most endocrine disorders will help decrease perioperative complications. Despite the best preoperative management, problems occur, which should be handled easily with proper preparations.

Glucometers should be used to follow blood sugar closely in diabetics to avoid hypoglycemia and ketoacidosis and to maintain serum glucose at 120 to 200 mg/dl. A continuous insulin infusion with the dose calculated by the following equation:

$$\text{Insulin IU/hour} = \frac{\text{plasma glucose (mg/dl)}}{150}$$

helps minimize large swings in blood glucose levels associated with IV insulin boluses. The incidence of protamine reactions is much higher in patients treated previously with either NPH or PZI insulin. For diabetics who are anticipated to have anticoagulation and to need heparin reversal with protamine, resuscitative drugs should be readily available.

Excess adrenocortical hormone is associated with diabetes mellitus, hypertension, decreased intravascular volume, and hypokalemic metabolic alkalosis. The patients will have a smoother intraoperative course if these problems are addressed preoperatively.

Potassium deficiency, depleted intravascular volume, and steroid deficit (if the adrenals are resected) are particular concerns in patients with hyperaldosteronism.

Close communication between surgeon, endocrinologist, and anesthesiologist is necessary to coordinate preoperative medical management with alpha-blockade, beta-blockade, and volume replacement for patients with pheochromocytoma. Histamine release, abdominal manipulation, and sympathetic stimulation should be minimized. Drugs must be available to treat the expected large intraoperative swings in blood pressure.

Validation (retrospectively) of adrenal insufficiency is done with the measurement of cortisol 30 and 60 minutes after synthetic ACTH is given intravenously. If steroid supplementation needs to be started before confirmation tests can be done, dexamethasone, which will not interfere with the ACTH stimulation test, is used. Replacement therapy should provide supplementation for any patient who has received steroids in the last year. One should never supplement with a lower dose than the patient has been receiving. For maximum stress (major surgery) 2/3 of the maximum daily steroid output (200 to 300 mg hydrocortisone equivalent) or about 200 mg is provided by giving 1/4 of the dose when the IV is started and the remainder by continuous infusion over 24 hours. For minor procedures, 100 mg of hydrocortisone equivalent will suffice, given as 1/4 when the IV is started and the rest as a continuous IV infusion over 24 hours. Volume status, electrolytes, and glucose will need close attention.

Elective surgery should be postponed until the hyperthyroid patient is chemically and clinically euthyroid. Antithyroid drugs take at least 2 weeks to achieve this goal. Heavy premedication, increased inhalational agent requirement, and accelerated drug metabolism are the main considerations. Sodium iodide, hydrocortisone, and beta-blockers are used to treat thyroid storm.

Elective surgery should also be postponed until the hypothyroid patient is chemically and clinically euthyroid. Gradual replacement usually takes weeks. Steroid replacement may be required if the patient is adrenally insufficient, as is often the case. Marked cardiac insufficiency, baroreceptor unresponsiveness, hypothermia, decreased intravascular volume, delayed gastric emptying time, and slow drug metabolism are considerations in hypothyroid patients.

Recommended Reading

Diabetes Mellitus

Bruno A, Cavallo-Perin P, Cassader M, Pagano G. Deflazacort vs prednisone. Arch Intern Med 1987;147:679.

Campbell DR, Hoar CS, Wheelock FC. Carotid artery surgery in diabetic patients. Arch Surg 1984;119:1405.

Campbell PJ, Bolli GB, Cryer PE, Gerich JE. Pathogenesis of the dawn phenomenon in patients with insulin-dependent diabetes mellitus. N Engl J Med 1985;312:1473.

Ciccarelli LL, Ford CM, Tsueda K. Autonomic neuropathy in a diabetic patient with renal failure. Anesthesiology 1986;64:283.

Elliott MJ, Gill G, Home PD, Noy GA, Holden MP, Alberti GMN. A comparison of two regimens for the management of diabetes during open heart surgery. Anesthesiology 1984;60:364.

Ewing DJ, Campbell IW, Clarke BF. The natural history of diabetic autonomic neuropathy. Q J Med 1980;193:95.

Gurri JA, Burnham SJ. Effect of diabetes mellitus on distal lower extremity bypass. Am Surg 1982;48:75.

Hjortrup A, Rasmussen BF, Kehlet H. Morbidity in diabetic and non-diabetic patients after major vascular surgery. Br Med J 1983;127:1107.

Johnson WD, Pedraza PM, Kayser KL. Coronary artery surgery in diabetics: 261 consecutive patients followed four to seven years. Am Heart J 1982;104:823.

Karhunen U, Summanen P, Laatikainen L. Concomitant problems to the anesthesia of diabetic vitrectomy patients. Acta Ophthalmol 1987:190.

Lloyd–Mostyn RH, Watkins PJ. Defective innervation of heart in diabetic autonomic neuropathy. Br Med J 1975;3:15.

McMurry JF. Wound healing with diabetes mellitus. Surg Clin North Am 1984;64:769.

Petty C, Cunningham NL. Insulin adsorption by glass infusion bottles, polyvinylchloride infusion containers and intravenous tubing. Anesthesiology 1974;40:400.

Salzarulo HH, Taylor LA. Diabetic "stiff joint syndrome" as a cause of difficult endotracheal intubation. Anesthesiology 1986;64:366.

Schade DS. Surgery and diabetes. Med Clin North Am 1988;72:1531.

Stewart WJ, McSweeney SM, Kellett MA, Faxon DP, Ryan TJ. Increased risk of severe protamide reactions in NPH insulin-dependent diabetics undergoing cardiac catheterization. Circulation 1984;70:788.

Stoelting RK, Dierdorf SF, McCammon RL. Anesthesia and co-existing disease, 2nd ed. New York: Churchill Livingstone, 1988:473.

Walsh DB, Eckhauser FE, Ramsburgh SR, Burney RB. Risk associated with diabetes mellitus in patients undergoing gallbladder surgery. Surgery 1982;92:254.

Wright RA, Clemente R, Wathen R. Diabetic gastroparesis: an abnormality of gastric emptying of solids. Am J Med Sci 1985;289:240.

Zaloga GP, Chernow B. Insulin and oral hypoglycemics. In: Chernow B, ed. The pharmacological approach to the critically ill patient. Baltimore: Williams & Wilkins, 1988:637.

Adrenal Disorders

Bittar DA. Innovar-induced hypertensive crises in patients with pheochromocytoma. Anesthesiology 1977;46:359.

Bone RC, Fisher CJ, Clemmer TP, Slotman GJ, Metz CA, Balk RA. A controlled clinical trial of high-dose methylprednisolone in the treatment of severe sepsis and septic shock. N Engl J Med 1987;317:653.

Bravo EL, Gifford RW. Pheochromocytoma: diagnosis, localization and management. N Engl J Med 1984;311:1298.

Chernow B, Vernoski B, Zaloga GP, et al. Dexamethasone causes less steroid-induced alkalemia than methylprednisolone or hydrocortisone. Crit Care Med 1984;12:384.

Chin R Jr. Corticosteroids. In: Chernow B, ed. The pharmacologic approach to the critically ill patient. 2nd ed. Baltimore: Williams & Wilkins, 1988:559.

Cousins MJ, Rubin RB. The intraoperative management of phaeochromocytoma with total epidural sympathetic blockade. Br J Anaesth 1974;46:78.

Cunningham SK, Moore A, McKenna J. Normal cortisol response to corticotropin in patients with secondary adrenal failure. Arch Intern Med 1983;143:2276.

Darowski MJ, Coutinho WBA, Power SJ, Jones RM. Vecuronium and phaeochromocytoma. Anaesthesia 1986;41:1225.

DeCoster R, Helmers JHJH, Noorduin H. Effect of etomidate on cortisol biosynthesis: site of action after induction of anesthesia. Acta Endocrinol 1985;110:526.

Fragen RJ, Shanks CA, Molteni A, Avram MJ. Effects of etomidate on hormonal responses to surgical stress. Anesthesiology 1984; 61:652.

Hanowell ST, Hittner KC, Kim YD, MacNamara TE. Anesthetic management of primary aldosteronism. Anesth Rev 1982;9(8):36.

Hull CJ. Phaeochromocytoma: diagnosis, preoperative preparation and anaesthetic management. Br J Anaesth 1986;58:1453.

Galletly DC, Yee P, Maling TJB. Anaesthetic management of combined caesarean section and phaeochromocytoma removal. Anaesth Intens Care 1983;11:249.

Garcia R, Jennings JM. Pheochromocytoma masquerading as cardiomyopathy. Am J Med 1972;29:568.

James MFM, Huddle KRL, van der Veen BW. Use of magnesium sulphate in the anaesthetic management of phaeochromocytoma in pregnancy. Can J Anaesth 1988;35:178.

Kaufman L. Use of labetalol during hypotensive anaesthesia and in the management of phaeochromocytoma. Br J Clin Pharmacol 1979;8:229.

Koch–Weser J. Withdrawal from glucocorticoid therapy. N Engl J Med 1976;295:30.

Lacoumenta S, Paterson JL, Myers MA, Hall GM. Effects of cortisol suppression by etomidate on changes in circulating metabolites associated with pelvic surgery. Acta Anaesthesiol Scand 1986;30:101.

Lampe GH, Roizen MF. Anesthesia for patients with abnormal function of the adrenal cortex. Anesthesiol Clin North Am 1987; 5:245.

McDonald WN, Doll WA, Schmidt N, Reynolds C. Intravenous nitroglycerin control of blood pressure during resection of phaeochromocytoma. Can Anaesth Soc J 1982;29:108.

Mihm FG. Pulmonary artery pressure monitoring in patients with pheochromocytoma. Anesthesiology 1982;57(93):a42.

Muldoon SM, Moss J, Freas W, Roizen MF. The effects of anaesthetics on the sympathoadrenal system. Clin Anaesth 1984;2:289.

Perry PJ, Tsuang MT, Hwang MH. Prednisolone psychosis: clinical observations. Drug Intell Clin Pharm 1984;18:603.

Rouby JJ, Gory G, Gaveau T, Glaser P, Viars P. Dangerous rise in pulmonary wedge pressure following aortography in a patient with a pheochromocytoma. Anesth Analg 1980;59:154.

Samaan NA, Hickey RC. Pheochromocytoma. Semin Oncol 1987; 14:297.

Schoenfeld Y, Gurewich Y, Gallant LA, Pinkhas J. Prednisone-induced leukocytosis. Am J Med 1981;71:773.

Shapiro JD, El-Ganzouri A, White PF, Ivankovich AD. Midazolam–sufentanil anaesthesia for phaeochromocytoma resection. Can J Anaesth 1988;35:190.

Stoelting RK, Dierdorf SF, McCammon RL. Anesthesia and co-existing disease, 2nd ed. New York: Churchill Livingstone, 1988:473.

Stonham J, Wakefield C. Phaeochromocytoma in pregnancy. Anaesthesia 1983;38:654.

Streck WF, Lockwood DH. Pituitary adrenal recovery following short-term suppression with corticosteroids. Am J Med 1979;66:910.

Sumikawa K, Amakata Y. The pressor effect of droperidol on a patient with pheochromocytoma. Anesthesiology 1977;46:359.

Symreng T, Karlberg BE, Kagedal B, Schildt B. Physiological cortisol substitution of long-term steroid-treated patients undergoing major surgery. Br J Anaesth 1981;53:949.

Weatherill D, Spence AA. Anaesthesia and disorders of the adrenal cortex. Br J Anaesth 1984;56:741.

Welborn LG. Pheochromocytoma in children and the anesthetic management. Middle East J Anesth 1987;9:109.

Ziment I. Steroids. Clin Chest Med 1986;7:341.

Thyroid Disorders

Amino N, Mori H, Iwatani Y, Miyai K. High prevalence of transient postpartum thyrotoxicosis and hypothyroidism. N Engl J Med 1982;306:849.

Becker C. Hypothyroidism and atherosclerotic heart disease pathogenesis, medical management, and the role of coronary artery bypass surgery. Endocrine Rev 1985;6:432.

Benson DW. Anesthesia for thyroid surgery. Semin Anesthesia 1984;3(2):168.

Cooper DS. Subclinical hypothyroidism. JAMA 1987;258:246.

Drucker D, Burrow GN. Cardiovascular surgery in the hypothyroid patient. Arch Intern Med 1985;145:1585.

Eriksson M, Rubenfeld S, Garber AJ, Kohler PO. Propranolol does not prevent thyroid storm. N Engl J Med 1977;296:263.

Feek CM, Sawers SA, Irvine WJ, Beckett GJ, Ratcliffe WA, Toft AD. Combination of potassium iodide and propranolol in preparation of patients with Graves' disease for thyroid surgery. N Engl J Med 1980;302:883.

Forfar JC, Muir AL, Sawers SA, Toft AD. Abnormal left ventricular function in hyperthyroidism. N Engl J Med 1982;307:1165.

Hamilton WFD, Forrest Al, Gunn A, Peden NR, Feely J. Beta-adrenoceptor blockade and anaesthesia for thyroidectomy. Anaesthesia 1984;39:335.

Ikeda S, Schweiss JF. Excessive blood loss during operation in the patient treated with propylthiouracil. Can Anaesth Soc J 1982;29:477.

Levelle JP, Jopling MW, Sklar GS. Perioperative hypothyroidism: an unusual postanesthetic diagnosis. Anesthesiology 1985;63:195.

Levine HD. Compromise therapy in the patient with angina pectoris and hypothyroidism. Am J Med 1980;69:411.

Murkin JM. Anesthesia and hypothyroidism: a review of thyroxine physiology, pharmacology, and anesthetic implications. Anesth Analg 1982;61:371.

Robson NJ. Emergency surgery complicated by thyrotoxicosis and thyrotoxic periodic paralysis. Anaesthesia 1985;40:27.

Roizen MF, Hensel P, Lichtor L, Schreider BD. Patients with disorders of thyroid function. Anesth Clin North Am 1987;5:277.

Saxe AW, Brown E, Hamburger SW. Thyroid and parathyroid surgery performed with patient under regional anesthesia. Surgery 1988;103:415.

Servin FF, Nivoche Y, Desmonts JM, Rice SA, Mazze RI. Biotransformation of halothane and enflurane in patients with hyperthyroidism. Anaesthesiology 1986;64:387.

Sherry KM, Hutchinson IL. Postoperative myxoedema. Anaesthesia 1984;39:1112.

Stoelting RK, Dierdorf SF, McCammon RL. Anesthesia and co-existing disease, 2nd ed. New York: Churchill Livingstone, 1988:473.

Weinberg AD, Brennan MD, Gorman CA, Marsh HM, O'Fallon M.

Outcome of anesthesia and surgery in hypothyroid patients. Arch Intern Med 1983;143:893.

Pituitary Disorders

Chan VWS, Tindal S. Anaesthesia for transsphenoidal surgery in a patient with extreme gigantism. Br J Anaesth 1988;60:465.

Hassan SZ, Matz GJ, Lawrence AM, Collins PA. Laryngeal stenosis in acromegaly: a possible cause of airway difficulties associated with anesthesia. Anesth Analg 1976;55:57.

Kitahata LM. Airway difficulties associated with anaesthesia in acromegaly. Br J Anaesth 1971;43:1187.

Stoelting RK, Dierdorf SF, McCammon RL. Anesthesia and co-existing disease, 2nd ed. New York: Churchill Livingstone, 1988:473.

Porphyria

Allen SC, Rees GAD. A previous history of acute intermittent porphyria as a complication of obstetric anaesthesia. Br J Anaesth 1980;52:835.

Bancroft GH, Lauria JI. Ketamine induction for caesarian section in a patient with acute intermittent porphyria and achondroplastic dwarfism. Anesthesiology 1983;50:143.

Kostrzewska E, Gregor A. Ketamine in acute intermittent porphyria: dangerous or safe? 1978;49:376.

Mastajoki P, Heinonen J. General anesthesia in the "inducible" porphyrias. Anesthesiology 1980;53:15.

Sergay SM. Management of neurologic exacerbations of hepatic porphyria. Med Clin North Am 1979;63:453.

Slavin S, Christoforides C. Thiopental administration in acute intermittent porphyria without adverse effect. Anesthesiology 1976;44:77.

Stoelting RK, Dierdorf SF, McCammon RL. Anesthesia and co-existing disease, 2nd ed. New York: Churchill Livingstone, 1988:473.

Hyperparathyroidism

Al-Mohaya S, Naguib M, Abdelatif M, Farag H. Abnormal responses to muscle relaxants in a patient with primary hyperparathyroidism. Anesthesiology 1986;65:554.

Hensel P, Roizen MF. Patients with disorders of parathyroid function. Anesth Clin North Am 1987;5:287.

Pyrtek LJ, Belkin M, Bartus S, Schweitzer R. Parathyroid gland exploration with local anesthesia in elderly and high-risk patients. Arch Surg 1988;123:614.

Stoelting RK, Dierdorf SF, McCammon RL. Anesthesia and co-existing disease, 2nd ed. New York: Churchill Livingstone, 1988:473.

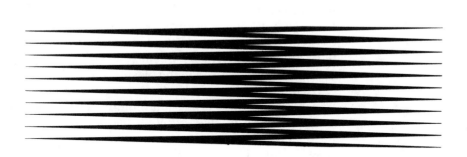

Anemia, Bleeding Disorders, and Transfusion Therapy

Robert N. Sladen

≡ Anemia

General Considerations

I. PATHOPHYSIOLOGY
   A. Anemia and Oxygen Delivery
      1. Hemoglobin (Hb) is essential for the transport of oxygen (O_2) in the blood. In a normal individual with an arterial oxygen content (Ca_{O_2}) of 20 ml/dl, 0.3 ml of O_2 is dissolved in the plasma and 19.7 ml is carried on Hb. At rest, the mean oxygen consumption by the tissues is 250 ml/minute. If Hb were completely absent, the resting cardiac output would have to be 85 L/minute to satisfy this demand! Anemia thus impairs ability to deliver O_2 to the tissues. For example, a decrease of Hb from 15 to 10 g/dl decreases Ca_{O_2} and usually causes an increase in cardiac output (CO) to maintain oxygen delivery.

$$\text{Oxygen delivery} = Ca_{O_2} \times CO$$

      2. Inadequate delivery of O_2 results in anaerobic metabolism and lactate production, leading ultimately to cell injury and death.
   B. Compensatory Mechanisms
      1. As Ca_{O_2} declines, there is a stimulus to 2,3-diphosphoglycerate (2,3-DPG) production in red cells, which shifts the oxyhemoglobin dissociation curve to the right and facilitates unloading of Hb at the tissues. This reduces mixed venous saturation and appears to be the most important compensatory mechanism in mild anemia (Hb 10–15 g/dl). Note that it is totally dependent on the adequacy of inorganic phosphate. Below an Hb of 10 g/dl, oxygen delivery is maintained by a progressive increase in cardiac output through increased heart rate or stroke volume.
      2. In addition, as the hematocrit decreases, decreased blood viscosity results in enhanced microcapillary circulation. Renal erythropoietin stimulates red blood cell (RBC) production in the bone marrow, reflected in an increased peripheral reticulocyte (immature red cell) count.
      3. Individual organs can compensate for decreased O_2 delivery by vasodilation of the supply vessels to in-

crease perfusion. However, the myocardium extracts virtually all the delivered O_2. Coronary sinus blood, with an oxygen tension of 23 mmHg, is the most desaturated in the body. Because extraction cannot increase further, the only mechanism for providing more O_2 to the myocardium is increased perfusion by means of coronary vasodilation.

4. Transport of dissolved O_2 in plasma becomes much more important in anemia. For example, if with breathing of 100% O_2, the arterial oxygen tension (PaO_2) is increased from 100 to 500 mmHg, Ca_{O_2} is increased by ($.003 \times 500$) or 1.5 ml/dl, which may make a significant difference to a patient with myocardial ischemia.

5. If anemia develops slowly enough, remarkably low levels of Hb may be tolerated without organ failure. Nonetheless, organs that are chronically nutritionally depleted and hypoxic—especially the myocardium—have little reserve to deal with anesthetic and surgical stress. Thus, whereas acute anemia may be relatively well tolerated in young, healthy individuals, in patients with cardiovascular, pulmonary, or cerebrovascular disease, organ ischemia or failure may quickly ensue.

II. PREOPERATIVE EVALUATION
  A. History
    1. The cause and chronicity of anemia should be established (Table 8-1).
    2. The symptoms of anemia and their severity should be elicited: fatigue, lassitude, loss of concentration or memory, dyspnea, presyncope or syncope, palpitations, loss of weight, amenorrhea, and new onset or exacerbation of angina.
    3. The severity of associated disease should be evaluated.
  B. Physical Examination
    1. Signs of anemia should be sought.
      a. Pallor of the mucous membranes and nailbeds
      b. Hyperdynamic circulation: tachycardia and wide pulse pressure (collapsing pulse) secondary to low systemic vascular resistance
      c. Cardiomegaly: displaced, forceful left ventricular apex
      d. Ejection (diamond-shaped) systolic murmur

Table 8-1. Causes of Anemia

Acute

Blood loss
 Major trauma, major surgery
Hemolytic reactions
 Mismatched transfusion, bacterial endocarditis, acute pancreatitis
Acute or chronic hemolytic anemia
 Sickle cell crisis, G6PD deficiency

Chronic

Blood loss (iron deficiency anemia)
 Gastrointestinal: peptic ulcer disease, varices, inflammatory bowel
  disease, carcinoma
 Genitourinary: menorrhagia, hematuria
Megaloblastic anemias
 Vitamin B_{12} deficiency (pernicious anemia), folate deficiency
Systemic diseases (multifactorial)
 Sepsis (e.g., bacterial endocarditis)
 Uremia (inadequate erythropoietin, uremic bone marrow depression,
  decreased RBC survival)
 Liver failure (chronic alcoholic nutritional depletion, folate deficiency,
  gastritis, hypersplenism)
 Chronic inflammatory disease (e.g., rheumatoid arthritis)
Hemolytic anemia
 Hereditary spherocytosis, G6PD deficiency, paroxysmal nocturnal
  hemoglobinuria
 Transfusion-induced hemolysis, prosthetic valve leaks
  (macroangiopathic hemolytic anemia)
Aplastic/hypoplastic anemia
 Blood dyscrasias (e.g., multiple myeloma); chemotherapy; irradiation;
  drug reactions (e.g., trimethoprim, chloramphenicol)
Hemoglobinopathies
 Sickle cell anemia
 Thalassemia

---

    e. Left ventricular gallop, tachypnea with basal crackles, ankle edema (high-output failure).

2. Any blood loss should be evaluated.

    a. Acute loss (hypovolemic anemia)

        1) Less than 10%: usually no clinical signs.

        2) 20% reduction: orthostatic hypotension (systolic blood pressure decreases by more than 15 mmHg with elevation of head, legs down); tachycardia.

        3) 40% reduction: resting tachycardia, hypotension, tachypnea, diaphoresis.

      b. Chronic loss (normovolemic anemia)
- **1)** Tachycardia and pallor usually found at Hb 9 to 10 g/dl.
- **2)** Dyspnea at Hb 7 to 8 g/dl.
- **3)** Weakness, lassitude at Hb 5 to 6 g/dl.
- **4)** Dyspnea at rest and congestive heart failure (CHF) at Hb less than 5 g/dl.
- **5)** With severe anemia, retinal hemorrhages or papilledema may be present.

  3. Signs of associated disease should be sought: hepatosplenomegaly (hereditary spherocytosis, sickle cell anemia, chronic liver disease), cachexia (cancer), arthritis (rheumatoid, connective tissue diseases), or uremia.

C. Laboratory Investigations

  1. Hb and hematocrit (Hct) define the severity of the anemia (Table 8-2). Note that Hct does not reflect RBC mass in acute blood loss until the plasma volume has reequilibrated (24–48 hours). Hematology indices help define the nature of the anemia: normochromic, normocytic anemia suggests acute blood loss or chronic inflammation; hypochromic, microcytic anemia suggests iron deficiency or chronic blood loss; megaloblastic anemia suggests folate deficiency or phenytoin toxicity. A peripheral smear is mandatory to evaluate cell size and evi-

Table 8–2. Normal Hematology Values (RBCs and Platelets)

Hemoglobin (Hb) (g/dl)	Males	13.6–17.2
	Females	12.0–15.0
Hematocrit (Hct) (%)	Males	39–49
	Females	33–43
RBC ($\times\ 10^9$/dl)	Males	4.3–5.9
	Females	3.5–5.0
Mean corpuscular volume (MCV) (fl)		80–98
Mean corpuscular hemoglobin (MCH) (ng)		27–31
Mean corpuscular Hb concentration (MCHC) (%)		32–36
Reticulocyte count (%)		0.5–1.5
Platelets (per μl)		150,000–450,000

(Courtesy of the Hematology Laboratory, Duke University Medical Center.)

dence of hemolysis, acute inflammation (Heinz bodies), or myeloproliferative disorders.

2. Hemolysis workup (if clinically indicated)

   a. The differential diagnosis of an acute hemolytic reaction includes transfusion of mismatched blood, severe sepsis, infection by hemolytic organisms, periprosthetic valve leak (microangiopathic hemolytic anemia), sickle cell crisis, hypersplenism, paroxysmal nocturnal hemoglobinuria, glucose-6-phosphate dehydrogenase (G6PD) deficiency, thrombotic thrombocytopenia purpura, and hemolytic uremic syndrome.

   b. Laboratory analysis includes peripheral smear (crenated, burr, helmet cells, sickle cells), reticulocyte count (less than 1–2% indicates RBC production defect; above 5% suggests hemolysis), haptoglobin (decreased below 100 mg/dl with increasing release of free Hb), Coombs test (if positive, suggests autoimmune hemolytic anemia), cold antibodies, and positive free plasma Hb. Unconjugated hyperbilirubinemia accompanies severe hemolysis and manifests as jaundice with dark urine.

3. Other laboratory investigations, as indicated by clinical evaluation: renal function tests (acute hemolysis, uremia), liver function tests, hemoglobin electrophoresis, bone marrow examination.

4. The ECG may indicate sinus tachycardia or other arrhythmias, left ventricular hypertrophy (LVH), or myocardial ischemia.

5. Chest radiography may demonstrate cardiomegaly or pulmonary congestion or edema.

III. INDICATIONS FOR PREOPERATIVE TRANSFUSION

   A. The primary advantage of preoperative restoration of Hb is increasing oxygen-carrying capacity and cardiovascular reserve. Transfusion is mandatory for patients with acute blood loss with hypovolemia. Anticipation of significant blood loss during the surgical procedure (e.g., major vascular or orthopedic surgery) favors preoperative transfusion. There is little scientific evidence that anemia worsens wound healing (which is affected by tissue O_2 tension rather than Hb), and resistance to infection may actually be diminished by the leukocyte depressant effect of homologous blood transfusion.

B. The traditional notion that the minimum acceptable preoperative Hb is 10 g/dl (Hct of 30%) should not be slavishly followed. Patients with normovolemic anemia who are otherwise healthy appear to tolerate surgery and anesthesia well with an Hb as low as 7 g/dl. On the other hand, in the presence of significant cardiac, pulmonary, cerebral, or renal disease, an Hb of at least 10 g/dl may be necessary to ensure adequate organ reserve.

C. Preoperatively, transfusion is not indicated in patients with chronic, stable normovolemic anemia, because the risks generally outweigh the benefits. These risks include fluid overload and pulmonary edema, mismatched transfusion, disease transmission, and suppression of the immune response.

D. In chronic renal failure, an Hct of around 28% is well tolerated because of increased 2,3-DPG production unless overzealous dialysis or aluminum hydroxide administration has induced hypophosphatemia. Preoperative transfusion is indicated only if the Hct is less than 25% and there has been recent acute blood loss or if there is associated cardiopulmonary disease. Because the patient's volume balance is precarious, transfusion should be provided during hemodialysis, preferably the day before surgery.

IV. ANESTHETIC MANAGEMENT

    A. Premedication

    Because of the limited cardiopulmonary reserve, premedication should be relatively light. Combinations of narcotics and benzodiazepines should be avoided, as they are more likely to cause respiratory depression and hypoxemia.

    B. Monitoring

        1. Patients should be closely monitored to ensure the adequacy of oxygenation and oxygen delivery. Pulse oximetry should be used for all cases.

        2. The threshold for deciding on invasive monitoring should be lowered. Arterial cannulation (close observation of blood pressure, frequent assessment of arterial blood gases) and a central venous pressure catheter should be considered when anemia is symptomatic, for surgery associated with fluid shifts, or when moderate cardiopulmonary or renal dysfunction is present.

3. In the presence of CHF, severe pulmonary or renal insufficiency, or sepsis or when significant blood loss is anticipated, a pulmonary artery catheter should be placed. This will allow serial assessment of intravascular volume, cardiac output, and O_2 delivery.

4. Continuous mixed venous oximetry provides an immediate and direct guide to the adequacy of O_2 delivery to the tissues. During anesthesia, the mixed venous oxygen saturation ($S\bar{v}O_2$) usually increases from the normal range of 75% to 85% to 90% because of a marked reduction in oxygen consumption. If tissue oxygenation is inadequate, the $S\bar{v}O_2$ will fall progressively below 75%. If this occurs in the face of a normal or increased cardiac output and PaO_2, it provides a very important indication for intraoperative or postoperative blood transfusion.

C. Choice of Anesthetic Technique
   1. Regional anesthesia
      a. Regional anesthesia should be provided carefully. The cardiovascular response to sympathetic block is compromised, but aggressive fluid loading prior to the block to prevent this may not be tolerated. Where possible, steps should be taken to reduce the rate of onset and distribution of sympathetic block (e.g., low, unilateral, or continuous spinal techniques; continuous rather than single-shot epidural anesthesia with small increments of local anesthetic). Oxygen must be administered at all times.
      b. Use of regional anesthesia does not reduce the indications for invasive monitoring. The risk of hypothermia (and postoperative shivering) is as great with regional as with general anesthesia.
      c. Rebound pulmonary edema is a potential postoperative complication in patients with anemic cardiomyopathy when venous return to the heart increases as the sympathetic block wears off.

2. Induction and maintenance of general anesthesia

    a. Preoxygenation with 100% O_2 may increase the dissolved O_2 concentration from 0.3 to 1.8 ml/dl, depending on lung function, and may enhance oxygen reserve during induction and intubation. End points of effective preoxygenation include an SaO_2 of 100% (pulse oximetry), sustained $\bar{S}vO_2$ exceeding 85% (mixed venous oximetry), or nitrogen washout (mass spectrometry).

    b. Nitrous oxide should be avoided in severe anemia to allow provision of 100% O_2 and to avoid cardiovascular depression.

    c. Myocardial depression must be avoided. Narcotic anesthetic techniques are preferred to volatile agents. Ketamine is a useful induction agent (e.g., at low doses such as 0.5–1.0 mg/kg together with a benzodiazepine such as midazolam, 0.2–1.0 mg/kg). If a volatile agent is chosen, isoflurane is preferred to halothane or enflurane because it has less negative inotropic effect.

    d. The solubility of volatile anesthetics is decreased in anemia because of a paucity of lipid-rich RBCs. Theoretically, this should lead to more rapid induction and emergence. However, this effect is offset by the increased cardiac output, and its clinical importance is uncertain.

    e. Acute respiratory alkalosis caused by overzealous ventilation during anesthesia must be avoided, as it causes cerebral vasoconstriction, hypokalemia (and cardiac arrhythmias), decreased O_2 supply (shifts the oxyhemoglobin dissociation curve to the left), and increased O_2 demand (stimulates glycolysis). Capnometry is an important guide to matching minute ventilation with the reduced CO_2 production induced by anesthesia.

D. Hypothermia: Significance and Prevention

    1. Hypothermia is a constant companion to anesthesia, because anesthesia abolishes two important mechanisms of heat preservation: piloerection and shivering. Another, peripheral vasoconstriction, is blunted by volatile anesthetics, vasodilator drugs, and regional anesthesia. General anesthetics alter central homeostatic mechanisms. Hypothermia occurs even more rapidly in patients at the extremes of life because of their inadequate subcutaneous fat and immature (geriatric) cardiovascular responses.

2. Hypothermia increases systemic vascular resistance (increased blood viscosity, vasoconstriction) and may further impair already-compromised cardiac function. The effects on the patient with sickle cell anemia may be disastrous. During emergence and recovery, hypothermia is followed by rebound rewarming and shivering. This markedly increases O_2 consumption and CO_2 production and induces vasodilation. The already-depleted cardiopulmonary reserve of the anemic patient is further taxed, causing hypotension, tachycardia, acidosis, and myocardial ischemia.

3. The following simple precautions can prevent hypothermia:

   a. The OR must be warmed before the patient arrives and the environment kept heated until the patient is induced, prepared, and draped. The OR is rewarmed at the end of the procedure before the patient is uncovered.

   b. All exposed surfaces of the patient should be covered. Woolen or plastic head wraps can markedly reduce heat loss, particularly in infants.

   c. A blood warmer is used for all fluids, not just blood. The OR nursing staff should warm all preparation and irrigation fluids.

   d. A heater–humidifier is used for inspired gas, and total gas flows are reduced to a minimum (e.g., 2 L/min) during maintenance of anesthesia.

   e. A heating blanket is used if available, although this is not as effective as the other methods described.

E. Intraoperative Transfusion

1. Transfusion should be guided by:

   a. The severity of the anemia

   b. The cardiovascular reserve of the patient

      c.   The degree of intraoperative blood loss

      d.   Close evaluation of the patient's status.

   2.   If the patient is barely compensated or has significant cardiopulmonary disease, intraoperative transfusion should be commenced promptly, as these patients may not tolerate the usual indication of a loss of 10% or more of blood volume. Changes in clinical status associated with rapid blood loss that indicate the necessity for intraoperative transfusion include tachycardia, hypotension, oliguria, arrhythmias, hypocarbia in the face of constant minute ventilation (i.e., decreased cardiac output), hypoxemia, and decreasing cardiac filling pressures, cardiac output, or $S\bar{v}O_2$.

F.   Emergence and Postoperative Care

   1.   Care should be taken to ensure full reversal of anesthesia prior to extubation. Extubated patients must be transported to the recovery room or intensive care unit with supplemental mask oxygen, preferably monitored by pulse oximetry.

   2.   In the postanesthetic care unit and intensive care unit, close attention should be paid to the avoidance of further hypothermia, which will stimulate shivering and increase oxygen consumption. Use of an overhead radiant heater is particularly useful. Hypovolemia and pain should be aggressively but carefully treated to minimize cardiovascular and metabolic stress.

   3.   Decisions to transfuse in the postoperative period should be based on the same rules as those used in the OR.

V.   SUMMARY OF ANESTHETIC CONSIDERATIONS

Hemoglobin is essential for the transport of oxygen; therefore, oxygen delivery to the tissues is compromised by anemia. Compensatory mechanisms for decreased arterial oxygen content are increased production of 2,3-PDG, increased cardiac output, peripheral vasodilation, and increased release of erythropoietin. Despite optimal compensation, dyspnea at rest, CHF, weakness, hypotension, and tachycardia can be seen at rest with severe anemia (Hb <5 g/dl). Preoperative evaluation and correction of the cause of anemia should be performed if time allows.

    Preoperatively, acutely anemic patients should be given transfusions to an Hct of at least 28% before major surgery to optimize intravascular volume and ensure adequate RBC reserve. Patients who are chronically anemic and normovolemic appear to tolerate surgery and anesthesia with an Hb as low as 7 g/dl if intraoperative fluid loss is minimal. Because of their limited cardiopulmonary reserve, premedication should be relatively light. Patients should be closely monitored to ensure the adequacy of oxygenation and oxygen delivery.

Regional anesthesia should be provided with special care for the anemic patient. Fluid loading to compensate for the cardiovascular response to a sympathetic block may not be well tolerated. Preoxygenation is especially important before induction because the increase in dissolved O_2 will help compensate for the decrease in the Hb oxygen content. Nitrous oxide should not be used in severe anemia, because it limits delivered oxygen concentration. Overventilating the patient should be avoided. Respiratory alkalosis may cause cerebral vasoconstriction, hypokalemia (cardiac arrhythmias), and decreased O_2 delivery (shifts the oxyhemoglobin dissociation curve to the left). Intraoperative blood transfusions should be started earlier in the anemic patient, because RBC reserve is lower. Vasoconstrictive drugs may be used transiently to support the blood pressure while blood volume is being restored.

Specific Causes of Anemia and Associated Problems

I.   ACUTE BLOOD LOSS
   A.   Acute hemorrhage may be encountered by the anesthesiologist preoperatively, intraoperatively, or postoperatively.
   B.   The basic principles in its management are:
      1.   Securing of the airway to ensure adequate oxygenation and ventilation.
      2.   Establishment of adequate access by placing two or more large (14-gauge) intravenous lines. Large-bore central lines are very helpful when peripheral access is limited, but their placement is hazardous during CPR, and subclavian catheters particularly may be relatively contraindicated in the presence of a severe coagulopathy. The femoral vein provides access that is safely achieved and maintained during CPR or with a coagulopathy. Surgical trauma units

routinely obtain major access by inserting sterile nasogastric sump tubes into large leg veins by surgical cutdown.

3. Rapidly administered blood should be passed through warmers to reduce viscosity, prevent cardiac cooling and arrhythmias, and facilitate unloading of oxygen from the transfused blood. At 8°C, the oxyhemoglobin dissociation curve is shifted so far left that the Hb is totally unable to give up O_2 at usual tissue O_2 tensions.

4. Hypothermia must be avoided. Once body temperature falls to 32°C or below, a profound and often irreversible coagulopathy ensues.

5. Intravascular volume status and arterial blood gases and electrolytes are assessed frequently. Ventilation should be controlled, and boluses of sodium bicarbonate (25–50 mEq) should be administered to maintain pH 7.25 or above to enhance responsiveness to endogenous and exogenous catecholamines. Noninvasive methods of measurement may not be accurate in this setting, and pulse oximetry often does not work in shocked, vasoconstricted patients. Capnometry may also be misleading: the alveolar–arterial CO_2 gradient widens markedly in the presence of low cardiac output, and a normal end-tidal CO_2 does not ensure a normal pH in the presence of metabolic acidosis. Hyperkalemia and hypocalcemia may occur during rapid blood transfusion (>150 ml/min).

6. Vasoactive drugs must be used judiciously. Drugs such as norepinephrine (Levophed) or phenylephrine (Neo-Synephrine) should be reserved for transient maintenance of blood pressure while blood volume is being restored during life-threatening hemorrhage. Inotropic agents such as dopamine (Intropin) or epinephrine (Adrenalin) may be indicated for associated cardiac failure but may induce tachyarrhythmias, especially in the presence of myocardial ischemia or acidosis.

II. MEGALOBLASTIC ANEMIA

A. General Characteristics
Megaloblastic anemia is a maturation disorder of red cells attributable to a deficit of essential nutrients (folate or vitamin B_{12}) and is characterized by macrocytic, hypo-

chromic red cells on the peripheral smear. Other bone marrow elements, such as polymorphonuclear leukocytes (hypersegmented) and platelets (giants), may also be affected. Therapy is simple replacement of the deficient nutrient. Precise identification of each disorder is required, however, as administration of folate in the presence of vitamin B_{12} deficiency will exacerbate the neurologic manifestations of vitamin B_{12} deficiency.

B. Folate Deficiency
Folate deficiency is a common disorder in critically ill patients, alcoholics, pregnant patients, and those receiving phenytoin (Dilantin). Its clinical features include a smooth tongue, hyperpigmentation, peripheral edema, peripheral neuropathy, and liver dysfunction.

C. Vitamin B_{12} Deficiency
  1. Vitamin B_{12} (cyanocobalamin) deficiency is much less common than folate deficiency. Simple nutritional deficiency can occur with abnormal diets, but the body stores are extensive.
  2. Pernicious anemia is caused by vitamin B_{12} deficiency secondary to autoimmune gastric mucosal atrophy and lack of secretion of intrinsic factor, which is essential for vitamin absorption in the ileum. Deficiency may also be caused by ileal disease or resection. The disease is characterized by a peripheral neuropathy with lateral and posterior column degeneration, resulting in loss of the sense of position and vibration.
  3. Spinal and epidural anesthesia are best avoided in the presence of peripheral neuropathy.
  4. Nitrous oxide inhibits the enzyme methionine synthetase by oxidizing cyanocobalamin. Prolonged use of N_2O (for example, to provide analgesia in intensive care units) may itself result in pernicious anemia.

III. HEMOGLOBINOPATHIES
  A. Classification
    1. A mutant hemoglobin is a qualitative or structural defect in Hb formation. The hemoglobin seen in sickle cell anemia (HbS) is an example.
      a. Normal Hb has a molecular weight of 68,000 and a hydrophobic heme pocket with a hydrophilic surface, dependent on globin–globin

binding. The Hb tetramer shifts with O_2 loading and unloading.

    b. More than 450 mutant hemoglobins are known. There is a wide range of manifestations:

      1) No abnormality of function

      2) An unstable, weakened tetramer (e.g., HbE, common in southeast Asia) resulting in oxidation of Hb, Heinz body formation, and hemolytic anemia

      3) Altered P50 (Hb O_2 affinity)

      4) Methemoglobinemia ("familial cyanosis," "brown blood")

      5) Sickle cell anemia.

  2. Thalassemia is a quantitative or production defect resulting in the formation of excess amounts of an impaired chain and hemolytic anemia.

B. Sickle Cell Anemia

  1. Incidence

Manifestations of sickle cell anemia depend on the inherited genotype, which occurs in a significant proportion of black people in the United States. The most severe anemia occurs with the homozygous form (SS) (0.1% to 1% of US blacks). More moderate variants include SC (sickle-target cell) and S/β-thalassemia. Sickle cell trait (AS) is asymptomatic and occurs in as many as 8% of US blacks. Multiple organ involvement is characteristic of people with sickle cell disease. The perioperative mortality rate is about 7.5%.

  2. Pathophysiology

    a. A mutation at the sixth amino acid on the Hb beta chain causes glutamate (a hydrophilic amino acid) to be replaced by valine (a hydrophobic amino acid), resulting in an "oily" spot on the surface of HbSS. There is no change in the P50. However, when the HbSS is deoxygenated, this hydrophobic spot binds with another to form strands of Hb that clump into tactoids (elongated crescents) and result in sickling of RBCs. The sickled cell is rigid and wedges in capillaries, resulting in increased viscosity and sludging, which promotes further sickling. Vascular obstruction ultimately leads to localized, then widespread, infarction and generalized organ dysfunction. Acute episodes of sickling are called sickle cell crises.

b. In homozygous sickle cell anemia (SS), 85% to 90% of Hb is HbS; the remainder is fetal Hb (HbF). In heterozygous sickle cell trait (AS), 30% to 50% of Hb is HbS; the remainder is HbA or HbA2, variably distributed among the RBC population. In SS, RBCs sickle at normally occurring $P\bar{v}O_2$ (40–60 mmHg); at a PO_2 of 20 mmHg, 100% of cells are sickled. In AS, RBCs sickle only at a PO_2 of less than 20 mmHg (SO_2 30%–40%).

c. Factors promoting sickling include hypoxemia (i.e., an increased concentration of deoxygenated Hb), increased blood viscosity (stasis, hypothermia, dehydration), and acidosis. Sickling inevitably occurs in venular rather than arteriolar blood. Fresh sickling is reversible, and simple hydration alone can desickle sickled cells. However, once the RBC membrane is damaged by the Hb polymers, sickling is irreversible; and blood viscosity remains increased even when SO_2 is restored. Increased RBC 2,3-DPG (a normal response to anemia) ironically predisposes to sickling by facilitating unloading of O_2 from Hb. Increased levels of HbF protect against sickling, leading to the clinical use of hydroxyurea, a cytotoxic drug that increases HbF levels.

3. Clinical features
   a. There is chronic hemolytic anemia (Hb 6–8 g/dl).
   b. Sickle cell crises are episodes of acute hemolysis and acute, often excruciating, pain caused by multiple organ ischemia. They are induced by stress, sepsis, pregnancy, hypovolemia, hypoxemia, and acidosis. Acute viral infections may precipitate an aplastic crisis (pancytopenia); a sequestration crisis implies massive trapping of RBCs by the reticuloendothelial system with hypovolemic shock.

c. Cerebrovascular accidents are common especially in children. Stroke is significantly reduced by a transfusion program of two units every 2 weeks. Stroke may be induced by hyperventilation (i.e., cerebral vasoconstriction secondary to acute respiratory alkalosis), severe anemia, infection, sickle cell crisis, or hypoxemia. In adults, the mortality rate is 50%; in children, it is around 15%.

d. Pulmonary involvement may be severe without being symptomatic. Chest radiography may also be normal, but vital capacity is reduced, and the lung scan is markedly abnormal: there is a "notched" perfusion scan and "patchy dropout" on a ventilation scan. Lung involvement is particularly common in SC. Pulmonary embolism and respiratory infection is common in the postoperative period.

e. Cardiac involvement is usually secondary to high-output failure (chronic anemia) or to cor pulmonale (pulmonary hypertension attributable to multiple pulmonary infarcts).

f. Renal abnormalities are established by the age of 5 to 8 years. The hypertonic medulla concentrates Hb and causes local sickling. As medullary nephrons infarct, there is loss of concentrating ability (obligatory hyposthenuria), further increasing the risk of dehydration. Hematuria results from renal infarcts, papillary damage, and necrosis.

g. Hepatic and splenic infarcts may be focal or diffuse and may lead to abscesses. Splenic paralysis predisposes to pneumococcal bacteremia (an important cause of death in children), necessitating prophylactic antibiotic therapy. Cholelithiasis and cholecystitis are relatively common. Hemochromatosis ensues with iron overload after multiple transfusions. Severe liver dysfunction can result in pseudocholinesterase deficiency.

h. White cell function is depressed (decreased chemotaxis and opsoninization), with decreased resistance to infection.

      i.   Aseptic necrosis of the femoral head and osteo-myelitis are common. Salmonella infection of small bones of the hand is characteristic. The skin of the lower extremities is susceptible to breakdown, resulting in ankle ulcers.

      j.   There is a marked increase in maternal and fetal morbidity and mortality rates during pregnancy and delivery: spontaneous abortion, placental insufficiency, increased sickle cell crises, stillbirth, and peripartum hemorrhage. However, SS newborns are protected by their high levels of HbF for several months.

      k.   Excessive use of narcotic analgesics to treat the acute and chronic pain may result in manipulative and dependent personality types and increased tolerance to narcotics.

4.   Sickle cell trait

Sickle cell trait is largely asymptomatic, so that the diagnosis may be missed at the time of surgery. Nonetheless, important complications may be precipitated by surgical stress, and the perioperative mortality rate is about 0.8%. Manifestations of AS include splenic infarction at high altitude, hyposthenuria, hematuria, bacteriuria and pyelonephritis (especially during pregnancy), stroke, and pulmonary embolism.

5.   Preanesthetic transfusion therapy

      a.   Transfusion of normal (HbA) RBCs may be simple, multiple (twice weekly), or exchange (50% replacement of blood volume). Hb polymer formation is proportional to intracellular HbS concentration; by reducing HbS to less than 50%, sickling is reduced. The goal of transfusion of HbA cells is to decrease venous blood viscosity and venooclusion and increase Hct, O_2-carrying capacity, and tissue oxygenation. However, if the Hct is increased above 35%, this advantage may be offset by increasing arteriolar viscosity.

      b.   Indications for transfusion include acute splenic sequestration, aplastic crises, recurrent strokes, priapism, and acute hypoxemia. Preoperative transfusion is generally indicated before major surgery.

    c.   Prophylactic transfusion during pregnancy significantly decreases the frequency of crises but does not appear to alter maternal or fetal outcome at delivery.

6.   Preoperative assessment and preparation

    a.   Existing organ dysfunction should be assessed.

    b.   Premedication that causes respiratory depression (hypoxemia, respiratory acidosis) should be avoided.

    c.   Aggressive preoperative hydration is essential. Added protection may be conferred by inducing mild hyponatremia (serum sodium approximately 130 mEq/L) by the intravenous administration of D-deamino-arginine vasopressin (DDAVP), 0.3 μg/kg.

    d.   Exchange transfusion can be used to reduce HbS to less than 50%.

7.   Intraoperative and postoperative management

    a.   Strict asepsis is maintained in the placement of all invasive catheters.

    b.   Supplemental O_2 is provided at all times, especially during preoperative preparation and postoperative transport.

    c.   High FI_{O_2} is used to enhance dissolved oxygen delivery and avoid hypoxemia. Pulse oximetry is used to monitor and ensure adequate arterial O_2 saturation, and capnometry is used to avoid acute respiratory alkalosis or acidosis.

    d.   Aggressive monitoring, maintenance, and restoration of intravascular volume status are imperative.

    e.   Hypothermia is avoided, and normal pH maintained.

    f.   The use of tourniquets is avoided. Note that sickling may result from the lactic acidosis induced by the unclamping of arteries during vascular procedures.

    g.   Spinal or epidural anesthesia is favored because the sympathetic blockade enhances perfusion and may even relieve a vascular crisis.

    h.   Cardiac surgery with cardiopulmonary bypass (hypothermia, acidosis) requires careful monitoring and aggressive transfusion.

    i.   In the postoperative period, the primary goals

are to maintain warmth, prevent and treat shivering (increased oxygen consumption, respiratory acidosis), and maintain oxygenation and hydration.

C. Thalassemia

1. Pathogenesis

The thalassemias are the most common of human hereditary disorders, particularly in people of Mediterranean, Asian, African, and South Pacific descent. There is a defect in globin chain synthesis, resulting in decreased normal Hb and chronic hemolysis.

2. Classification

a. Alpha-thalassemia is a defect in α-chain synthesis.

The manifestations depend on the number of abnormal (α) or normal (N) genes (four in all, on chromosome 16).

1) $\alpha\alpha\alpha\alpha$: homozygous (hydrops fetalis, fatal)

2) $\alpha\alpha\alpha$N: HbH disease (nonfunctional Hb, made up of β chains only)

3) $\alpha\alpha$NN: α-trait (iron-deficiency anemia)

4) αNNN: silent carrier.

b. Beta-thalassemia is a defect in β-chain synthesis.

There are two controlling genes on chromosome 11. β is a genetic deletion; β^+ is an abnormal β gene, and N is a normal gene. Different gene combinations can result in the following:

1) β/β: Major (Cooley's anemia; no β chains—increased HbF and HbA2)

2) β^+/β^+: Intermedia

3) β/β^+ or β^+/N: Minor

4) β (HPFH: genetic deletion with persistent fetal hemoglobin).

3. Clinical features and anesthetic management

a. Beta-thalassemia major (Cooley's anemia) is the most important entity. It is characterized by a severe hemolytic anemia, folate deficiency, and hypersplenism and therefore thrombocytopenia. Bone marrow hyperplasia results in facial abnormalities and potentially difficult intubation; occasionally, spinal cord compression occurs. The requirement for multiple transfusions inevitably results in hemo-chromatosis (liver, spleen, heart), with death from CHF in the second decade.

    b. Preoperative assessment of the degree of ane-mia, hemolysis, coagulopathy, and hemo-chromatosis is essential. A difficult airway should be anticipated. Preoperative transfu-sion is indicated when anemia is severe (Hb <6–8 g/dl). Intraoperative management should be as previously discussed, with special precautions to monitor for and prevent CHF.

D. Hemolytic Anemias

    1. Hereditary spherocytosis

In this condition, an abnormal RBC membrane al-lows sodium and water absorption, resulting in swollen cells (spherocytes), which are readily lysed by the spleen. This results in a chronic mild hemo-lytic anemia, reticulocytosis, and unconjugated hy-perbilirubinemia. Hemolysis may be increased by the stress of infection and by advanced age. Chronic hemolysis results in bile pigment calculi and chole-cystitis (the most common surgical presentation). Patients may also present for elective splenectomy, which virtually eliminates hemolysis, although it increases susceptibility to pneumococcal infections.

Anesthetic management is similar to that pro-vided for other patients with anemia. There are no special considerations.

    2. Paroxysmal noctural hemoglobinuria

        a. Pathogenesis

            1) The underlying defect is a membrane ab-normality that results in sensitivity of RBCs, granulocytes, and platelets to com-plement-mediated damage. This process presents in young adults as a chronic he-molytic anemia with acute exacerbations and is characterized by early morning he-moglobinuria. Neutropenia, thrombocy-topenia, and jaundice are variable.

            2) Platelet abnormality may cause increased bleeding tendency or venous thrombosis, resulting in renal impairment, episodes of abdominal pain, and occasional hepatic, portal, or cerebral vein obstruction. There is an increased incidence of postoperative thrombosis.

b. Anesthetic management

1) Preoperative transfusion with packed washed RBCs is indicated if anemia is severe and may reduce the incidence of postoperative thrombosis, but there is always a risk that it will activate complement and so exacerbate hemolysis. The latter consideration also applies to the intraoperative transfusions of plasma and platelets, which must therefore be given judiciously.

2) The use of spinal or epidural anesthesia (peripheral vasodilation) and analgesia (early mobilization) is favored unless contraindicated by thrombocytopenia or severe anemia.

3) Protamine used to reverse perioperative heparin forms a heparin–protamine complex, which may activate complement. If necessary, heparin reversal can be accomplished with hexadimethrine bromide (Polybrene).

4) Strict asepsis must be used for all invasive catheters. Aggressive maintenance of intravascular volume is important to preserve renal function and prevent thrombosis.

5) Postoperatively, prophylactic measures should be taken to avoid venous thrombosis, including low-dose subcutaneous heparin and early mobilization.

E. Erythrocyte Enzyme Defects

1. Glucose-6-phosphate dehydrogenase deficiency is the most common hereditary RBC enzyme defect. It is sex linked and occurs in 8% to 11% of black males in the US. Mediterranean and Asian forms also exist and are more severe. Drug-induced peroxidation of Hb results in the formation of superoxide radicals and hydrogen peroxide (H_2O_2). Normally, G6PD allows the generation of nicotinamide adenine diphosphate (NADP) via the hexose monophosphate

shunt. NADP promotes the regeneration of glutathione, which scavenges superoxide radicals and H_2O_2. G6PD deficiency therefore results in oxidant-induced red cell damage and hemolysis.

2. Patients are usually asymptomatic unless stressed by infections, diabetic ketoacidosis, or renal failure. Also, a variety of oxidative drugs may trigger hemolysis, including antimalarials, quinidine, sulfonamides, nitrofurantoin, penicillin, acetaminophen, isosorbide dinitrate, and methylene blue. However, oxidative agents used in anesthesia that increase formation of methemoglobin, such as prilocaine and sodium nitroprusside, do not appear to cause hemolysis in G6PD deficiency and are not contraindicated.

3. The primary anesthetic consideration is to avoid the use of known precipitants in the perioperative period.

F. Acquired (Immune) Hemolytic Anemias
1. Pathogenesis and diagnosis
    a. Damage to the RBC is induced by an antigen–antibody reaction at the RBC membrane.
    b. The diagnosis is made by the Coombs test. Coombs antiserum is antibody to human immunoglobulin G (IgG). In the direct test, the antiserum is added to the patient's blood; in the indirect test, the antiserum is added to the plasma of the patient with which RBCs of known antigenicity have been combined. Clumping of RBCs indicates the presence of IgG (i.e., antibodies to RBC membrane) and is a positive result.
2. Etiology
    a. Drug-induced (uncommon): high-dose penicillin, alpha-methyl dopa, levodopa.
    b. Hypersplenism. This may occur whenever there is splenomegaly (e.g., cirrhosis, Felty's syndrome) and is associated with destruction of all blood components (pancytopenia).
    c. Hemolytic disease of the newborn (erythroblastosis fetalis) occurs when Rh antigens from an Rh-positive mother (or Rh-positive blood transfusion) cross the placenta into an Rh-negative fetus and induce the formation of Rh anti-

bodies, which subsequently cause hemolysis. If the reaction is severe, intrauterine death (hydrops fetalis) or severe neonatal jaundice with cerebral damage (kernicterus) may occur. It is entirely preventable by the administration of Rh immune globulin (RhoGAM) to the mother within 72 hours of delivery.

    d.   Mismatched transfusion.

IV.   SUMMARY OF ANESTHETIC CONSIDERATIONS

Acute perioperative blood loss can cause marked hypotension from loss of intravascular volume. Rapid administration of blood should always be through warmers to reduce RBC viscosity, prevent cardiac cooling and arrhythmias, and facilitate oxygen unloading. Hyperkalemia and hypocalcemia may occur with rapid blood transfusion. Use of vasopressors may be required transiently to maintain the blood pressure until intravascular volume is restored.

One of the frequently encountered hemoglobinopathies that can significantly affect anesthetic and operative outcome is sickle cell anemia, which is most often seen in black people. The most severe anemia occurs with the homozygous form (SS). Sickling will occur at normal venous O_2 concentration. Any decrease in arterial O_2 concentration will greatly exacerbate sickling and could precipitate a sickle cell crisis. Patients with sickle cell disease (>90% HbS) should receive an exchange transfusion to reduce HbS concentration to less than 50%. This should minimize sickling, decrease viscosity, and improve oxygen-carrying capacity. Providing supplemental oxygen is very important for the sickle cell patient, as it is with any anemic patient.

General or regional anesthesia may be safely used in most patients with anemia. However, regional anesthesia should be avoided in patients with anemia and peripheral neuropathy from B_{12} deficiency.

≡ Bleeding Disorders

I.   NORMAL COAGULATION

    A.   Vasculature

       The vessel wall provides some measure of hemostasis by contracture. More important, exposure of the endothelium stimulates activation and adhesion of platelets and activation of the coagulation cascade.

B. Platelets

    1. Platelet adhesion

        When endothelial integrity is broken, collagen is exposed. Von Willebrand's factor (VWF) produced in the endothelium links a glycoreceptor protein on the platelet surface to the subendothelial collagen.

    2. Platelet aggregation

        a. Platelet adhesion stimulates platelet aggregation. At first, aggregation is easily stimulated but reversible and may be followed by disaggregation.

        b. A second, irreversible, phase follows when aggregation induces the release of platelet granules. Alpha granules contain fibrinogen, cationic proteins, and platelet factors 3 and 4. Dense granules contain serotonin, calcium, and adenosine diphosphate (ADP), which further promotes aggregation. Release of platelet factor 3 activates the coagulation cascade.

    3. Platelet mediators (eicosanoids: 20-carbon fatty acids)

        a. Thrombin, collagen, and endogenous catecholamines stimulate phospholipase A_2, an enzyme present on lipid membranes, which transforms arachidonic acid into prostaglandins.

        b. Thromboxane A_2 (TxA_2) is an eicosanoid synthesized within platelets that induces platelet contraction, release of platelet granules, and vasoconstriction.

        c. Prostacyclin (PGI_2) is a closely related eicosanoid produced by endothelial cells that inhibits platelet aggregation and induces vasodilation. PGI_2 also increases cyclic adenosine monophosphate (cAMP) levels within platelets, which inhibits phospholipase and TxA_2 production.

        d. The balance between TxA_2 and PGI_2 plays an important role in modulating platelet function. Acetylsalicylate (aspirin) irreversibly inactivates prostaglandin synthetase and, by markedly decreasing TxA_2 production, inhibits platelet aggregation and increases bleeding time for the life of the platelet (7–10 days).

C. Coagulation Cascade

1. The preceding interrelated events result in formation of a platelet plug and provide a surface for activation of the coagulation cascade. This is a biologic amplification system whereby a relatively small stimulus results in the production of a large amount of fibrin, which stabilizes the hemostatic plug formed by platelets.

2. The cascade is composed of circulating serine proteases, most of which are produced by the liver.

   a. The intrinsic pathway of the cascade is triggered by a substance intrinsic to the blood: factor XII (Hagemann factor). Factor XII is activated by contact with an abnormal (damaged, artificial) endothelial surface and, in turn, triggers a cascade of procoagulant activation (factors XI, IX, VIII).

   b. The extrinsic pathway is triggered by (extrinsic) tissue thromboplastins released from damaged cells, including endothelium, platelets, or leukocytes.

   c. Both pathways culminate in the formation of a thromboplastic complex under the influence of factors V and X, calcium, and platelet factor 3, which enters the final common pathway and culminates in the formation of a stable fibrin clot.

3. The mechanisms promoting clot formation simultaneously generate mechanisms that oppose it to prevent overwhelming coagulation.

   a. Antithrombin III is an α_2-globulin whose generation specifically antagonizes the procoagulants of the intrinsic pathway (factors XII, XI, IX, VIII) (i.e., it acts as a physiologic anticoagulant).

   b. Factor XII simultaneously triggers fibrinolysis by stimulating tissue plasminogen activator, which acts on plasminogen to form plasmin. Plasmin lyses fibrin; fibrin degradation products (FDP) directly inhibit the serine proteases and thrombin formation.

        c.   Protein C is a vitamin K-dependent factor that is activated by thrombin, thrombomodulin, and protein S. Activated protein C inactivates factors V and VIII and inhibits tissue plasminogen inactivators, thereby promoting fibrinolysis.

    4.   In this way, the body maintains a balance between clot formation and clot breakdown. Imbalance results in excessive bleeding or excessive clot formation. For example, factor VIII deficiency results in abnormal bleeding (hemophilia), whereas antithrombin III or protein C deficiency results in a hypercoagulable state and recurrent thrombosis.

II.   LABORATORY EVALUATION

    A.   Platelets

        1.   Platelet count

            The normal platelet count is between 150,000 and 400,000/μl. Spontaneous bleeding seldom occurs until thrombocytopenia is severe (<20,000 platelets/μl). However, to ensure surgical hemostasis, a count of at least 80,000 platelets/μl is required.

        2.   Ivy bleeding time

            a.   The Ivy bleeding time (BT) is an attempt to quantitate the effect of abnormal platelet function (thrombocytopathy) or thrombocytopenia on clot formation. An arm blood-pressure cuff is inflated to a pressure midway between diastolic and systolic. A small cut is made in the skin of the antecubital fossa, and blood is gently soaked up with a filter paper until a stable clot allows no further absorption. The normal Ivy BT is 3 to 8 minutes.

            b.   A prolonged BT implies either abnormal platelet function (if the platelet count is >100,000/μl) or an absolute or effective reduction in functioning platelets below 100,000. The BT will be normal despite coagulation cascade abnormalities if there are adequate functioning platelets (in contrast, if thrombocytopenia is severe, all coagulation pathways are prolonged). The following equations are used to estimate the number of effective platelets on the basis of the BT and platelet count (PC):

$$BT \text{ (min)} = 30.5 - [(PC)/3850]$$

Example:
If PC = 50,000, BT = 17.5 min

$$\text{Effective PC} = (30.5 - BT) \times 3850$$

Example:
If BT = 17.5 min, effective PC = 50,000

    c.   The BT is a subjective test that should be performed by a trained technician. Precise quantitation of platelet function requires platelet aggregation studies, which are costly and time consuming. A prolonged BT does not necessarily imply increased surgical bleeding.

  3.   Thrombocytopathy is most frequently induced by antiplatelet drugs such as acetylsalicylate (aspirin) or dipyridamole (Persantin) used in the prophylaxis of arterial thrombosis and will increase the BT. Thrombocytopathy is also frequently seen with von Willebrand's disease (deficit of VWF and factor VIII) and uremia (inhibition of release of VWF/VIII complex from endothelium).

B. Intrinsic Pathway

  1.   Activated partial thromboplastin time (aPTT)

      a.   The intrinsic and common pathways are tested by the aPTT. Cephalin (partial thromboplastin), a platelet-substitute standardized phospholipid preparation, and kaolin, a surface activator, are added to citrated plasma. The time to clot formation following the addition of an excess of calcium is compared with a normal control (approximately 30 seconds).

      b.   A prolonged aPTT indicates abnormal intrinsic or common pathway function. It is the most sensitive method of measuring the anticoagulant effect of heparin, which thereby is precisely dosed. However, its high sensitivity impairs its specificity. Very small decreases in intrinsic factor activity, as with low-dose heparin therapy, may prolong the aPTT without an increase in clinical bleeding.

2. Activated clotting time (ACT)

    a. A small amount of whole blood (2 ml) is placed in a tube with a given amount of diatomaceous earth, which activates factor XII. The time to initiation of clot formation is measured either manually or automatically. The commonly used Hemachron system consists of glass tubes with cylindrical magnets and Celite activator. When the magnet becomes enmeshed in fibrin, the timer stops and automatically gives the ACT in seconds.

    b. The ACT is used primarily to monitor heparinization and its reversal by protamine during and after cardiopulmonary bypass (CPB). A baseline ACT is obtained before heparinization (normal: 80–120 seconds), which serves as a control. Prolongation of the ACT to greater than 480 seconds by heparin is generally accepted as safe anticoagulation for CPB. Below 400 seconds, there is the danger of formation of fibrin monomer and deposition of fibrin and platelets on the extracorporeal circuit, which could lead to disseminated intravascular coagulation (DIC).

    c. The ACT becomes markedly prolonged below 32°C and loses its relation with increasing heparin effect beyond 500 seconds. Conversely, the ACT may decrease rapidly during rewarming. Sophisticated nomograms have been generated in an attempt precisely to quantitate the heparin dose required for anticoagulation and the protamine dose required for reversal. However, most institutions use a simple trial-and-error method of frequently repeating the ACT until the desired end points are achieved. The end point for protamine reversal of heparin is to achieve an ACT at or close to the control value.

    d. The ACT is not a sensitive indicator of platelet abnormalities or factor deficiencies: it provides no information on fibrin–platelet interaction, clot retraction, or lysis. The ACT may be prolonged despite adequate protamine reversal of heparin in the presence of hypothermia or hypofibrinogenemia. The ACT provides a more useful (and much more rapid) clinical guide to the need for additional protamine to reverse heparin than the oversensitive aPTT. In the presence of bleeding, a normal ACT suggests that it is not caused by heparin, even if the aPTT is prolonged.

C. Extrinsic Pathway

   1. Prothrombin time (PT)

      a. The PT tests the extrinsic and final common pathway. Tissue thromboplastin is added to citrated plasma, and the time to clot formation is compared with a control (normal approximately 10 seconds).

      b. Prolongation of the PT is associated with deficiencies of factors VII (proconvertin), X, V, II, and fibrinogen; a combination of these factors; or the presence of an inhibitor. It is the most important indicator of warfarin (Coumadin) therapy, vitamin K deficiency, and liver failure.

   2. Prothrombin and proconvertin time (P&P)

   The presence of a small amount of heparin interferes with the PT in a nonquantitative manner, which is important after cardiac surgery and residual heparinization. This interference may be overcome by diluting the sample and adding a stabilizer. The P&P test is a more reliable indicator of extrinsic pathway dysfunction after cardiac or vascular surgery.

D. Final Common Pathway

   1. Thrombin time (TT)

      a. The final common and intrinsic pathways are tested by the thrombin time (TT), in which exogenous thrombin is added to citrated plasma, and the time to clot is compared with a normal control (approximately 12 seconds).

      b. A prolonged TT indicates an abnormality of intrinsic pathway function and is an excellent clinical guide to heparin effect (i.e., it more closely approximates clinical bleeding secondary to heparin than does the aPTT). It is also prolonged if fibrinogen is deficient or abnormal (e.g., DIC, severe liver disease).

2. Reptilase time (RT)

Reptilase is a thrombin-like substance obtained from snake venom that is capable of triggering the final common pathway but which is not inhibited by heparin. Normal RT is approximately 15 to 18 seconds. The RT is particularly useful to distinguish bleeding attributable to heparin from that caused by DIC. If the TT is prolonged but the RT is normal, bleeding is attributable to heparin. If both the TT and the RT are prolonged, bleeding is secondary to DIC (although there may be a coexistent heparin effect, which cannot be excluded).

3. Fibrinogen level

Normal fibrinogen concentration is 150 to 400 mg/dl. Hypofibrinogenemia may occur with severe peripartum hemorrhage or DIC. Because the hepatic capacity for fibrinogen regeneration is extremely great, fibrinogen levels may not decrease in the early stages of consumptive coagulopathy.

4. Fibrin split products (FSP) and tests of fibrinolysis

a. FSP or fibrin degradation products (FDP) are released by fibrinolysis and themselves inhibit coagulation through interference with the coagulation cascade. FSP levels are expressed as titers: 1:32 (mild elevation), 1:128 (moderate), 1:>320 (severe).

b. Although FSP levels are characteristically elevated in DIC, this finding is not specific. Moderate elevation of FSP is found whenever there are large hematomas undergoing spontaneous lysis.

c. The euglobulin clot lysis time is a quantitative measure of fibrinolysis. It is much more sensitive to primary than to secondary fibrinolysis.

d. The D-dimer assay (Dimertest) measures a degradation fragment of polymerized fibrin. A positive test indicates secondary (i.e., DIC) rather than primary fibrinolysis.

E. Total Coagulation Testing

1. Thromboelastography (TEG)

a. TEG provides a qualitative measure of the viscoelastic clot strength (shear elasticity) and, as such, measures the total, interdependent process of coagulation and fibrinolysis rather than isolated pathways. Although invented in 1948, TEG has only recently achieved credibility among anesthesiologists and surgeons. It provides a rapid and reliable bedside guide to coagulation and the use of blood products in patients with severe blood loss. TEG has been used successfully in patients undergoing liver transplantation.

b.   A small (0.35-ml) fresh (<3 minutes) sample of whole blood is placed in a continuously rotating mirror-polished stainless steel crucible, in which a piston is suspended (Fig. 8–1). As fibrin strands form, the rotational motion is transferred from the crucible to the piston, which is amplified to a strip recorder that dis-

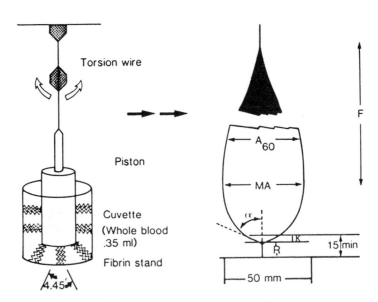

Figure 8–1   Principle of the thromboelastogram (*left*), as described in the text. Characteristic coagulation profile (*right*): R = reaction time, K = K value, α angle = clot formation rate, MA = maximum amplitude, A_{60} = amplitude 60 minutes after MA, A_{60}/MA = whole blood clot lysis index, F = whole blood clot lysis time. Normal values and diagnostic indications are given in Table 8-3. (*Tuman KJ et al. Effects of progressive blood loss on coagulation as measured by thromboelastography. Anesth Analg 1987; 66:856*)

plays a characteristic tracing or coagulation profile (Fig. 8–2). A number of specific parameters can be derived from the profile that reveal characteristic patterns in the presence of certain types of coagulopathy, especially thrombocytopenia, thrombocytopathy, factor deficiencies, fibrinolysis, or hypercoagulable states (Table 8-3).

c.   Abnormalities of the TEG bear a more predictable relation to clinical bleeding than do the standard tests. TEG is also useful in identifying hypercoagulable states (surgical stress, cancer). It is now being applied to other procedures associated with significant blood loss

TEG Tracings – Examples

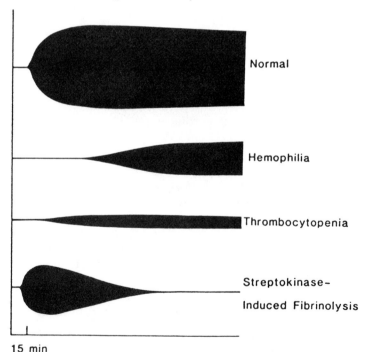

Normal

Hemophilia

Thrombocytopenia

Streptokinase–
Induced Fibrinolysis

15 min

Figure 8–2 Examples of normal and abnormal thromboelastographic profiles. *(Spiess BD and Ivankovich AD: Thromboelastography: a coagulation-monitoring technique applied to cardiopulmonary bypass. In: Ellison N, Jobes DR, eds. Effective hemostasis in cardiac surgery. WB Saunders, Philadelphia, 1988:163)*

Table 8–3. Thromboelastogram Parameters

Parameter	Definition	Process	Normal Range	Abnormality
R	Reaction time start 1 mm	Initial fibrin formation	7.5–15 min 15–30 mm	Prolonged: procoagulant deficiency, heparin, hypofibrinogenemia
K	Coagulation time R-20 mm amplitude	Speed of clot formation	3–6 min 6–12 mm	Decreased K, α°, MA: thrombocytopenia, hypofibrinogenemia
α°	Upslope from R	Speed of clot formation	45–50°	
MA	Maximum amplitude	Maximum clot strength	50–60 mm	Small MA: DIC, uremia
A_{60}	Amplitude 60 min after MA	Clot retraction, lysis		Decreased A_{60}: fibrinolysis

such as cardiac surgery and total hip replacement. After CPB, TEG accurately predicts 80% of postoperative bleeding v 50% for the ACT and coagulation profile alone or in combination. False positives occur in 20% of cases, but bleeding almost never occurs without a TEG abnormality. The TEG is very sensitive to heparin but is not useful for quantifying its dose. Other possible indications include assessment of the effect of aspirin and antiplatelet therapy, or the effect of DDAVP on platelet function, to guide epsilon-aminocaproic acid (EACA) therapy in DIC and fibrinolysis, and monitoring the effect of thrombolytic therapy.

2. Sonoclot

The Sonoclot is similar to the TEG and also measures the viscoelastic properties of clots. This device utilizes a plastic vibrating probe (200 Hz), which is placed in 0.4 ml of either plasma or whole blood. The impedance exerted by the clot is proportional to its viscosity, and the measurement is transformed into a characteristic tracing or signature. This technique appears to be most sensitive to changes in platelet count and function. It may also have the advantage of being able to quantitate heparin dosage.

III. COAGULOPATHIES

   A. Hereditary Disorders

      1. Hemophilia A (classic hemophilia)

         a. Classic hemophilia is transmitted as a sex-linked recessive trait and therefore rarely affects females. The biochemical abnormality is abnormal formation of procoagulant factor VIII (VIII:C), and the clinical severity depends on the deficit of normal VIII:C. Spontaneous bleeding usually does not occur until levels are less than 5% of normal. Levels below 25% of normal result in bleeding after surgery or trauma.

         b. Clinical presentation is a lifelong history of easy bruising and ecchymosis (petechiae and purpura are instead associated with platelet problems) and gingival bleeding after dental manipulation or extraction. Spontaneous hemarthrosis and progressive joint deformity is characteristic of severe hemophilia. Pericardial or intracerebral hemorrhage may be devastating.

         c. The diagnosis is based on history and laboratory evaluation. The aPTT is prolonged, but BT and PT are normal.

         d. Treatment is based on VIII:C replacement, as either cryoprecipitate or VIII:C concentrate. One pooled adult dose of cryoprecipitate contains 80 units of VIII:C. Multiple doses are required, because the in vivo half-life of VIII:C concentrate is only 8 to 12 hours. There is a high risk of transmission of hepatitis and human immunodeficiency virus (HIV). Before screening for HIV was introduced, a tragically large number of hemophiliacs were infected with AIDS during the early 1980s.

         e. Patients with severe hemophilia A are at obvious risk for surgery. The minimum acceptable VIII:C level depends on the degree of anticipated blood loss; for major surgery, it should be raised to at least 35% to 50% of normal. Because VIII:C disappears quickly, frequent transfusions of cryoprecipitate or VIII:C concentrate are necessary during long procedures and multiple transfusions, as well as after surgery.

1) Cryoprecipitate dose calculation (based on 80 units VIII:C/unit cryoprecipitate)

$$\text{units of cryoprecipitate} = \frac{\text{desired VIII:C (\%)} \times \text{plasma vol (ml)}}{100 \times 80}$$

2) Factor VIII concentrate dose calculation Replacement is based on the number of units in the VIII:C concentrate. At least one unit of VIII:C activity is given per milliliter of plasma volume.

f. Intramuscular injections must be avoided to prevent hematoma. The use of antiplatelet agents compounds bleeding problems because platelets are so important for hemostasis in hemophiliacs. Bleeding from dental procedures is particularly problematic because of the vascularity of the delicate oral mucosal and salivary plasmin. Perioral hematomas may cause tracheal compression. Use of EACA (Amicar) has been advocated to inhibit salivary plasmin, but 50% to 70% of normal VIII:C activity should be ensured prior to extraction.

g. Mild hemophilia responds to the administration of DDAVP (see section on uremia), which transiently increases the level of circulating VIII:C. It is inadequate in severe hemophilia or for major surgical procedures.

2. Hemophilia B (Christmas disease)

a. Hemophilia B, transmitted as a homozygous sex-linked trait, is a deficiency of factor IX (Christmas factor). The clinical presentation and perioperative considerations are the same as for hemophilia A.

b. Cryoprecipitate does not contain factor IX. Specific factor concentrates such as Proplex or Konyne, which contain activated factors II,

VII, IX, and X, must be used. Rapid transfusion causes acute hypotension; in the presence of severe liver dysfunction, coagulation factors are not deactivated and may cause DIC. Transmission of viral disease is an important risk because each unit of concentrate is pooled from more than 400 donors.

3. Von Willebrand's disease

    a. This disorder is transmitted as an autosomal dominant with variable expression and is therefore equally distributed between the sexes. There are three components: (1) low VIII:C procoagulant activity, (2) defective release of VWF/VIII complex from capillary endothelium, which leads to (3) abnormal platelet aggregation.

    b. Clinically, bleeding problems are less severe than in patients with hemophilia A, though they may still be formidable. Epistaxis, easy bruising, and bleeding after dental extractions are common.

    c. The diagnosis is based on history and laboratory evaluation. The aPTT is prolonged, but in contrast to hemophilia, the BT is also abnormal, and there is decreased platelet aggregation in response to ristocetin.

    d. Patients may be treated with transfusions of cryoprecipitate, which contains VIII:C plus von Willebrand factor; VIII:C concentrates alone are not useful. DDAVP, by enhancing the release of VWF/VIII complex from endothelium and circulating VIII:C, may be extremely useful prior to surgical procedures and reduces the risk of transfusion-associated diseases caused by frequent cryoprecipitate administration. However, the response of the BT to DDAVP in von Willebrand's disease is variable and may even be worsened in one subtype of the disease. Therefore, a test dose should be given 1 or 2 weeks prior to elective surgery.

B. Acquired Abnormalities

    1. Renal failure

        a. Chronic uremia (BUN >60 mg/dl) causes a coagulopathy characterized by normal PT, aPTT, platelet count but abnormal platelet function.

The BT is prolonged because of a qualitative platelet factor defect, which may involve platelet factor 3 and altered membrane phospholipids, resulting in decreased adherence to subendothelium and aggregation. An important component appears to be defective release of VWF/VIII, which is essential for platelet aggregation, from the capillary endothelium.

b. Because of this coagulopathy, uremic patients may present with gastrointestinal bleeding (uremic gastroenteritis), cerebral hemorrhage (hypertension), and hemorrhagic pericardial effusion. Aspirin and other antiplatelet agents are contraindicated. The risk of surgical bleeding is markedly increased.

c. Administration of platelets does not correct the coagulopathy because it is a defect of milieu. Although regular dialysis may diminish uremic coagulopathy by reducing the BUN, dialysis does not eliminate the problem. Hemodialysis is best performed the day prior to elective surgery to achieve the advantages of correction of fluid status and acid–base and electrolyte abnormalities with decreased risk of dysequilibrium and residual anticoagulation. It is important to check the BT prior to surgery and to consider specific corrective measures if it is longer than 15 minutes.

d. The administration of 10 units of cryoprecipitate, which contains VWF/VIII complex, shortens the BT within 12 hours. This benefit lasts about 24 to 36 hours but is effective in only about 50% of patients and exposes them to a high risk of disease transmission.

e. DDAVP (desmopressin acetate, Stimate) has become established as a safe, effective, and reliable means of improving platelet function in uremia.

1) DDAVP is a synthetic derivative of arginine vasopressin (AVP) in which L-arginine is replaced by D-arginine, resulting in a vasodilator rather than a vasoconstrictor effect. The deamination prolongs its action from 4 to 24 hours. Von

Willebrand factor is a large polymeric glycoprotein (subunit MW 230,000), synthesized by endothelium and platelets, which forms bridges at the platelet–platelet and platelet–endothelium interface. VWF is covalently bound to VIII:C (procoagulant VIII) to form VWF/VIII complex required for normal platelet adhesion and BT. DDAVP appears to promote endothelial release of VWF/VIII multimers, which enhance platement aggregation and endothelial binding. It is not effective in severe thrombocytopenia.

2) The recommended IV dose is 0.3 μg/kg given as 4 μg/ml diluted in 50 ml of glucose over 15 to 20 minutes. Rapid administration may result in hypotension. The BT returns toward normal 1 to 2 hours after infusion and remains so for 8 to 12 hours. Tachyphylaxis occurs with repeated dosing, presumably because the endothelium becomes depleted of VWF/VIII multimers. A normal response after tachyphylaxis may be restored by withdrawing DDAVP for 3 to 4 days.

2. Liver failure
   a. Coagulopathy of liver failure
      1) Factors II (prothrombin), VII, IX, and X are dependent on hepatic production. The PT is a sensitive index of liver synthetic function and is the first clotting test to become abnormal with increasing liver impairment. Ultimately, the aPTT and TT become prolonged as well.
      2) Although fibrinogen is also synthesized by the liver, the hepatic reserve is enormous, and it will be affected only by end-stage liver failure, although the fibrinogen synthesized may become progressively abnormal.
      3) VIII:C synthesis is extrahepatic in the endothelium so that the aPTT is usually preserved until a very late stage of liver disease.

       4)   Thrombocytopenia occurs secondary to hypersplenism and frequent bleeding episodes. Platelet function is not directly affected.

       5)   Hepatic coagulopathy is exacerbated by a poor nutritional state (vitamin K deficiency). There is capillary fragility and loss of skin turgor (it may become paper thin). Patients commonly present with severe bleeding from esophageal, gastric, and rectal varices; ulceration occurs in 25% of patients with cirrhosis.

    b.   Treatment of severe hepatic coagulopathy is extremely difficult. The PT is resistant to correction by transfusion of fresh frozen plasma (FFP); as many as 10 units may not achieve complete correction. Platelets and cryoprecipitate should be administered as indicated by the platelet count and fibrinogen level. Anticoagulants and antiplatelet agents are contraindicated.

3.   Thrombocytopathy and antiplatelet drugs

    a.   Cyclooxygenase inhibition will inhibit platelet function. Blockade of conversion of arachidonic acid to cyclic endoperoxides, including TxA_2, promotes platelet aggregation. Examples of drugs with this effect are aspirin (irreversible acetylation, lasts 7–10 days; i.e., the lifespan of platelets), indomethacin, and other nonsteroidal anti-inflammatory agents (NSAIA).

    b.   Phosphodiesterase inhibitors such as dipyridamole (Persantin) will produce an elevation of intracellular cAMP.

    c.   Adenylate cyclase stimulation by prostacyclin or halothane will also increase intracellular cAMP levels. This, in turn, activates protein kinase, causing phosphorylation (inactivation) of the enzymes catalyzing platelet activation.

4.   Effect of cardiopulmonary bypass

    a.   Abnormalities of platelet number and function comprise the single most important coagulopathy after CPB. However, postoperative bleeding does not always occur when the platelet count is low, nor for that matter when the BT is prolonged.

  b. Hemodilution directly decreases the platelet count, but platelet function is disproportionately impaired.

  c. The fibrinogen-coated surface of the extracorporeal circuit (ECC) triggers platelet activation and aggregation, with release of cytoplasmic granules containing adenosine diphosphate (ADP) and serotonin. Both thrombocytopenia and thrombocytopathy result.

  d. Platelet damage is exacerbated by prolonged bubble oxygenation, cardiotomy suction, and deep hypothermia.

5. Drug-induced thrombocytopenia

  a. Drugs incriminated in thrombocytopenia include antibiotics, diuretics, heparin, protamine, and quinidine. Thrombocytopenia is seldom clinically significant with these drugs.

  b. Heparin-induced thrombocytopenia (HIT)

   1) Mild thrombocytopenia frequently occurs with heparin therapy. Severe thrombocytopenia associated with thrombosis (HIT) occurs in as many as 5% of patients. It carries an 80% morbidity and a 20% mortality rate as a result of deep vein thrombosis (DVT), myocardial infarction, stroke, mesenteric infarcts, and peripheral ischemia.

   2) HIT appears to be an IgG–heparin immune-complex disorder because of the identification of heparin-dependent platelet aggregating factor. Bovine lung heparin appears to be responsible more commonly than that derived from porcine mucosa. Heparin may act as a hapten for antibody formation, which activates platelets. This process may also damage endothelium, predisposing to thrombosis. Identification has been difficult because heparin has variable molecular weight (4,000–20,000 daltons) and thus variable antigenicity.

   3) The diagnosis is made when severe

thrombocytopenia ($<100,000/\mu l$) occurs after 6 to 12 days of heparin therapy (or immediately on reexposure with previous sensitization). HIT may occur even with subcutaneous dosing or use of heparin flush in IV lines. Important signs include apparent tachyphylaxis to heparin and development of thrombosis.

4) The diagnosis is confirmed by a positive platelet aggregation test (increase in light transmission, serotonin release with heparin) or the identification of platelet-associated IgG antibodies.

5) HIT responds to withdrawal of heparin therapy. Use of low-MW heparin may be helpful, but HIT still occurs in 20% to 40% of sensitized patients. Platelet aggregation requires TxA_2 activation; therefore, HIT is inhibited by aspirin, but not in all patients. Because thrombotic complications are most common when the platelet count rises after heparin withdrawal, use of oral antiplatelet agents is mandatory. However, it may take days to weeks before platelet function returns to a level than ensures surgical hemostasis. Elective surgery should be postponed until platelet counts have returned toward normal. Platelet transfusion is not indicated and may exacerbate thrombosis.

6) The obligatory anticoagulation for CPB presents a special problem, especially for emergency cardiac surgery. Iloprost is a synthetic derivative of PGI_2 (prostacyclin) that is 10 times as potent but more stable chemically and less vasoactive than PGI_2, with a plasma half-life of 15 minutes. Its use, either alone or together with heparin, prevents platelet aggregation and has facilitated safe application of CPB in this situation. Iloprost infusion is started at induction of anesthesia. Platelet aggregation with ADP is measured prior to heparin administration. Once it is clear that the addition of

heparin does not induce aggregation, full heparinization is effected. Iloprost infusion is discontinued after protamine reversal of heparin following CPB.

6. Platelet adsorption

Platelets are absorbed onto any prosthetic material that is not heparin coated, such as pulmonary artery catheters (earlier devices) or an intra-aortic balloon pump (IABP).

7. Idiopathic thrombocytopenic purpura (ITP)

a. ITP is an IgG autoimmune thrombocytopenia that follows viral infections in children and young adults. Patients present with petechiae or purpura, usually over the upper body, or bleeding (e.g., epistaxis). The majority of children recover spontaneously; in untreated adults, ITP becomes chronic, with long periods of remission and sudden exacerbations. Drug-induced thrombocytopenia (quinidine, sulfamethoxazole–trimethoprim) may be indistinguishable from ITP.

b. Laboratory evaluation reveals decreased platelet count, increased BT, anemia proportional to blood loss, normal leukocyte counts, and a normal or increased number of normal megakaryocytes in the bone marrow.

c. Treatment consists of high-dose steroids and, if there is no response in 2 to 4 weeks, splenectomy. Platelet transfusions are confined to life-threatening hemorrhage or perioperative coverage. Perioperative concerns include adequate steroid coverage and consideration of platelet transfusion. Platelet antibodies are common because of frequent transfusion, so that HLA-matched platelets must be used.

8. Thrombotic thrombocytopenic purpura (TTP)

a. TTP is much more sinister than ITP. It usually affects young women, who present with petechiae and purpura, jaundice, fever, hemolysis, thrombocytopenia, and decreasing renal and neurologic function. The etiology is unknown.

b. Treatment modalities include high-dose steroids, antiplatelet agents, exchange transfusion, plasmapheresis, and splenectomy. Elective surgery should be postponed until a period of remission.

   c. Perioperative care of these patients includes the usual precautions for anemia, plus preservation of compromised renal and neurologic function and control of bleeding. Hypovolemia is common because of increased insensible losses attributable to fever. Consideration should be given to preoperative exchange transfusion or plasmapheresis. HLA-matched platelet transfusions are indicated for platelet counts below 50,000/μl.

9. Disseminated intravascular coagulation

   a. Pathogenesis

     1) DIC results from diffuse microvascular thrombin generation and clot formation. The most common cause is shock, with tissue stasis, hypoxia, and acidosis. As lactic acidosis increases, arterioles dilate, allowing capillary flow into beds obstructed at their venular ends by cellular debris. Hydrostatic pressure increases, driving plasma into the interstitial space. The residual blood becomes increasing viscous, and platelets layer out and aggregate. Extrinsic pathway activation occurs with the release of tissue thromboplastin from damaged cells; the intrinsic pathway is activated by contact of factor XII (Hageman factor) with altered capillary endothelium or its activation by proteolysis or hemolysis.

     2) In septic and anaphylactic states, complement-mediated damage to leukocytes results in the release of proteolytic enzymes that activate coagulation in the systemic circulation (septic shock) or pulmonary circulation (adult respiratory distress syndrome; ARDS). In certain disease states, such as acute promyelocytic leukemia, amniotic fluid embolism, or diffuse malignancy, there is direct release of tissue thromboplastin into the circulation. In liver failure, activated pro-

coagulants are not cleared from the circulation.

3) The net result of these processes is that microvascular coagulation obstructs capillary flow to vital organs, exacerbating the ischemic insult of shock; consumes available clotting factors, resulting in a consumption coagulopathy that may or may not manifest as clinical bleeding; and triggers various degrees of secondary fibrinolysis that exacerbates any current bleeding.

4) DIC probably exacerbates organ damage in shock, especially to the kidney, lung, brain, and periphery. It is an unequivocal indicator of a profound disturbance of the microcirculation and a barometer of the severity of shock.

b. Diagnosis

1) Thrombocytopenia is pathognomonic of DIC; indeed, the diagnosis should not be made in the presence of a normal platelet count (although sharp decreases within the normal range should not be missed).

2) All clotting tests are prolonged: aPTT, PT, TT, and RT.

3) Fibrinogen levels may be maintained, even though consumption is high, by a dramatic increase in production by the liver. A low fibrinogen level is an important sign of severe DIC, but a normal fibrinogen level does not exclude it.

4) Secondary fibrinolysis may be revealed clinically by the presence of diffuse oozing. Laboratory findings include a progressive increase in FSP to a titer above 1:320, a positive Dimertest, or an abnormally rapid clot dissolution on TEG.

c. Treatment and perioperative management

1) The fundamental approach to the treatment of DIC is to reverse the underlying cause: to reestablish capillary perfusion, restore tissue oxygenation, and correct metabolic acidosis. DIC invariably re-

solves as the severity of shock recedes and is an important marker of improvement.

2) Blood products (platelets, FFP, cryoprecipitate) should not be given unless there is clinical bleeding or a fresh surgical wound because they may simply fuel microvascular coagulation. Also, they are unlikely to correct the coagulopathy until the shock state itself is corrected. When administered, specific products should be given to achieve specific ends such as RBCs to correct a low Hct, platelets to correct thrombocytopenia, FFP to correct prolonged PT, or cryoprecipitate to correct hypofibrinogenemia.

3) Low-dose heparin (to inhibit microvascular coagulation) is controversial, because it may exacerbate bleeding or thrombocytopenia. Its use is generally confined to specific situations such as acute promyelocytic leukemia. Epsilon-aminocaproic acid, an antifibrinolytic agent, is contraindicated alone because it may provoke unimpeded coagulation. It has been administered concomitantly with heparin when secondary fibrinolysis is marked.

4) The kidneys and the lungs are at special risk during DIC, presumably because of microvascular obstruction. Because both acute renal failure and pulmonary edema may occur, there is obviously a conflict between keeping the patient "dry" (which would help pulmonary function but exacerbate renal ischemia) or "wet" (which would protect the kidney but exacerbate pulmonary edema). However, the morbidity and mortality rate of postoperative acute renal failure (60% to 90%) substantially outweighs that of postoperative acute respiratory failure (20%). On this basis, it appears rational to support renal perfusion aggressively by maintaining adequate intravascular volume, together

with the use of vasodilators and osmotic and loop diuretics (low-dose dopamine, mannitol, furosemide) and to plan for a period of postoperative mechanical ventilatory support. After all, if renal function is preserved, there should be no problem in inducing diuresis to mobilize sequestered fluid once the patient has become hemodynamically stable after surgery.

IV.   ANTICOAGULANT THERAPY

   A.   Heparin

      1.   Heparin inhibits activated factors IIa (thrombin), IXa, Xa, and XIa, and its action is evaluated by prolongation of the ACT, aPTT, and TT. The PT may be abnormal, especially with higher doses, but the effect is unpredictable and nonlinear.

      2.   Antithrombin III is part of the normal circulating anticoagulation mechanism. Its primary activity is to inhibit thrombin. Heparin acts as an anticoagulant by accelerating the binding of antithrombin III to thrombin. Most heparin preparations are a mixture of heparins of variable MW from 4000 to 20,000. As lower-MW heparin binds more avidly to antithrombin III, preparations may differ in their anticoagulant properties, depending on the distribution of MW. In the presence of decreased levels of antithrombin III, heparin will appear to be less effective, and administration of FFP to replace antithrombin III may be required for adequate heparinization.

      3.   The half-life of heparin is 90 minutes at normothermia and increases as the body temperature decreases. Smokers have increased clearance.

      4.   Heparin resistance may be secondary to continuing coagulation, antithrombin III deficiency, prior heparin therapy, intravenous nitroglycerin, or advanced age.

   B.   Protamine

      1.   The finding that protamine neutralizes the effect of heparin, which ushered in the era of anticoagulant therapy, was completely serendipitous. In 1937, Chargaff and Olson were attempting to prolong the effect of heparin by the addition of protamine (in a manner they hoped was analogous to protamine–zinc insulin) but found instead that protamine completely antagonized heparin action.

2. Heparin–protamine is essentially an acid–base reaction between the polyanion sulfate, heparin, and the polycation, arginine-rich protamine.

3. Although it is rapidly cleared from plasma, excessive administration of protamine (twice the normal dose) itself causes anticoagulation, probably through its competition with antithrombin III for binding with thrombin, which it inhibits.

4. Protamine dose and "heparin rebound" is variable, depending on the total dose of heparin administered and, perhaps more important, the type of heparin. For example, beef lung heparin, which has strong anti-IIa activity, is more easily neutralized than pork mucosal heparin, which has strong anti-Xa activity.

5. Continued monitoring of bleeding and ACT is more important than precise determination of the exact amount of protamine required to neutralize heparin. Although small ratios (e.g., 0.3 mg of protamine/100 units of heparin) may be sufficient to reverse heparin, the incidence of rebound is greater.

C. Protamine Reactions

1. Dose related (predictable)
Systemic hypotension is produced by rapid injection secondary to vasodilation, probably on the basis of histamine release.

2. Idiosyncratic (unpredictable)
   a. Anaphylaxis (pulmonary and systemic vasodilation, capillary leak).
   b. Pulmonary vasoconstriction (acute right-sided heart failure), possibly secondary to complement activation, sequestration of leukocytes and platelets, and an acute inflammatory response.
   c. Noncardiogenic pulmonary edema (ARDS).

3. "Risk factors," none of which has been substantiated, include vasectomy, fish allergy, diabetes controlled with protamine–zinc insulin, and previous exposure to protamine.

4. Prevention of protamine reactions includes slow administration of diluted preparation, arterial or left-sided injection, or simultaneous injection of calcium

chloride. Of these, the first is the most reliable in preventing hypotensive responses.

D. Warfarin sodium (Coumadin)

   1. Warfarin blocks the synthesis of vitamin K-dependent factors (II, VII, IX, X) and is monitored by its effect on the PT. The goal of maintenance anticoagulant therapy is usually to increase the PT to 1.5 times normal.

   2. The effect of warfarin may be increased by vitamin K deficiency (noteworthy in critically ill patients receiving broad-spectrum antibiotics), liver disease (especially in chronic alcoholics), hypermetabolic states, advanced age, and drugs such as trimethoprim–sulfamethoxazole. Bleeding complications are increased by concomitant administration of drugs with anticoagulant effects (aspirin). Warfarin may be rendered less effective by hepatic microsomal enzyme induction (barbiturates, glutethamide). The half-life of warfarin ranges from 1 to 4 days, depending on dietary vitamin K, hereditary resistance, or individual differences in pharmacokinetics.

   3. The effects of warfarin can be reversed within 12 to 16 hours by the administration of vitamin K (10 mg subcutaneously) or immediately by the administration of FFP. Caution must be exercised in patients with prosthetic valves. For procedures that may involve significant blood loss, warfarin may be stopped 3 to 5 days prior to surgery and a heparin infusion started, which can be discontinued 3 to 4 hours preoperatively.

E. Aspirin

   1. The effect of aspirin on platelet function has already been discussed. The drug is commonly prescribed to patients with coronary artery and cerebrovascular disease as an antiplatelet agent and appears to decrease significantly the risk of arterial thrombosis.

   2. Although a single dose of aspirin can affect platelet function for 7 to 10 days, the correlation between aspirin therapy, BT, and perioperative bleeding is not established.

   3. Aspirin should be discontinued 7 days before elective surgery to ensure adequate platelet function. If this is not possible, the BT may be helpful in evaluating platelet function. However, the finding of a prolonged BT does not correlate directly with a certainty of excessive surgical bleeding and is not an indication for prophylactic platelet transfusion. DDAVP may enhance aspirin-inhibited platelet function, but more studies are needed.

4. Platelet transfusion should be considered for excessive perioperative bleeding in patients who have taken aspirin within a week of surgery.

V. FIBRINOLYTIC (THROMBOLYTIC) THERAPY

   A. Fibrinolytic Enzyme System
   When thrombin catalyzes the cleavage of fibrinogen into polymerized monomers and their stabilization by factor XIII, plasminogen and plasminogen activators are adsorbed onto the fibrin clot. Plasminogen is converted to plasmin. Plasmin in the clot transforms insoluble fibrin to soluble peptides, but free plasmin is inactivated by circulating alpha$_2$ antiplasmin, confining thrombolysis to the fibrin clot.

   B. Plasminogen Activators
   Plasminogen activators include urokinase (specific for plasminogen) and streptokinase (SK, produced by beta-hemolytic streptococci). SK indiscriminately activates both fibrin-bound and free plasminogen to plasmin, and once alpha$_2$ antiplasmin is exhausted, the enzyme digests procoagulants II, V, VIII, resulting in a bleeding diathesis. Systemic thrombolysis and bleeding is not appreciably reduced by using intracoronary SK (100,000–300,000 units) v intravenous SK (1–1.5 million units). SK may induce anaphylaxis; anti-SK antibodies preclude retreatment for several months.

   C. Complications of Fibrinolysis

   1. The main complication is hemorrhage (10%–25% of cases with SK), especially in the elderly. Bleeding occurs because of the rapid breakdown of both new and formed clots (e.g., catheter sites, surgical wounds).

   2. The incidence is less with tissue plasminogen activator (tPA), which preferentially activates the thrombolytic system adjacent to a fibrin clot.

   D. Management of Bleeding after Administration of Fibrinolytic Agents

   1. Diagnosis of thrombolysis is made by euglobulin lysis time (euglobulin fraction—fibrinogen, plasminogen and plasminogen activator; normal >80 minutes) or decreased A$_{60}$ on TEG. Other tests (TT,

PT, aPTT) may become prolonged because of pro-coagulant depletion.

    2. Cryoprecipitate or FFP is used as indicated by fibrinogen level or PT. EACA may be used if hemorrhage persists. If possible, surgery is delayed for 24 hours.

VI. ANESTHETIC CONSIDERATIONS FOR PATIENTS WITH COAGULOPATHY

    A. Preoperative Correction

        1. As far as possible, the coagulopathy should be corrected prior to surgery along the guidelines provided in the discussion of each entity.

        2. Elective surgery should not be performed in the presence of an active uncorrected coagulopathy. For emergency surgery, attempts to correct the coagulopathy should be ongoing during the procedure.

    B. Precautions with Invasive Monitoring

        1. Careful precautions should be taken with central line placement. The external jugular and femoral veins are preferred because hematomas may be directly compressed. The internal jugular vein should be used with great caution, and the subclavian vein is contraindicated because of the potential for exsanguination from a perforated subclavian artery. The risk of fatal hemorrhage from a pulmonary artery catheter is greatly increased, and care should be taken to avoid excessive advancement and overwedging.

        2. Nasotracheal intubation is contraindicated because of the danger of inducing epistaxis, which may be disastrous: acute airway obstruction and asphyxiation can occur. Nasogastric tubes and nasopharyngeal temperature probes also can cause alarming epistaxis. The oral route should be used for intubation.

        3. Anticipation of perioperative bleeding

            a. Adequate intravenous access is secured with large (14 g or 16 g) IV catheters. Blood warmers are prepared, and adequate supplies of crossmatched blood are made available in the OR suite.

            b. Careful consideration should be given to the use of invasive monitoring even though the risk may be increased because of the potential for rapid fluid shifts caused by hemorrhage and the need for administration of large quantities of blood products.

    c.   The blood bank and the hematologist (if available) should be notified of the potential problem to expedite coagulation studies and the provision of blood and blood products during the case.

VII. SUMMARY OF ANESTHETIC CONSIDERATIONS

Hemostasis is maintained by vasculature contracture, platelet aggregation and activation, and activation of the coagulation cascade. Platelet counts greater than 80,000/µl are needed to ensure surgical hemostasis. Preoperative platelet function can be quantitated with the Ivy bleeding time.

The coagulation cascade consists of intrinsic and extrinsic pathways, which culminate in a final common pathway. The intrinsic and final common pathways can be tested with aPTT and thrombin time. Prothrombin time and prothrombin proconvertin time are used to evaluate the extrinsic and final common pathways. Thromboelastography (TEG) is a rapid and reliable method of testing the entire coagulation system. Characteristic TEG tracings are seen with thrombocytopenia, thrombocytopathy, factor deficiencies, fibrinolysis, or hypercoagulable states.

Common inherited coagulation disorders are hemophilia A (classic hemophilia); hemophilia B (Christmas disease), a factor IX deficiency; and von Willebrand's disease. Fresh frozen plasma or cryoprecipitate can be used preoperatively to increase factor VIII and von Willebrand's factor to at least 35% of normal. Factor IX deficiency can be corrected preoperatively with fresh frozen plasma or specific factor concentrates such as Proplex and Konyne.

Chronic uremia may cause a coagulopathy by inhibiting the release of von Willebrand factor and factor VIII from endothelial cells. There is decreased production of factor II, VII, IX, X, and fibrinogen with liver failure. Both of these acquired coagulation disorders may be corrected with fresh frozen plasma and cryoprecipitate.

Thrombocytopathy from uremia or after cardiopulmonary bypass may respond to DDAVP. Platelet transfusions are usually limited to patients who are actively bleeding with low platelet counts (<50,000/µl) or to patients with thrombocytopenia before operations that are associated with significant blood loss.

Disseminated intravascular coagulation is best treated

by correcting the underlying cause (i.e., septic shock). Blood products should not be given unless there is excessive bleeding.

Whenever feasible, administration of blood products should be guided by appropriate coagulation testing.

Patients on anticoagulant therapy should have their coagulation status corrected prior to surgery. Heparin can be stopped 4 to 6 hours prior to surgery or be neutralized with protamine immediately before surgery. The effects of warfarin can be reversed within 12 to 16 hours by the administration of vitamin K or immediately with fresh frozen plasma. Coagulation can also be normalized if warfarin is discontinued 3 to 5 days before surgery.

≡ Transfusion Therapy

I.   BLOOD CROSS-MATCHING
   A.   Type and Screen
      1.   Blood is typed for ABO and Rh group and tested for A, B, and D (Rh) antigens and anti-A and anti-B antibodies. This procedure takes approximately 45 minutes.
      2.   The antibody screen tests the patient's serum for unexpected hemolytic or cytotoxic antibodies.
      3.   If the antibody screen is negative, type-specific blood can be administered after an abbreviated cross-match (5 minutes) to the patient with assurance of 99% safety.
   B.   Full Cross-match
      Patient serum is added to donor cells to verify ABO compatibility and detect antibodies to low-incidence antigens. This procedure takes approximately 45 minutes.
   C.   Donor Testing
      1.   Donor blood is tested for ABO, Rh group, and antibodies.
      2.   Disease transmission screening includes hepatitis B surface antigen (HBsAg), non-A, non-B hepatitis, antibody to hepatitis B core antigen (anti-HBc), alanine aminotransferase (ALT), syphilis, and human immunodeficiency virus (HIV).

II. **BLOOD TRANSFUSION**
  A. Whole Blood
    1. The primary indication for intraoperative transfusion of whole blood (WB) is hypovolemic anemia, evidenced by circulatory instability.
      a. Estimated blood loss exceeding 750 ml in an adult (i.e., more than 15% of estimated blood volume) associated with a decrease in systolic blood pressure (SBP) by 20% or below 100 mmHg.
      b. Increase in heart rate (HR) above 100/minute or orthostatic changes in blood pressure or HR.
    2. Most WB is stored using citrate–phosphate–dextrose (CPD) preservative, giving a maximum shelf life of 21 days at 1–6°C. Blood should not be reissued once its temperature exceeds 10°C (30 minutes at room temperature). One unit of RBCs should increase Hb by 1 g/dl.
    3. Citrate acts as an anticoagulant, phosphate as a buffer, and dextrose (glucose) as an energy source. After 1 day of storage, leukocyte and platelet function is negligible. After 2 weeks, levels of factors V and VIII decrease to 50%; however, this is generally sufficient for surgical hemostasis. Characteristics of 21-day-old CPD-preserved WB include a viability 24 hours after transfusion of about 80%, pH 6.84, 2,3-DPG 23% of normal, P_{50} 17 mmHg, serum potassium 21 mEq/L, plasma Hb 19.1 mg/dl. Shelf life may be prolonged to 35 days by the addition of adenine for ATP (CPDA-1) or to 42 days by the addition of other preservatives such as AS-1 (Adsol) or AS-3 (Nitricel).
  B. Packed Red Blood Cells
    1. Packed RBCs can be prepared from WB at any time during the storage period. They essentially provide the O_2-delivery benefits of WB with a decreased risk of volume overload. Reduction in anti-A and anti-B antibodies allows O-negative packed RBC transfusion when ABO-identical blood is not available.
    2. The hematocrit of a unit preserved in CPDA-1 is approximately 70%, and for a unit preserved in Adsol, 60%. The Hct is expected to increase 3% with transfusion of each unit of packed RBCs (Table 8-4).
    3. Use of packed RBCs for extensive transfusion requires supplementation with FFP, which is not the case with WB.

Table 8–4. Recommendations for Perioperative Red Blood Cell Administration (1988)

1. Available evidence does not support the use of a single criterion for transfusion such as hemoglobin concentration of less than 10 g/dl. No single measure can replace good clinical judgment as the basis for decision making regarding perioperative transfusion.
2. There is no evidence that mild to moderate anemia contributes to perioperative morbidity.
3. Perioperative transfusion of homologous red blood cells carries documented risks of infection and immune changes. Therefore, the number of homologous transfusions should be kept to a minimum.
4. A number of promising alternatives to homologous transfusion are being developed. These alternatives will reduce the use of homologous transfusion to some extent, and their development should be encouraged. However, in the foreseeable future, homologous blood transfusion will continue to be the therapeutic mainstay. Therefore, primary attention should be devoted to the promotion of safe and effective transfusion from carefully selected volunteer donors.
5. Future research is necessary to define the best indications for red blood cell transfusion and the safest methods of blood conservation and delivery.

(National Institutes of Health Consensus Conference: Perioperative red blood cell transfusion. JAMA 1988;260:2700.)

III. COMPLICATIONS
   A. Transfusion Reactions
      1. Acute intravascular hemolysis (ABO incompatibility)
         a. Transfusion of improperly cross-matched blood is most often attributable to a clerical or identification error.
         b. The ABO antigens of the transfused cells react with the patient's anti-A or anti-B antibodies, resulting in complement activation and intravascular hemolysis. Cell lysis liberates hemoglobin and cell stroma, which may trigger DIC and precipitate acute renal failure.
         c. The severity of hemolysis depends on the volume and duration of mismatched blood transfusion and extent of delay in treatment, but hemolysis can occur with as little as 20 ml of blood.

     d.   Acute symptoms include burning along the vein, chills, and low back or chest pain. The patient may become febrile and severely hypotensive. Later sequelae include oozing in the surgical field, petechiae, ecchymoses, hematuria (hemoglobinuria), and anuria secondary to DIC, hemolysis, and renal failure.

     e.   The transfusion should be stopped immediately upon recognition of the reaction. Treatment is supportive. Aggressive volume administration with crystalloids or colloids and mannitol (12.5–25 g over 10–20 minutes) and furosemide (10–40 mg IV) should be given in an attempt to preserve urine output and renal function. Vasopressor or inotropic agents may be needed temporarily to support the blood pressure. If DIC and coagulopathy is severe, patients may require further transfusion and other blood products.

     f.   Samples of donor and recipient blood should be cross-matched again to confirm mismatching. Bacterial cultures of donor blood should be obtained. The patient's blood and urine should be sent for free hemoglobin measurement, and blood should be sent for serum haptoglobin, bilirubin, BUN, and DIC screen (platelets, PT, PTT, fibrinogen, and FDP).

2.   Delayed intravascular hemolysis (other RBC antigens and antibodies)

     a.   Delayed hemolytic reactions occur 2 to 21 days after transfusion and present as a declining hematocrit with hemolytic jaundice (unconjugated hyperbilirubinemia) and hemoglobinuria.

     b.   These reactions are attributable to low levels of recipient antibody missed by cross-matching or which develop after transfusion. Although the reactions are usually of low grade, subsequent transfusion may precipitate an acute hemolytic reaction.

3.   Urticarial reactions (transfused protein antigens)

     a.   Diffuse urticaria, occasionally with facial edema, is symptomatic of this response.

     b.   If there is no evidence of hemolysis (fever, hypotension, DIC), blood transfusion may be continued. Treatment consists of simple measures (e.g., H1-histamine blockers such as diphenhydramine) only.

4. Febrile reactions (leukoagglutinins, platelets)

a. Chills, fever, and occasionally hypertension or hypotension, without evidence of hemolysis, developing about 1 hour after transfusion, are characteristic.

b. Usually, the reaction is attributable to recipient antibodies to donor leukocytes or platelets. It responds to supportive measures.

c. Repeated episodes may be an indication for future use of leukocyte-poor RBCs.

B. Complications of Extensive Transfusion

1. Coagulopathy

a. Dilution (transfusional) coagulopathy usually requires rapid transfusion of one to two blood volumes.

1) Thrombocytopenia is the earliest, the most common, and the most predictable consequence of dilutional coagulopathy. Nonetheless, platelet administration should be based on a rapidly declining platelet count rather than on the total number of units of blood transfused.

2) Procoagulants
Labile factors V and VIII become depleted after 24 hours of storage. However, because only 10% to 30% of normal levels are sufficient to maintain surgical hemostasis, procoagulant depletion is seldom an important cause of dilutional coagulopathy. The traditional practice of giving two units of FFP for every four units of blood is no longer tenable; FFP should be administered only if there is active bleeding associated with a prolonged PT.

b. Disseminated intravascular coagulation

c. Hemolytic transfusion reaction

2. Hypocalcemia

a. Ionized calcium is chelated by citrate in preserved blood. However, significant ionized hypocalcemia is caused only with very rapid blood administration, such as one unit every 5 minutes.

    b. Occasionally, and especially immediately after CPB, hypocalcemia may contribute to myocardial depression, necessitating supplemental calcium chloride (10–20 mg/kg IV).

3. Citrate toxicity

Citrate accumulates only in the presence of severe liver disease or hypothermia. Citrate acidosis is relatively common during liver transplantation.

4. Potassium imbalance

    a. Hyperkalemia is uncommon even though the measured potassium concentration in old, stored blood may reach 21 mEq/L. Potassium is rapidly moved intracellularly when blood is transfused and accumulates only in severe shock with acidosis or in small children receiving extensive transfusion.

    b. Hypokalemia is much more common, usually occurring 24 to 48 hours after transfusion when the citrate load has been metabolized to bicarbonate (one unit of blood releases 15 mM citrate, converted to 15 mM bicarbonate), resulting in metabolic alkalosis.

5. Acid–base imbalance

    a. Metabolic acidosis attributable to transfusion per se is uncommon despite the citrate and lactic acid accumulation in old, stored blood. Metabolic acidosis is generally related to the degree of shock rather than to the size of the transfusion.

    b. Metabolic alkalosis is common and predictable 24 to 48 hours after transfusion (see above). It may cause clinical problems (hypokalemia, arrhythmias, decreased ventilatory drive) and require treatment with potassium chloride and acetazolamide.

6. Hypothermia

    a. Hypothermia (core temperature below 34°C) may have devastating effects and severely impair attempts at resuscitation of the patient in hemorrhagic shock.

    b. Hypothermic coagulopathy is difficult to assess because laboratory tests are conducted at

37°C. Platelet aggregation is markedly impaired because TxA_2 release is diminished by hypothermia (note that the Ivy BT is sensitive to the temperature of the limb on which it is performed; i.e., if the limb is cold, the BT is prolonged even if the core is warmer with better platelet function). During severe hypothermia (below 30°C), platelets become sequestered in the liver, and the total platelet count falls as well.

c. Rapid infusion of cold blood into a central line may cause acute myocardial hypothermia, precipitating myocardial depression, ventricular dysrhythmias, and even cardiac arrest.

d. The $Hb-O_2$ dissociation curve is markedly left shifted in cold blood. At 8°C, the $S\bar{v}O_2$ of blood is 100% (i.e., Hb is totally unable to release O_2 to the tissues). Cold blood is essentially an inert volume expander, incapable of participating in O_2 transport. Before it can, it must be warmed by the patient's own heat, further increasing O_2 demand and exacerbating the potential for tissue ischemia.

e. The use of blood warmers is absolutely mandatory during rapid blood transfusion.

C. Transfusion-transmitted Disease
  1. Hepatitis (7%–10% of all transfusions)
    a. Because of routine testing for HBsAg, only 10% of cases of post-transfusion hepatitis today are hepatitis B. Hepatitis A is extremely rare.
    b. Non-A, non-B hepatitis causes 90% of cases, of which 75% are anicteric and identified by laboratory studies rather than clinical presentation. However, about 50% of patients develop chronic active hepatitis, and 10% to 20% of these go on to cirrhosis. Elevated ALT, anti-HBc, and anti-hepatitis C have emerged as useful markers of the presence of non-A, non-B hepatitis, which may help to reduce its incidence in the future.
  2. Acquired immunodeficiency syndrome (AIDS)
    a. The incidence of transmission of HIV is approximately 1 in 100,000 units, depending on the region of donor source. Blood product

recipients account for about 2% of all AIDS cases.

    b. Since 1985, all donor blood has been tested routinely for HIV antibody. However, there is a "window" of about 2 to 3 months between donor exposure and the development of HIV antibody, so that a small incidence of HIV-infected blood will remain in the foreseeable future.

    c. In the first years of the AIDS pandemic, a very large number of hemophiliac patients were infected. However, lyophilized concentrates of factors VIII and IX are heat treated, which markedly reduces the risk of HIV transmission. Unfortunately, FFP and cryoprecipitate lose their effectiveness if heat treated.

  3. Other infections

    a. Cytomegalovirus (CMV) and Epstein-Barr virus (EBV) may be transmitted in leukocytes and can cause fatal infections in immunocompromised patients.

    b. Spirochetal and bacterial sepsis are possible with platelet transfusion, as these units are stored at room temperature.

    c. Rarely, parasitic infections such as malaria, trypanosomiasis, and toxoplasmosis are transmitted.

IV. COMPONENT THERAPY

Blood component therapy has become popular among blood bankers over the last two decades because it enables discrete components to be separated from a single unit of WB and used for many patients. Although this is cost effective (and perhaps profitable, some cynics might suggest), there is increasing sentiment among surgeons and anesthesiologists for a return to the use of WB for massive transfusion because of decreased procoagulant depletion and FFP requirement.

  A. Fresh Frozen Plasma

    1. Each unit of FFP is separated from a single unit of whole blood within 6 hours of phlebotomy and frozen at $-18°C$ for up to a year (Table 8-5). Once thawed, it should be used within 24 hours, preferably within 2 hours for maximum benefit. It should be ABO compatible, but cross-matching is not necessary. Single-donor plasma (SDP) is plasma sepa-

Table 8–5. Recommendations for Administration of Fresh Frozen Plasma (1985)

1. The administration of fresh frozen plasma (FFP) has risen dramatically in recent years despite the paucity of definitive indications for its use and in the presence of mounting evidence of its potential risks, which include viral hepatitis and possibly acquired immunodeficiency syndrome. Many patients who receive FFP can be managed more effectively and safely with alternative modalities. Appropriate use of FFP must be justified on clinical grounds until better evidence is available. Research to develop safer FFP and alternative therapies is encouraged.
2. There is no justification for the use of FFP as a volume expander or as a nutritional source. Safer alternative therapies exist.
3. FFP is indicated for some documented coagulation protein deficiencies as well as for selected patients who require massive transfusions. It is indicated for patients with multiple coagulation defects as in liver disease, in conjunction with therapeutic plasma exchange for thrombotic thrombocytopenic purpura, for infants with protein-losing enteropathy, and for selected patients with other immunodeficiencies. Its use in most other cases should be discouraged.
4. Innovative educational efforts are needed to encourage appropriate use.

(National Institutes of Health Consensus Conference: Administration of fresh frozen plasma. JAMA 1985;253:551.)

rated from whole blood after 6 hours and thus deficient in the labile factors V and VIII.

2. FFP contains all coagulation factors but no platelets. Generally, two to three units is sufficient to achieve the 10% to 40% of the normal plasma concentration of clotting factors required for surgical hemostasis.
3. Indications
    a. Isolated factor deficiencies (II, V, VII, VIII, IX, XI, XII) when specific components are not available.
    b. Liver disease when PT is prolonged.
    c. Rapid warfarin reversal based on prolongation of PT.
    d. Significant surgical bleeding when PT is prolonged (not for prophylaxis).
    e. Massive transfusion with continued severe bleeding (factors V and VIII are labile, with

half-lives of <12 hours in whole blood, but dilutional thrombocytopenia is more common).

    f.   Antithrombin III deficiency manifested by heparin resistance.

  4.   Complications

    a.   Transfusion reactions are unlikely because red cells are removed, the unit is ABO-compatible, and carriers of major antibodies are usually eliminated from the donor pool.

    b.   The risks of transmission of viral disease are identical to those of transfusion of WB or RBCs.

    c.   Acute anaphylactoid responses with profound capillary leak syndrome resulting in hypotension and ARDS may occur. A causal relation to FFP has not been definitively established because other blood products are so often in concomitant use, but this does appear to be a real entity.

  5.   Contraindications

    a.   Treatment of prolonged PT (especially if <12.5 seconds) in the absence of bleeding

    b.   Prophylaxis (e.g., after CPB)

    c.   Simple volume expansion or "nutrition." The incidence of life-threatening reactions with FFP is 0.1% compared with 0.003% with human albumin.

B. Cryoprecipitated Antihemophilic Factor (Cryoprecipitate)

  1.   One unit of FFP thawed at 4°C yields 10 to 15 ml of cryoprecipitate. It may be stored at −18°C for 1 year but should be administered within 6 hours of thawing. Cryoprecipitate contains anti-A and anti-B antibodies, so ABO compatibility is preferred.

  2.   It contains fibrinogen, fibronectin, VIII:C, von Willebrand's factor, and factor XIII. One unit contains 20% to 50% of the factors present in FFP in 2% to 4% of the volume; usually, 10 or more units are pooled.

  3.   Indications

    a.   Hemophilia A (VIII:C deficiency), von Willebrand's disease, and fibrinogen (<100 mg/dl) or factor XIII deficiency.

    b.   Cryoprecipitate also helps correct prolonged

bleeding times (>15 seconds) in uremic patients. After administration of 10 units, bleeding times decrease maximally within 1 to 2 hours after transfusion and return to baseline levels by 24 hours. Cryoprecipitate may enhance platelet function after CPB and uremia by providing VIII:C/VWF complex. However, DDAVP is preferred in both these situations because it does not carry the risk of disease transmission.

    c. Cryoprecipitate is often used in liver transplantation because of the frequent development of VIII:C and fibrinogen deficiency.

    d. It can be used as topical "glue" in cardiac procedures, but bovine topical thrombin is preferred.

    e. Cryoprecipitate is not indicated in hemophilia B because it does not contain factor IX.

  4. Complications

    a. Disease transmission is enhanced because a single dose (10 units) of cryoprecipitate is pooled from ten donors.

    b. Anaphylactic reactions are rare but possible.

C. Platelets

  1. Platelets are stored at 20° to 24°C for a maximum of 5 days, but their effectiveness falls off rapidly after 48 hours. Storage at room temperature increases the risk of infection transmission (especially syphilis). A "storage lesion" impairs their function for 3 to 4 hours after transfusion. Cold-stored platelets (at 4°C) have more normal function immediately after transfusion but a much shorter in vivo life span. Platelets should be transfused via a standard 170-μm filter.

  2. One random-donor unit of platelets should increase the platelet count by approximately 10,000/μl if there is no ongoing platelet destructive process. ABO cross-matching is not required, but only Rh-negative units should be given to Rh-negative women of childbearing potential.

  3. Single-donor apheresis collection provides the same amount of platelets as is obtained from five to eight WB donations and can be matched for HLA type.

The risk of alloimmunization and disease transmission is markedly reduced, but this process is complex and expensive.

4. Indications for perioperative platelet transfusion (Table 8-6)

a. Preoperative platelet count below 50,000/µl. However, if the thrombocytopenia is chronic, a BT should be performed. Platelet transfusion is indicated only if the BT is more than twice normal.

Table 8–6. Recommendations for Platelet Transfusion (1986)

1. Patients with thrombocytopenia (less than 50,000/µl) or an abnormality of platelet function or both who have significant bleeding should receive platelets if the platelet disorder is likely to be causing or contributing to bleeding.
2. A bleeding time of less than twice the upper limit of the reference range is usually not an indication for transfusion of platelets, unless there are other conditions that interfere with hemostasis.
3. Preparation for invasive procedures in thrombocytopenic or thrombocytopathic patients might include prophylactic administration of platelets. Transfusion of enough platelets to correct the bleeding time is logical, but there are few, if any, pertinent studies.
4. Dilutional thrombocytopenia occurs in patients receiving multiple transfusions to replace blood lost through hemorrhage and may lead to generalized microvascular bleeding. Following replacement of one blood volume, 35% to 40% of the platelets usually remain. The majority of patients who receive rapid replacement of one or two blood volumes do not develop microvascular bleeding as a result of thrombocytopenia. Therefore, platelets should not be administered in the absence of documented thrombocytopenia and clinically abnormal bleeding.
5. Controlled prospective studies examining postoperative blood loss and outcome have demonstrated no correlation between platelet counts and bleeding after cardiopulmonary bypass and no detectable benefit from the prophylactic administration of platelets to such patients.
6. Efforts to overcome the problems associated with alloimmunization to platelets are imperative. A major step in this regard would be the establishment of a national network to facilitate transfusion of HLA-matched platelets to selected patients.
7. Infections transmitted by platelets remain a major concern. Elimination of bacterial growth in platelet concentrates stored at room temperature warrants special attention.

(National Institutes of Health Consensus Conference: Platelet transfusion therapy. JAMA 1987; 257:1777.)

        b. Preoperative thrombocytopathy documented by a prolonged BT. However, uremic thrombocytopathy is best corrected by the use of DDAVP.

        c. Active bleeding with rapidly falling platelet count. During extensive blood transfusion (>10 units), platelet administration may be considered even if the platelet count is still "normal" (e.g., rapid decrease from 250,000 to 110,000/μl).

        d. Active bleeding after CPB despite correction of heparin effect with protamine, especially if CPB time exceeds 2 hours. Because thrombocytopathy is common and the most likely cause of coagulopathy in this situation, platelet transfusion is reasonable. However, there is no justification for the prophylactic administration of platelets after CPB.

    5. Complications

        a. Alloimmunization to HLA-A and HLA-B is common with repeated platelet transfusion and probably is caused by leukocytes present in the concentrates. Rapid platelet destruction is avoided by the use of HLA-matched platelets, but in one-third of cases, even this is ineffective.

        b. Disease transmission is enhanced by the use of pooled concentrates from six to ten donors for each platelet transfusion. Virus transmission risk includes the same spectrum as for red cells; because of room temperature storage, there also is a small but important risk of transmitting bacterial infection.

V. SUMMARY OF ANESTHETIC CONSIDERATIONS
Estimated blood loss of 15% or greater is usually associated with a decrease in systolic blood pressure, increase in heart rate, and orthostatic changes in blood pressure or heart rate. Red blood cell transfusion is usually necessary to stabilize hypovolemic anemia. Transfusion of one unit of whole blood or packed RBCs will increase the hematocrit approximately 3%. Blood warmers should always be used during rapid transfusions.

    Acute intravascular hemolysis is usually seen with transfusion of ABO-incompatible blood. Patients often become febrile and hypotensive and have diffuse bleeding. Blood transfusions must be immediately discontinued, and aggressive measures are needed to maintain blood pressure and renal function. Less serious are urticarial and febrile reactions. Usually, hemolysis is not seen, and transfusion can be continued with supportive measures for fever, chills, nausea, and itching.

Hepatitis is seen with 7% to 10% of all transfusions. Non-A, non-B hepatitis causes 90% of cases, of which 75% are anicteric. The incidence of transmission of HIV is approximately 1 in 100,000 units. Cytomegalovirus and Epstein-Barr virus may be transmitted in leukocytes and cause fatal infection in immunocompromised patients. Spirochetal and other bacterial infection is possible with platelet transfusion, because these units are stored at room temperature. Rarely, parasitic infections such as malaria, trypanosomiasis, and toxoplasmosis have been transmitted.

Dilutional coagulopathy may occur with transfusions. Usually, it is secondary to thrombocytopenia after transfusion of one or more total-body blood volumes. Significant dilution of procoagulants is less common, as only 10% to 30% of normal levels is needed to maintain surgical hemostasis. Hypocalcemia, citrate toxicity, potassium imbalance, acid–base imbalance, and hypothermia may be associated with rapid infusion of large amounts of blood.

Fresh frozen plasma, once thawed, should be used within 24 hours but preferably within 2 hours. FFP contains all the coagulation factors but no platelets. Generally, two to three units is sufficient to achieve the 10% to 40% of the normal plasma concentration of clotting factors required for surgical hemostasis.

One unit of FFP thawed at 4°C yields 10 to 15 ml of cryoprecipitate. Cryoprecipitate has high concentrations of fibrinogen, VIII:C, von Willebrand's factor, factor XIII, and fibronectin. Cryoprecipitate is most useful for patients with deficiencies in factor VIII:C, von Willebrand complex, factor XIII, and fibrinogen. It may also be useful in patients with platelet dysfunction. Serial coagulation tests should be done when administering blood products.

Preoperative platelet transfusion is indicated if the platelet count acutely decreases to less than 50,000/μl. If thrombocytopenia is chronic, a bleeding time test should be performed. If the time is more than twice normal, platelet transfusion is indicated. Transfusion of one unit of platelets will usually increase count by 10,000/μl. Often, thrombocytopathy from uremia or cardiopulmonary bypass can be treated effectively by DDAVP.

Recommended Reading

Baer RW, Vlahakes GJ, Uhlig PN, Hoffman JI. Maximum myocardial oxygen transport during anemia and polycythemia in dogs. Am J Physiol 1987;252:H1086.

Caravalho AC. Bleeding in uremia: a clinical challenge. N Engl J Med 1983;308:38.

Clause LH, Camp PC. The regulation of hemostasis: the protein C system. N Engl J Med 1986;314:1298.

Consensus conference: administration of fresh frozen plasma. JAMA 1985;253:551.

Consensus conference: platelet transfusion therapy. JAMA 1987;257:1777.

Consensus conference: perioperative red blood cell transfusion. JAMA 1988;260:2700.

Ellison N, Jobes DR. Effective hemostasis in cardiac surgery. In: A Society of Cardiovascular Anesthesiologists Monograph. Philadelphia: WB Saunders, 1988.

Jansen PA, Tubeliver SJ, Weinstein MJ, Deykin D. The treatment of the bleeding tendency in uremia with cryoprecipitate. N Engl J Med 1980;303:1318.

Kang YG, Mortin DJ, Marqueg J, et al. Intraoperative changes in blood coagulation and thromboelastographic monitoring in liver transplantation. Anesth Analg 1985;64:888.

Kappa JR, Fisher CA, Cottrell ED, et al. Heparin-induced platelet activation in 16 surgical patients: diagnosis and management. J Vasc Sur 1987;5:101.

Kappa JR, Horn MK III, Fisher CA, et al. Efficacy of iloprost (ZK 36374) vs. aspirin in preventing heparin-induced platelet activation during open heart surgery. J Thorac Cardiovasc Surg 1987; 94:405.

Kelton JG, Sheridan D, Santos A, et al. Heparin-induced thrombocytopenia: laboratory studies. Blood 1988;72:925.

Kobrinsky NL, Israels ED, Gerrard JM, Chaeng MS, Watson CM, Bishop AJ, Shroeder ML. Shortening of bleeding time by L-deamino-8-D-arginine vasopressin in various bleeding disorders. Lancet 1984;1:1145.

Koshy M, Burd L, Wallace D, et al. Prophylactic red-cell transfusions in pregnant patients with sickle cell disease: a randomized cooperative study. N Engl J Med 1988;319:1447.

Kreiger JN, Hilgartner MW, Redo SF. Surgery for patients with congenital disorders of blood coagulation. Ann Surg 1977;185:290.

Lambert CJ, Marenzo–Rowe AJ, Leveson JE, et al. The treatment of postperfusion bleeding using ϵ-aminocaproic acid, cryoprecipitate, fresh frozen plasma and protamine sulfate. Ann Thorac Surg 1979;28:440.

Lerman J, Gregory GA, Eger EI. Hematocrit and solubility of volatile anesthetics in blood. Anesth Analg 1984;63:911.

Mannucci PM, Canciani MT, Rota L, Donovan BS. Response of factor VIII/von Willebrand's factor to DDAVP in healthy subjects and patients with hemophilia A and von Willebrand's disease. Br J Haematol 1981;47:283.

Mannucci PM, Remuzzi G, Pusineri F, et al. Deamino-8-D-arginine vasopressin shortens the bleeding time in uremia. N Engl J Med 1983;308:8.

Marengo–Rowe AJ, Lambert CJ, Leveson JE, Thiele JP, Geisler GF, Adam M, Mitchel BF Jr. The evaluation of hemorrhage in cardiac patients who have undergone extracorporeal circulation. Transfusion 1979;19:426.

Miller RD, Robbins TO, Tong MJ, Barton SL. Coagulation defects associated with massive blood transfusions. Ann Surg 1971;174:794.

Reed RL, Ciavarella D, Heimbach DM, et al. Prophylactic platelet administration during massive transfusion. Ann Surg 1986;203:44.

Roy RC, Stafford MA, Hudspeth AS, et al. Failure of prophylaxis with fresh frozen plasma after cardiopulmonary bypass. Anesthesiology 1988;69:254.

Shanberg JN, Murato M, Quattrociocci–Longe T, et al. Heparin–protamine complexes in the production of heparin rebound and other complications of extracorporeal bypass procedures. Am J Clin Pathol 1987;87:210.

Smith CL, Snouder SL. Anesthesia and glucose-6-phosphate dehydrogenase deficiency. Anaesthesia 1987;42:281.

Taylor MB, Whitwam JG, Worsley A. Paroxysmal nocturnal haemoglobinuria: perioperative management of a patient with Budd-Chiari syndrome. Anaesthesia 1987;42:639.

Tourbof KD, Bethizole RE, Zizzi JA, Subramaniam S, Andersen MN. Coronary bypass in a patient with hemophilia B, or Christmas disease. J Thorac Cardiovasc Surg 1979;77:562.

Wilkerson DK, Rosen AL, Gould SA, Sehgal LR, Sehgal HL, Mass GS. Oxygen extraction ratio: a valid indicator of myocardial metabolism in anemia. J Surg Res 1987;42:629.

CHAPTER 9

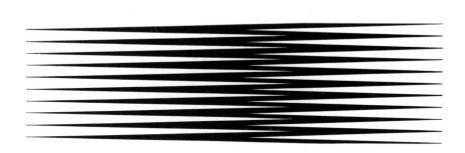

Malignancies

Raymond L. Sabon
Eugene Y. Cheng

Age-adjusted incidence rates for cancer continue to show a slow but steady increase in the United States. Cancer patients frequently require elective or emergency surgery. Knowledge of the primary malignancy, associated paraneoplastic syndromes, and the impact of anticancer therapies is necessary for proper anesthetic management of these patients.

I.   INCIDENCE, TREATMENT, AND PROGNOSIS OF SOLID TUMORS
   A. Lung Cancer
      1. Lung cancer kills more men and women than any other form of malignancy. The four principal histologic types of bronchogenic carcinoma are squamous, small cell or oat cell, adenocarcinoma, and large cell.
      2. Squamous cell carcinoma accounts for approximately 50% of bronchogenic carcinomas. Small cell, adenocarcinoma, and large cell types account for 20%, 15%, and 15% of bronchogenic tumors, respectively. A link to smoking has been shown for all principal cell types.
      3. Therapy is based on the cell type.
         a. The definitive treatment for non-small-cell bronchogenic carcinoma is surgical resection. Radiation may be of benefit for patients with involved hilar or mediastinal lymph nodes. Adjuvant chemotherapy is experimental.
         b. Small-cell carcinoma is usually considered to be widespread when discovered and generally is not resected. Chemotherapy is used to induce remission. Radiation therapy is delivered to the brain of patients in remission to prevent isolated relapse at this site. Chest irradiation and surgical resection of the primary tumor are experimental.
      4. The overall 5-year survival rate is only 30% to 50%, even in patients with apparently localized disease at presentation.
   B. Breast Cancer
      1. Breast cancer is the most common malignancy in women. It is estimated that as many as 10% of all women will develop this disease.
      2. Recent studies suggest that subtotal mastectomy followed by irradiation may be as effective as total

mastectomy in patients with tumors smaller than 4 cm.

3. Patients with positive axillary nodes are considered to have systemic micrometastases and therefore receive adjuvant chemotherapy.

4. The presence of estrogen or progesterone receptors in the tumor favorably influences prognosis. In such patients, endocrine manipulation such as oophorectomy, hypophysectomy, bilateral adrenalectomy, tamoxifen, or aminoglutethimide may be used.

5. Overall 5-year survival rates range from 80% for patients with localized disease to 10% for those with disseminated disease.

C. Colorectal Cancer

1. The primary treatment for colorectal adenocarcinoma is surgical resection. The prognosis is directly related to the extent of disease.

2. In patients with highly invasive rectal carcinoma and a high likelihood of local recurrence, postoperative chemotherapy plus radiation may improve survival.

3. In patients with metastatic disease, the liver is the only site of metastasis more than 50% of the time. Intravenous or direct hepatic arterial infusion of chemotherapy has not been shown to prolong survival dependably.

4. A tumor marker, carcinoembryonic antigen (CEA), is frequently followed postoperatively. Progressively rising levels usually indicate recurrent disease.

5. Overall 5-year survival rates range from 90% in well-localized disease to 5% in metastatic disease.

D. Prostate Cancer

1. Adenocarcinoma of the prostate is the third leading cause of cancer-related death in men.

2. Localized stages can be treated by radical prostatectomy or primary irradiation.

3. Patients with contiguous or metastatic spread of disease beyond the prostate receive irradiation and hormonal manipulation for palliation of symptoms. Surgical orchiectomy is the hormonal method of choice, with estrogenic drugs such as DES a less-favorable alternative.

4. Prostatic acid phosphatase and prostate-specific an-

tigen levels are often elevated in patients with advanced disease, and these levels can be followed to monitor the response to hormonal manipulation. At present, chemotherapy is experimental.

5. Patients with localized disease have approximately a 50% 10-year survival rate, whereas patients with metastatic disease have a 58% 5-year survival rate.

E. Testicular Cancer

1. Testicular carcinoma is one of the most common causes of cancer death for males in their second and third decades of life. Seminomas account for approximately 40% of testicular tumors and often are confined to the testicle at the time of diagnosis. Nonseminomatous tumors include teratomas, embryonal carcinomas, choriocarcinomas, endodermal sinus tumors, and mixed tumors.

2. Staging is performed by inguinal orchiectomy and radiologic study (seminoma) or lymph node dissection (nonseminomatous tumors). Treatment of local stages is by inguinal orchiectomy and irradiation of retroperitoneal lymph nodes (for seminoma) or lymphadenectomy (for nonseminomatous tumors).

3. Recent developments in combination chemotherapy allow the induction of long-term remission in 80% or more of patients with disseminated disease. Relapses are often controlled by similar chemotherapy.

4. The circulating tumor markers beta-human chorionic gonadotropin (β-HCG) and alpha-fetoprotein (AFP) are followed during remission, with progressive rises usually indicating recurrent disease.

5. Patients with nonseminomatous tumors have an overall 5-year survival range from 70% to 100%. The 5-year survival rate in patients with seminomas ranges from 93% in patients with localized disease to 20% in patients with distant disease.

F. Hodgkin's Disease

1. Hodgkin's disease is a lymphomatous cancer that typically presents as a palpable cervical mass frequently associated with systemic symptoms such as fever, weight loss, and night sweats. With advances in staging and therapy, it is possible to cure as many as 80% of patients, with better results being obtained with younger cases.

2. After noninvasive staging procedures, patients without evidence of bulky or disseminated disease undergo staging laparotomies with splenectomy. Patients with local disease then undergo definitive radiation therapy, combination chemotherapy, or both.

3. Initial combination chemotherapy is used on patients with disseminated disease. Subsequent radiation therapy is experimental. Complications of therapy include acute nonlymphocytic leukemia, which is most common in patients over the age of 40 who have received both chemotherapy and radiation.

4. The overall 10-year survival rate is 75% to 80%.

G. Ovarian Cancer

1. Epithelial carcinoma accounts for approximately 90% of all ovarian cancers, with germ cell tumors accounting for approximately 5%.

2. Epithelial carcinoma usually occurs in women over the age of 50 years. The prognosis is related to tumor stage, histologic grade, and the extent of residual tumor after resection.

3. Combination chemotherapy or whole-abdomen and pelvic irradiation may be indicated in patients with poorly differentiated or advanced-stage tumors.

4. Germ cell tumors usually occur in women less than 25 years of age and are often unilateral. Like the testicular germ cell tumors, they may secrete the tumor markers AFP, β-HCG, or both.

5. Dysgerminomas are the female analog of seminomas and are very radiosensitive. Other germ cell tumors are usually curable with combination chemotherapy.

6. The 5-year survival rate for epithelial carcinomas ranges from 60% in localized disease to 3% in extensive disease.

H. Cervical Cancer

1. The incidence of carcinoma of the cervix is related to the age at first intercourse and first pregnancy, the number of sexual partners, and venereal disease. In particular, Herpes simplex virus Type 2 is related to, but not a proved etiologic agent of, carcinoma of the cervix.

2. The principal histologic types of cancer of the cervix are squamous cell carcinoma, accounting for 80%;

adenocarcinoma, accounting for 18%; and sarcoma, accounting for 2%.

3. The most localized stage is carcinoma in situ, and this can be treated by either conization or hysterectomy. More extensive disease is treated by radiation therapy, pelvic exenteration, or both.

4. Five-year survival rates range from 95% to 100% for carcinoma in situ to 5% for extensive disease.

I. Uterine Cancer

1. Cancer of the uterus is most commonly found in women over the age of 50 years. The principal histologic types are endometrial adenocarcinoma, accounting for 70%; adenoacanthoma, accounting for 20%; and adenosquamous carcinoma, accounting for 10%.

2. The tumor is confined to the body of the uterus approximately 75% of the time. The lungs are the most frequent site of metastasis.

3. Treatment for local stages is total abdominal hysterectomy, radiation therapy, or both. More extensive stages are managed by radiation by implantation and external-beam irradiation. Progestins may also be used. Chemotherapy is experimental.

4. The overall 5-year survival rate ranges from 75% for local stages to 10% for extensive disease.

II. INCIDENCE, TREATMENT, AND PROGNOSIS OF HEMATOLOGIC MALIGNANCIES

A. Acute Lymphocytic Leukemia

1. This acute leukemia is primarily a disease of children but accounts for nearly 15% of adult acute leukemias. Leukemic central nervous system (CNS) involvement is common, as are lymphadenopathy, splenomegaly, anemia, and susceptibility to serious infection. Liver involvement is possible, resulting in impaired metabolism of many drugs.

2. Induction of remission is by combination chemotherapy. CNS prophylaxis after remission is usually by cranial irradiation and intrathecal methotrexate.

3. Remission requires maintenance chemotherapy. The value of autologous or allogenic bone-marrow transplantation is being studied.

4. The overall median survival time in adolescents and adults is approximately 2 years. Children may have up to a 50% to 60% cure rate.

B. Acute Nonlymphocytic Leukemia
  1. This disease accounts for most adult acute leuke-mias. Acute myelocytic leukemia is the most common type, followed by myelomonocytic, promyelocytic, and erythroleukemic types.
  2. The principal clinical manifestations result from marrow involvement causing pancytopenias with weakness, infection, and bleeding. Acute promyelocytic leukemia is commonly associated with disseminated intravascular coagulation prompted by the release of procoagulant from lysed cells. Heparin may be lifesaving.
  3. Definitive treatment is by combination chemotherapy. Hyperuricemia is common and can be profound following institution of chemotherapy. Renal impairment is a not-infrequent occurrence with high levels of uric acid. CNS involvement requires intrathecal administration of chemotherapeutic agents.
  4. Median survival is 12 to 24 months for patients who achieve complete remission.
C. Chronic Granulocytic Leukemia
  1. This type of leukemia is primarily found in young and middle-aged adults. Clinical presentation usually includes splenomegaly, excessive bruising and bleeding, weakness, fatigue, and weight loss.
  2. Leukocytosis and anemia can be marked, and platelet counts may be elevated early in the disease.
  3. Treatment may consist of splenectomy, oral alkylating agents, local irradiation to the spleen, or whole-body irradiation with ^{32}P.
  4. The Philadelphia chromosome is a balanced translocation from chromosome 22 to chromosome 9, and its presence is an important prognosticator. Median survival in Ph^1-positive patients is 30 to 45 months versus 9 to 15 months in patients without the chromosome.
D. Chronic Lymphocytic Leukemia
  1. This type of leukemia tends to pursue a more benign course than the granulocytic variety. It constitutes approximately 25% of all leukemias.
  2. Severe splenomegaly and leukocytosis are usually present along with a variable degree of anemia and thrombocytopenia. Massive lymphadenopathy may encroach on the airway, making adequate ventila-

tion difficult. Autoimmune hemolytic anemia may be present and complicate cross-matching.

3. The basal metabolic rate can be elevated as much as a third above normal, causing increased oxygen consumption.

4. Treatment is with chemotherapy, most often alkylating agents.

5. Median survival in patients with limited disease is longer than 12 years compared with 1.5 years in patients with extensive disease.

E. Polycythemia Vera

1. Polycythemia vera is a myeloproliferative disorder in which there is unregulated proliferation of leukocytes, erythrocytes, and platelets. The median age of onset is between 55 and 60 years.

2. Patients are at increased risk for both thrombosis and bleeding. Thrombosis is thought to result from increased viscosity and marked thrombocytosis. The bleeding tendency is thought to be related to the increased ratio of erythrocytes to fibrin, the vascular engorgement, and, possibly, abnormal platelet function. Hyperuricemia and gout are common in these patients because of the increased production and destruction of cells.

3. Treatment is by repeated phlebotomies and short courses of oral alkylating agents.

4. The median survival in treated patients is 8 to 15 years.

F. Multiple Myeloma

1. This disease is caused by a neoplastic proliferation of plasma cells that causes bone marrow failure and osseous destruction.

2. Large quantities of a single type of immunoglobulin are produced at the expense of normal immunoglobulins. This results in an increased susceptibility to infection. In addition, the excess light chains are filtered by the glomeruli and damage the renal tubules. Marked hypercalcemia can be present, usually because of an osteoblast-activating factor. Rarely, a sensorimotor polyneuropathy is present and can precede the diagnosis of myeloma by several months. Severe osseous destruction results in osteoporosis and osteolysis often complicated by pathologic fractures and bone pain. Occasionally,

high serum protein levels result in a hyperviscosity syndrome causing visual disturbances, heart failure, and a bleeding diathesis.

3. Oral alkylating agents and steroids are the usual treatment. Radiation is useful for the treatment of painful osteolytic lesions.

4. In patients with a large tumor mass and a poor response to therapy, the median survival is 0.5 to 3 years. Patients with a small tumor mass have a median survival of 3.5 to 10 years.

III. PARANEOPLASTIC SYNDROMES

Many pathophysiologic disturbances are commonly associated with cancer. Their importance to the anesthesiologist relates to their ability to alter the responses to medications and to require or contraindicate specific perioperative therapies and techniques (Table 9-1).

A. Cachexia

Anorexia, weight loss, negative nitrogen balance, and hypoalbuminemia are common in cancer patients. Some tumors stimulate normal macrophages to produce the hormone cachectin (tumor necrosis factor), which can cause the above clinical findings. Dosages of medications should be appropriately changed for decreased lean body mass, intravascular protein, and altered volumes of distribution. Wound healing will be impaired. If possible, patients should receive at least 2 weeks of nutrition prior to surgery to help restore nutritional balance.

B. Fever

Fever in a cancer patient may indicate an underlying infection, and this should always be ruled out prior to any surgical procedure. However, fever may be secondary to the malignancy itself, as is most commonly found with Hodgkin's disease, renal cell carcinoma, and hepatic metastases. Tumor cells stimulate normal monocytes to produce interleukin-1, which may be responsible for the elevated temperature. Fever itself is often associated with dehydration and an elevated metabolic rate. Increased intravenous fluid infusions may be required to maintain adequate volume status, and an increased F_{IO_2} may be needed to maintain normal oxygenation.

C. Tumor Hypoglycemia

Tumor hypoglycemia is most commonly associated with retroperitoneal tumors, hepatomas, adrenocortical carcinoma, and carcinoma of the gastrointestinal tract. Its

Table 9–1. Paraneoplastic Syndromes

Clinical Manifestation	Proposed Mediator	Commonly Associated Tumor Site or Types
Cachexia	Cachectin	Any
Fever	Interleukin-1, cachectin	Hodgkin's disease, renal cell carcinoma, hepatic metastases
Hypoglycemia	Nonsuppressible insulin-like factors	Retroperitoneal tumors, hepatoma, adrenocortical carcinoma
Cushing's syndrome	ACTH, CRF	Lung (small cell), pancreas (non-islet-cell), thymoma, neural crest lesions
Hyponatremia	ADH	Lung (small cell)
Hypercalcemia	PTH-like factors, osteoclast-activating factors	Lung, head and neck (squamous), renal cell, breast, ovary, multiple myeloma
Erythrocytosis	Erythropoietin	Renal cell carcinoma, cerebellar hemangio-blastomas, adrenal cortical carcinomas, hepatomas
Lactic acidosis		Lymphoma, lymphocytic leukemia, hepatic or bone marrow metastases
Hypocalcemia		Thyroid (medullary) osteoblastic metastases
Thrombocytopenia		Adenocarcinoma of lung, pancreas, colon
Hypercoagulability		Gastric, pancreas, lung, colon, prostate, ovary
Disseminated intravascular coagulation		Prostate, acute promyelocytic leukemia
Adrenal insufficiency		Any
Hyperuricemia		Leukemia
Nephrotic syndrome		Hodgkin's disease
Neuromuscular abnormalities		Lung (small cell), gastrointestinal adenocarcinoma
Myasthenic syndrome		
Dermatomyositis		

Table 9–1. Paraneoplastic Syndromes (*continued*)

Clinical Manifestation	Proposed Mediator	Commonly Associated Tumor Site or Types
Myasthenia gravis		
Pericardial effusion and tamponade		Lymphoma, melanoma, breast, lung
Spinal cord compression		Any
Brain metastases		Lung, breast, melanoma
Obstructive uropathy		Retroperitoneal tumors, lymphoma, sarcoma, prostate, rectum, cervix, bladder
Superior vena caval obstruction		Lung (small cell), lymphoma, breast, testis

presence is revealed by fasting hypoglycemia. The most likely mechanisms include a nonsuppressible insulin-like factor, interference with glycogenolysis or gluconeogenesis, or hepatic destruction. Treatment may be frequent small feedings, corticosteroids, a glucose infusion, or glucagon, as well as therapy against the primary tumor.

D. Cushing's Syndrome

Ectopic ACTH from small cell carcinoma of the lung is responsible for more than 50% of the cases of Cushing's syndrome. Other sources of ACTH are carcinoids, thymomas, non-B islet-cell tumors of the pancreas, and neural crest lesions. Ectopic corticotropin-releasing factor (CRF) is a much less common cause. Clinical presentation is most often with hypertension, hypokalemia, hyperglycemia, edema, and muscle weakness. The typical features of Cushing's syndrome (central obesity, moon facies, and abdominal striae) are rarely seen. Therapy is best directed against the primary tumor. Alternative treatment is by drugs that impair steroid synthesis such as mitotane, metyrapone, and aminoglutethimide.

E. Lactic Acidosis

Cancer patients with lactic acidosis usually present with hyperventilation, malaise, decreased mental status, anorexia, and vomiting. Laboratory findings include elevated serum lactate levels, decreased pH, and an increased anion gap. Acidosis is most often seen in patients with uncontrolled lymphocytic leukemia or lymphomas. It is rarely associated with solid tumors, and when it is, it often signifies extensive liver or bone marrow involvement. The response to bicarbonate therapy is poor unless combined with successful therapy for the primary malignancy. Animal studies have shown that elevated lactate levels, even in the presence of a normal pH, are associated with decreased myocardial contractility, reduced glucose utilization in the ischemic myocardium, and decreased exercise tolerance.

F. Syndrome of Inappropriate Antidiuretic Hormone Secretion (SIADH)
SIADH is diagnosed by the presence of hyponatremia, a serum osmolality less than 280 mOsm, and a urine osmolality greater than 300 mOsm in patients who do not have underlying adrenal or renal disease. It is most commonly associated with small cell carcinoma of the lung, cerebral disorders, and pulmonary infections. In addition, vincristine, barbiturates, and opiates may stimulate antidiuretic hormone (ADH) release. A metabolite of cyclophosphamide can mimic the actions of ADH on the kidney. The symptoms are related to the rapidity of the fall in serum sodium as well as to the absolute value. They include confusion, headache, nausea, vomiting, anorexia, irritability, lethargy, and seizures. The usual treatment is to restrict water intake to less than 1 L per day. Severe cases with CNS symptoms warrant treatment with furosemide and 3% saline. Chronic therapy is with demeclocycline or lithium, which interfere with the action of ADH on the collecting ducts.

G. Hypercalcemia of Malignancy
Hypercalcemia is found in 10% to 20% of all patients with malignancy. The most common associated malignancies are lung, breast, renal, and head and neck carcinomas and multiple myeloma. It is now well established that parathyroid hormone is rarely responsible for non-parathyroid hypercalcemia. The mechanisms of hypercalcemia in solid tumors are usually circulating humoral factors. Hematologic malignancies cause hypercalcemia through local bone destruction by cytokines released from malignant cells.

Clinical findings may include anorexia, nausea and vomiting, polyuria and polydipsia, pancreatitis, and confusion. The ECG can show shortening of the P-R and Q-T intervals. Therapy should include intravascular volume expansion and furosemide. Corticosteroids and mithramycin can also be used but may take 36 to 48 hours for effect. A safe serum Ca^{2+} level for the commencement of anesthesia is considered to be less than 14 mg/dl.

H. Hypocalcemia

Hypocalcemia is commonly associated with medullary cancer of the thyroid, increased calcium uptake by osteoblastic metastases, malabsorption, renal failure, hypomagnesemia, and cancer chemotherapeutic agents. Uncorrected hypocalcemia may compromise cardiac contractility and diaphragm function and lead to muscle spasm or seizures.

I. Anemia and Polycythemia

Anemia in the cancer patient can be secondary to red blood cell loss by bleeding, hypersplenism, or autoimmune hemolytic anemia. It may also be caused by decreased cell production secondary to malignant bone marrow infiltration, chemotherapy, radiation therapy, or nutrient deficiencies.

Polycythemia is often associated with elevated erythropoietin levels and is often asymptomatic. Commonly associated malignancies include renal cell carcinoma, hepatoma, cerebellar hemangioblastoma, ovarian carcinoma, and adrenocortical carcinoma.

J. Thrombocytopenia

Thrombocytopenia is usually related to cancer therapy, although unexplained thrombocytopenia may signal an occult adenocarcinoma of the lung, pancreas, or colon. Malignant thrombocytopenia also may be related to hypersplenism or disseminated intravascular coagulation (DIC).

K. Coagulopathies

There is an increased incidence of deep venous thrombosis (DVT) and other thromboembolic phenomena in association with cancer of the stomach, pancreas, lung, colon, prostate, and ovary. In these patients, consideration should be given to the use of DVT prophylaxis in the perioperative period. Aspirin and minidose heparin have been so used. If there is a high risk of bleeding or if anticoagulation is contraindicated, a vena caval umbrella should be placed.

Disseminated intravascular coagulation may be associated with cancer of the prostate, mucin-producing adenocarcinomas, and acute promyelocytic leukemia. Coagulation defects may also be caused by mithramycin or L-asparaginase therapy.

L. Adrenal Insufficiency
More than 90% of the adrenal gland must be replaced by tumor to cause clinical hypoadrenalism. Adrenal metastases cause less than 1% of all cases of adrenal insufficiency but are present in more than 9% of cancer patients at necropsy. More common causes of adrenal insufficiency include mitotane, aminoglutethimide, ketoconazole, withdrawal of chronic steroid therapy, overwhelming infection, and cytomegalovirus adrenalitis. The stress of the perioperative period may unmask latent adrenal insufficiency. Clinical findings can include fatigue, dehydration, oliguria, and cardiovascular collapse. Laboratory findings include hyperkalemia, metabolic acidosis, and hyponatremia. Preoperative assessment with the ACTH stimulation test should be done on patients suspected of having adrenal insufficiency. Therapy is intravenous fluids and steroid supplementation.

M. Hyperuricemia
Hyperuricemia is most often associated with a leukemia and a large tumor mass that undergoes rapid destruction by chemotherapeutic agents. Uric acid levels above 15 mg/dl often cause acute renal failure. Therapy should include allopurinol, intravenous fluids, and alkalinization of the urine.

N. Nephrotic Syndrome
Hodgkin's disease is the malignancy most frequently associated with the nephrotic syndrome. Renal biopsy shows minimal-change disease in 80% of these patients. Patients who have a carcinoma associated with the nephrotic syndrome are usually found to have membranous glomerulonephritis on biopsy. Immune complexes are felt to be the mechanism of renal injury in this latter group.

O. Neuromuscular Abnormalities
  1. The most common neuromuscular abnormality in cancer patients is the Eaton–Lambert syndrome (myasthenic syndrome). It is closely associated with small cell carcinoma of the lung and causes weakness and fatigue of the pelvic girdle and thigh musculature. Extraocular muscles are involved in rare

cases, and the deep tendon reflexes in the lower extremities are often depressed. These patients show a remarkable sensitivity to nondepolarizing muscle relaxants that is exacerbated by aminoglycoside antibiotics. Reversal is typically difficult with anticholinesterase agents. Response to depolarizing muscle relaxants is increased above normal, although to a lesser degree. Preoperative treatment with guanidine may be helpful.

2. Dermatomyositis is a disorder of the skin and muscles that presents with progressive proximal muscle weakness and elevated creatinine phosphokinase (CPK) levels. Respiratory weakness is frequent, increasing the chance of pulmonary aspiration. It is associated with adenocarcinoma of the gastrointestinal tract, and its presence in a man over 50 years of age suggests an occult neoplasm. It probably is associated with an increased sensitivity to neuromuscular blockers.

3. Myasthenia gravis occurs in 50% of patients with thymoma and is also associated with small cell carcinoma of the lung and with lymphoma. It usually presents as cranial nerve palsies that worsen with repetitive movements. These patients show an increased sensitivity to nondepolarizing muscle relaxants and a characteristic resistance to depolarizing muscle relaxants with an early appearance of Phase II block.

P. Pericardial Effusion and Tamponade
Metastatic involvement of the pericardium occurs most commonly with lymphoma, melanoma, and carcinomas of the breast and lung. Paroxysmal atrial fibrillation may be the presenting finding. Tamponade develops when the effusion develops rapidly or is large. The most sensitive and specific noninvasive test is echocardiography. Effusions usually respond readily to chemotherapy or radiation. Sclerosal therapy with tetracycline is occasionally used after drainage of the effusion. Recalcitrant effusions may require a pericardial window.

Q. Spinal Cord Compression
Spinal cord compression results from tumor invasion of the epidural space or from vertebral collapse secondary to osseous destruction. The presenting symptoms are back pain followed by numbness, parasthesia, and weak-

ness. A myelogram or metrizimide CT scan are necessary if the symptoms and plain radiographs suggest spinal cord compression. Treatment is by radiation therapy, corticosteroids, or surgical laminectomy. Once complete motor loss has developed, laminectomy is rarely successful in restoring sensory and motor function.

R. Brain Metastases

Between 10% and 20% of patients with widespread malignancies have brain metastases. The most commonly associated malignancies are carcinoma of the lung and breast and melanoma. Diagnosis is best accomplished by CT scan, with posterior fossa lesions possibly better evaluated by MRI scan. Treatment is usually with steroids followed by radiation. In a patient with reasonable life expectancy in whom the primary malignancy is under control, resection of a solitary cranial metastasis may be beneficial.

S. Obstructive Uropathy

Ureteral obstruction usually is unilateral and is asymptomatic unless renal failure ensues. It is most commonly associated with retroperitoneal tumors, lymphoma, sarcoma, or carcinoma of the prostate, rectum, cervix, and bladder. Bladder outlet obstruction becomes symptomatic at an earlier stage, with oliguria and bladder distention. It is most commonly secondary to prostatic carcinoma or benign prostatic hyperplasia. Significant obstruction is easily detected with abdominal ultrasound. Upper tract obstruction often is managed by percutaneous drainage. Urethral obstruction generally is handled by prostatic surgery.

T. Superior Vena Caval Obstruction

Most patients with neoplastic-related superior vena caval obstruction do not have a history of malignancy at the time of presentation. Presenting symptoms include facial plethora and edema, dyspnea, headache, and visual disturbances. Approximately 75% of these obstructions are related to carcinoma of the lung, usually the small cell type. Lymphoma, breast, and testicular malignancies are occasionally responsible. Treatment is radiation therapy or chemotherapy, depending on the tumor type. Emergency radiation or chemotherapy is needed only if there is evidence of cerebral dysfunction, impaired cardiac output, or upper airway obstruction. Intubation may be necessary to protect the airway while waiting for the tumor to respond to therapy.

IV. CANCER TREATMENT
Treatment of cancer may involve chemotherapy, radiation therapy, or surgery, each of which may entail special concerns for anesthetic and perioperative management. Most chemotherapeutic agents exert their effect by acting on the enzymes or their substrates involved in the synthesis of DNA. Combination chemotherapy involves the simultaneous use of several agents that act at different steps in DNA synthesis to increase overall cytotoxic activity. These agents are not selective for neoplastic cells, but rather any cells that are rapidly proliferating. Predictable toxicities include pancytopenias, alopecia, gastrointestinal mucosal ulceration, nausea, vomiting, diarrhea, and dermatitides. The most common dose-limiting toxicity is myelosuppression, which usually is reversible when chemotherapy is discontinued.

Chemotherapeutic drugs can be classified as alkylating agents, antimetabolites, plant alkaloids, antibiotics, nitrosoureas, enzymes, and miscellaneous. The actions, interactions, and toxic effects of each agent can be specific to the drug or its class or be common to all agents (Table 9-2).

A. Alkylating Agents
The cytotoxic effects of alkylating agents are directly related to the alkylation of components of DNA. Bone-marrow suppression is the dose-limiting side effect and is especially profound with busulfan, where it may last for several months. Increased skin pigmentation and hemolytic anemia may occur. Alkylating agents can cause a tumor lysis syndrome by inducing rapid destruction of susceptible tumor cells and marked hyperuricemia. There is a 2.5% to 10% incidence of pneumonitis and pulmonary fibrosis with these drugs. Busulfan has been associated with hypocalcemia. A metabolite of cyclophosphamide acts on the kidney to produce an SIADH-like syndrome. Thiotepa, mechlorethamine, and cyclophosphamide irreversibly inhibit plasma cholinesterase. This effect has been associated with prolonged responses to succinylcholine. In addition, use of these agents would be expected to prolong the effect of cocaine and ester local anesthetics.

B. Antimetabolites
Antimetabolites are structural analogs of normal metabolites required by cells. They are most effective against rapidly proliferating cells, particularly bone marrow and gastrointestinal epithelial cells. Thus, predictable tox-

Text continues on p. 495

Table 9-2. Chemotherapeutic Agents and Their Effects

Type of Agent	Name	Therapeutic Use	Common Side Effects
Vinca Alkaloids			
	Vinblastine	Hodgkin's disease Non-Hodgkin's lymphomas Breast Testis	Immunosuppression, peripheral and autonomic nervous system toxicity
	Vincristine	Acute lymphocytic leukemia Neuroblastoma Lung (small cell) Hodgkin's disease Non-Hodgkin's lymphomas	Immunosuppression, peripheral and autonomic nervous system toxicity
Antibiotics			
	Dactinomycin	Choriocarcinoma Testis Wilms' tumor Kaposi's sarcoma Rhabdomyosarcoma	Thrombocytopenia, leukopenia, anemia
	Daunorubicin	Acute granulocytic leukemia Acute lymphocytic leukemia	Thrombocytopenia, leukopenia, anemia
	Doxorubicin	Sarcomas Hodgkin's disease Non-Hodgkin's lymphoma Breast Thyroid Lung Gastric Neuroblastic	Cardiac toxicity, leukopenia, stomatitis

Drug	Indications	Toxicity
Bleomycin	Testis Head and neck Skin Lung Esophagus GI tract Hodgkin's disease Non-Hodgkin's lymphoma	Pulmonary toxicity, stomatitis
Mithramycin	Testis Bone metastases	Thrombocytopenia, leukopenia, coagulation defects
Mitomycin C	Gastric Cervix Colon Breast Pancreas Bladder Head and neck	Thrombocytopenia, leukopenia, anemia
Miscellaneous		
Cisplatin	Testis Ovary Bladder Head and neck Lung Thyroid Osteogenic sarcoma Endometrium Neuroblastoma Hodgkin's disease	Renal toxicity, CNS toxicity, peripheral nervous system toxicity
Procarbazine		Thrombocytopenia, leukopenia, MAO inhibitor

(continued)

Table 9–2. Chemotherapeutic Agents and Their Effects (continued)

Type of Agent	Name	Therapeutic Use	Common Side Effects
Nitrosoureas			
	BCNU	Hodgkin's disease Non-Hodgkin's lymphomas Multiple myeloma Melanoma Primary brain tumors	Anemia, leukopenia, thrombocytopenia
	CCNU	Hodgkin's disease Non-Hodgkin's lymphomas Lung (small cell) Primary brain tumors	Anemia, leukopenia, thrombocytopenia
	Methyl-CCNU	Primary brain tumors Gastric Colon	Anemia, leukopenia, thrombocytopenia
	Streptozocin	Malignant carcinoid Malignant pancreas insulinoma	Hepatic toxicity, renal toxicity, hypoinsulinism
Alkylating Agents			
	Mechlorethamine	Hodgkin's disease Non-Hodgkin's lymphoma Acute lymphocytic leukemia Chronic lymphocytic leukemia	Thrombocytopenia, leukopenia, plasma cholinesterase inhibitors
	Cyclophosphamide	Hodgkin's disease Non-Hodgkin's lymphoma Lymphoma Multiple myeloma Neuroblastoma	Immunosuppression, plasma cholinesterase inhibitor, leukopenia

Drug	Indications	Toxicity
Melphalan	Breast Ovary Lung Wilms' tumor Rhabdomyosarcoma Multiple myeloma	Plasma cholinesterase inhibitor, leukopenia, hemolytic anemia
Chlorambucil	Breast Ovary Chronic lymphocytic leukemia Non-Hodgkin's lymphoma Macroglobulinemia	Anemia, leukopenia, thrombocytopenia
Busulfan	Chronic lymphocytic leukemia	Anemia, leukopenia, thrombocytopenia
Dacarbazine	Melanoma Hodgkin's disease Soft-tissue sarcomas	Anemia, leukopenia, thrombocytopenia
Thiotepa		Plasma cholinesterase inhibitor, anemia, leukopenia

Antimetabolites

Drug	Indications	Toxicity
Methotrexate	Acute lymphocytic leukemia Choriocarcinoma Breast Head and neck Lung Osteogenic sarcoma	Immunosuppression, stomatitis, hepatic toxicity
5-Fluorouracil	Breast Colon Gastric Pancreas Ovary Head and neck Bladder	Immunosuppression, stomatitis, hepatic toxicity

(continued)

Table 9–2. Chemotherapeutic Agents and Their Effects (*continued*)

Type of Agent	Name	Therapeutic Use	Common Side Effects
	Cytarabine	Acute lymphocytic leukemia Acute granulocytic leukemia	Immunosuppression, stomatitis, hepatic toxicity
	6-Mercaptopurine	Acute lymphocytic leukemia Acute granulocytic leukemia Chronic granulocytic leukemia	Immunosuppression, stomatitis, hepatic toxicity
	Thioguanine	Acute lymphocytic leukemia Acute granulocytic leukemia Chronic granulocytic leukemia	Immunosuppression, stomatitis, hepatic toxicity
	5-Azathioprine		Immunosuppression, stomatitis, hepatic toxicity
Enzymes	L-Asparaginase	Acute lymphocytic leukemia	Immunosuppression, hepatic toxicity

icities are buccal mucosal ulceration, stomatitis, diarrhea, hemorrhagic enteritis, and, possibly, intestinal perforation. Renal tubular necrosis is also a possibility. Cerebellar ataxia has been noted occasionally with 5-fluorouracil. Reversible liver dysfunction may occur, and hepatic fibrosis is associated with daily oral methotrexate. Methotrexate is also associated with a delayed pulmonary toxicity with peripheral eosinophilia that may lead to pulmonary fibrosis. Intrathecal methotrexate has been associated with an acute paralysis, probably secondary to demyelination, and, when combined with radiation therapy or cytarabine, may cause chronic encephalopathy.

C. Plant Alkaloids

Plant alkaloids are cell-cycle–specific agents that bind to tubulin and disrupt the microtubules, causing cell division to be arrested in metaphase. Bone marrow suppression is a significant side effect manifested predominantly by leukopenia. Neurologic toxicity may be in the form of encephalopathies, peripheral neuropathies, or autonomic neuropathies. The peripheral neuropathy is a mixed sensory and motor lesion and is associated with loss of deep tendon reflexes and muscle weakness. Cranial nerve palsies are uncommon, although weakness involving the larynx can occur. Autonomic neuropathies are associated with constipation, ileus, and, occasionally, bowel perforation. Orthostatic hypotension also may occur. These agents can also cause inappropriate release of ADH for as long as 10 days after the initial drug administration.

D. Antibiotics

Anthracycline antibiotics form stable complexes with DNA. They cause moderate bone-marrow suppression but are most noted for their cardiac toxicity. The cardiac toxicity takes two forms: a dose-related congestive heart failure (CHF) and relatively benign and transient ECG changes. The incidence of CHF is approximately 1.8% but may be as high as 25% in patients who have received doxorubicin in doses of more than 550 mg/m^2. Those at increased risk are patients with prior radiation therapy involving the heart, concurrent cyclophosphamide therapy, or prior heart disease. These agents cause a loss of myocardial cells, and the CHF is typically resistant to the usual doses of inotropic agents. Early diagnosis is best made by echocardiography. There is a 10% incidence of ECG changes that include premature ventricular and supraventricular rhythms, left-axis deviation, decreased QRS voltage, and nonspecific ST-T changes. Most ECG changes except the decreased voltage resolve over 1 to 2 months after the cessation of therapy.

The cytotoxic effect of bleomycin relates to its ability to cause fragmentation of the DNA molecule. The most serious side effect is pulmonary toxicity, which occurs in 10% to 25% of patients, causing death in 1% to 2%. Risk factors include age over 70, total dose greater than 450 units, prior chest radiation, and existing pulmonary disease. Evidence suggests that a high F_{IO_2} under anesthesia may exacerbate the toxicity. It is recommended that the F_{IO_2} be limited if possible to 0.22 to 0.25 and that intravenous fluids be limited, with colloids given preferentially. Failure to follow these recommendations has been associated with fatal postoperative adult respiratory distress syndrome (ARDS), whereas reported series following these recommendations have had no cases of ARDS.

Presentation is usually with a nonproductive cough, fever, dyspnea, and bibasilar rales. Laboratory findings include hypoxia, hypocapnia, diminished diffusing capacity, restrictive flow pattern, and basilar interstitial pneumonitis progressing to fibrosis. Serial pulmonary function tests have not been predictive as an index of toxicity.

Mucocutaneous reactions occur in approximately 45% of patients. Manifestations include stomatitis, hyperesthesia of the hands, hyperkeratosis, vesiculation, and ulcerating lesions over pressure areas of the body.

Mithramycin is extremely toxic to the gastrointestinal tract and the bone marrow. A fatal hemorrhagic diathesis occurs in 1% to 5% and is related to impaired clotting factor synthesis, thrombocytopenia, and increased fibrinolysis. It can also cause reversible hypocalcemia, hypokalemia, and hypophosphatemia.

Mitomycin C causes DNA alkylation. The principal toxicity is myelosuppression. Interstitial pneumonitis leading to fibrosis may occur. Glomerular damage causing renal failure has been noted.

E.   Nitrosoureas

The nitrosoureas are effective as cancer chemotherapeutic agents by virtue of their alkylation and carboxylation of nucleic acids. Pulmonary toxicity can occur and has a presentation similar to that of bleomycin toxicity. Risk factors include age, prior lung disease, and total dose greater than 1500 mg/m². Myelosuppression also occurs and is associated with a late thrombocytopenia that may begin after the leukopenia has abated. Renal or hepatic toxicity occurs in almost 67% of patients treated with streptozocin but is usually reversible. Streptozocin is also associated with hyperglycemia because of its selective destruction of pancreatic beta cells, causing hypoinsulinism.

F. Enzymes

L-Asparaginase acts by destroying extracellular supplies of L-asparagine, causing death of tumor cells that lack the ability to synthesize this amino acid. The drug is associated with hepatotoxicity in 50% and usually causes marked elevation of blood ammonia. Mild myelosuppression and a coagulopathy may also be noted. Hemorrhagic pancreatitis occurs in 5% and may be associated with impaired insulin secretion. L-Asparaginase is also associated with an altered mental status, including depression, lethargy, somnolence, or coma.

G. Miscellaneous Agents

Cisplatin acts by forming platinum complexes that react with DNA to form intrastrand and interstrand cross-links. Myelosuppression and nephrotoxicity are the dose-limiting side effects. Nephrotoxicity is usually reversible when acute, but chronic use can lead to renal failure secondary to tubular necrosis. Hypomagnesemia and hypocalcemia are frequent and can persist long after the drug has been stopped. Neurotoxicity also occurs, manifested as seizures, loss of tasting sense, tinnitus and high-frequency hearing loss, and a stocking–glove peripheral neuropathy.

H. Radiation Therapy

Radiation therapy is effective against cancer by interacting with tissue to produce free radicals, which cause damage to DNA and, ultimately, cell death.

    1. Several forms of radiation therapy are available.

        a. External-beam irradiation involves projecting the radiation source at the desired site and varying the voltage to adjust the depth of penetration.

        b. Internal irradiation may be in the form of

brachytherapy or systemically administered ^{131}I or ^{32}P. Brachytherapy involves the placement of the radioactive source within a body cavity or tissue. Because the peripheral margins of the tumor may be inadequately irradiated, brachytherapy is often combined with external-beam therapy.

2.   Factors associated with an increased incidence of adverse effects from radiotherapy include increased age, large radiation fields, simultaneous administration of radiation-potentiating chemotherapy, and a compromised vascular supply.

    a.   Acute side effects occur within a few weeks and are the result of injury to rapidly proliferating cells. Examples are alopecia, nausea, vomiting, and diarrhea (Table 9-3).

    b.   Subacute side effects occur 2 to 6 months after therapy and are the result of injury to slowly recovering tissues. Examples are radiation pneumonitis and pericarditis. Late complications of fibrosis, fistulas, edema, necrosis, and secondary neoplasms appear months to years after therapy and are the result of damage to vascular and connective tissues.

3.   Wound healing may be compromised if surgery takes place in the radiation field. In addition, hormonal dysfunction may occur if the radiation ports include endocrine glands.

V.   PERIANESTHETIC MANAGEMENT

A.   Planning the optimal anesthetic for the patient with cancer first requires a thorough history.

1.   The type of cancer and its extent should be identified.

2.   The modality of cancer treatment (surgery, radiation, chemotherapy) should be known. Specifics should be sought regarding these therapies; for example, which chemotherapeutic agents were used, their cumulative doses, when the last dose was given, and the results. Questions should be directed toward identifying symptoms related to adverse effects from therapies.

3.   Signs and symptoms of those paraneoplastic syndromes commonly associated with the primary cancer should not be overlooked.

Text continues on p. 502

Table 9–3. Adverse Effects of Cancer Radiotherapy*

Site	Acute or subacute reactions (rad)[†]	Subacute or late reactions (rad)
Systemic (typically radiation to brain or abdomen)	Fatigue, anorexia: A Decreased libido: A	Fibrosis: L Sarcomas—all tissues: L
Skin	Dry desquamation: A (5000) Moist desquamation: A (6000) Hair loss: A (2000)	Atrophy, telangiectasia, fragility, induration, ulcer: L (5500) Skin cancer: L
Head and neck		
Eyes	—	Xerophthalmia: S, L (3000) Iridocyclitis: S, L (5000) Cataract: L (1000) Decreased visual acuity, blindness: L (5000)
Ears, tongue	Otitis media: A (3000) Loss of taste: A, S (3000)	Deafness: L (<6000) Meniere's syndrome: L (6000)
Mouth, salivary glands	Decreased saliva: A, S (2000) Acute painful sialitis: A (1000) Painful mucositis: A (4000)	Xerostomia, permanent: L (6000) Mucosal ulcer, severe fibrosis: L (6000)
Jaw	—	Osteonecrosis: S, L (6000)
Larynx	—	Persistent edema, cartilage necrosis: S, L (6500)
Cardiopulmonary		
Lung	Pneumonitis: S (2000)	Pulmonary fibrosis: L (3000)
Heart	Pancarditis, Pericarditis: S (4000)	Pericardial stricture or effusion, myocardiopathy: L (5000)
Aorta, arteries	—	Atherosclerosis: L

(continued)

Table 9–3. Adverse Effects of Cancer Radiotherapy* (continued)

Site	Acute or subacute reactions (rad)†	Subacute or late reactions (rad)
Gastrointestinal		

Alimentary canal	Nausea, vomiting: A
	Diarrhea: A (2000)
	Esophagitis: A (3000)
	Proctitis with tenesmus: A (4000)
	Proctitis with bleeding: A (5000)
		—
		Strictures, ulcers, perforation, fistulas of
		  Stomach or bowel: L (4500)
		  Esophagus or rectum: L (5500)
		Chronic proctitis: L (6000)

Liver	Hepatitis: S (2500)	Liver failure, ascites: L (3500) Biliary tract stricture: L
Pancreas	—	Exocrine insufficiency: L
Genitourinary		
Kidneys	Nephritis: S (2000)	Chronic nephritis, nephrosclerosis: L (<2000) Hypertension: S, L (2000)
Ureters	—	Stricture with obstruction: L (7500)
Bladder	Cystitis: A (4000)	Chronic cystitis; ulcer, contracture: L (6500)
Prostate	—	Impotence: S, L (6000)
Vagina	—	Ulcer, fistula: L (9000)
Uterus	—	Necrosis, perforation: L (>10,000)
Endocrine		
Pituitary	—	Hypopituitarism: L (4500)
Thyroid	—	Hypothyroidism: L (4500)
Adrenal	—	Hypoadrenalism: L (<6000)
Testes, ovaries	Sterility, temporary amenorrhea: A, S (300)	Sterility, permanent amenorrhea: L (1500)

Central Nervous

Brain	Cerebritis, somnolence syndrome: S	Brain necrosis: L (5500)
Spinal cord	Lhermitte's syndrome: S (4500)	Transverse myelitis: L (5000)

Other

Lymphatics	—	Lymphedema: L (5000)
Breast	—	Atrophy, induration: L (5000)
Muscle	—	Atrophy: L (>10,000)
Bone, cartilage	—	Necrosis, fracture: L (6000)
Bone marrow	Leukopenia, thrombocytopenia: A	Marrow hypoplasia: L (2000)
	Immunodeficiency: A, S	Leukemia: L
Fetus	Death: A, S (200–450)	

* Acute (A) reactions occur within a few weeks, subacute (S) ones 2 to 6 months after radiotherapy, late (L) ones several months to years after radiotherapy.

† The threshold (or tolerance) doses listed here (in rad) are the minimal doses that will result in a significant complication within normal tissue in 1% to 3% of patients within a 5-year period after treatment (TD3/5).

(Modified with permission from Rubin P, Poulter C. Principles of radiation oncology and cancer radiotherapy. In Rubin P, ed. Clinical oncology for medical students and physicians. 5th ed. New York: American Cancer Society, 1978.)

501

B. Physical examination should include a review of the patient's vital signs. Fever may indicate an opportunistic infection. Tachypnea may reveal underlying pulmonary disease. Examination of the skin and mucosal membranes may reveal petechiae or hemorrhage, indicating thrombocytopenia or coagulopathy. A musculoskeletal examination should attempt to identify any deformities. Cervical immobility or instability may be sufficient to make airway management difficult. Likewise, lumbosacral disease may preclude the use of spinal anesthetics. Cardiac examination should attempt to identify the presence of dysrhythmias or CHF. Hepatomegaly may indicate impaired hepatic metabolism. A neurologic examination should document any alterations in mental status and the presence of peripheral or autonomic neuropathies.

C. Laboratory tests should be directed by the findings of the history and physical examination. These tests often include a complete blood count, platelet count, coagulation profile, serum electrolytes, BUN, creatinine, glucose, liver function tests, chest radiograph, ECG, and urinalysis. Serum calcium, magnesium, albumin, and uric acid levels may be specifically indicated. Pulmonary function tests and arterial blood gases should be included, especially if bleomycin or other chemotherapeutic agents with potential pulmonary toxicity have been used. A MUGA scan or echocardiography to quantitate cardiac function should be obtained if doxorubicin has been used or if cardiomyopathy is suspected.

D. Specific Anesthetic Considerations

    1. Preoperative concerns

        a. Most patients with neoplastic disease should be considered immunocompromised and possibly infected with opportunistic organisms. For patient and physician safety, all procedures should be conducted with strict aseptic technique.

        b. Malnutrition and dehydration is not uncommon in patients with cancer. Preinduction hydration should be considered in patients who have had very poor oral intake, especially if they are febrile.

        c. Patients who have recently undergone chemotherapy or radiation therapy may have mark-

edly depressed leukocyte counts. Elective surgery should be postponed until the count
begins to normalize.

    d. Anemia or polycythemia is a potential prob-
lem in many cancer patients. Anemic patients
should receive transfusions to an Hct of 30%
prior to any major surgery. Patients who have
an Hct exceeding 55% have an increased incidence of bleeding and thrombosis and should
undergo phlebotomy to an Hct below 50%
prior to surgery.

2. Premedication

    a. Oral medications may not be well tolerated or
absorbed because of gastroparesis from the
primary disease or nausea and vomiting from
chemotherapy or radiation therapy.

    b. Many patients will be malnourished and debil-
itated. These patients will usually need less
medication.

    c. Cancer patients with chronic pain are often
treated with large amounts of opiates or sedatives. Much higher doses of opiates or sedatives
may therefore be needed for premedication,
induction, or maintenance of anesthesia.

    d. Steroids are often incorporated into chemo-
therapeutic regimens, so stress coverage
should be used. Usually, 150 mg of hydrocortisone or a steroid equivalent given in several
doses over a 24-hour period will provide adequate supplemental coverage.

3. Induction

    a. Rapid-sequence induction should be consid-
ered for all patients with nausea and vomiting
or ileus from the primary malignancy or its
treatment.

    b. Use of muscle relaxants should be monitored
with a nerve stimulator, especially in certain
situations.

        1) Alkylating agents (thiotepa, mechlor-
ethamine, cyclophosphamide) can irreversibly inhibit plasma cholinesterase
and prolong the response to succinylcholine.

        2) Patients with small cell bronchogenic

carcinoma or gastrointestinal adenocarcinoma may develop myasthenic syndrome.

3) Patients with kidney or hepatic disease, whether from therapy or malignancy, can have delayed excretion of muscle relaxants such as d-tubocurarine and pancuronium.

c. Preoxygenation may be used for most patients. Oxygen supplementation is not recommended for patients who have had bleomycin unless hypoxemia is present on room air, in which case, pulse oximetry should be used to guide supplementation.

d. Special attention should be paid to coagulation status if nasal intubation or a regional technique is being considered, as many neoplastic disease states and their treatments are associated with thrombocytopenia and coagulopathy.

4. Regional anesthesia
Spinal and epidural anesthesia should be avoided in patients with primary or metastatic disease to the spine or with a coagulopathy. Patients with brain metastases must be carefully evaluated for increased intracranial pressure if a spinal anesthetic is being considered. The presence of peripheral neuropathy or focal neurologic deficit is not a contraindication to regional anesthesia. However, peripheral nerve deficits should be documented thoroughly prior to any regional anesthetic technique.

5. Maintenance anesthesia
a. Careful titration of inhaled anesthetic agents is necessary. Pericardial effusions from metastases or radiation will compromise cardiac output. Congestive heart failure is frequently associated with doxorubicin, especially doses in excess of 550 mg/m^2.

b. Titration of intravenous anesthetics is also necessary. The debilitated cancer patient will have decreased serum protein, leading to increased free drug and an altered volume of distribution. This usually means an initially increased potency and longer elimination half-life. Renal and hepatic dysfunction also complicate the use of intravenous agents.

   c.   Abnormalities in glucose, potassium, calcium, and magnesium associated with some paraneoplastic syndromes should be normalized preoperatively. Glucose and potassium may have to be checked intraoperatively in patients whose levels were difficult to control preoperatively.

   d.   Patients who have had bleomycin chemotherapy should not receive an FIo_2 greater than 0.25, as greater concentrations increase the risk of pulmonary pneumonitis and ARDS.

  6. Emergence

   a.   Resolution of muscle relaxant effect should be established prior to extubation, especially in patients with myasthenic syndrome or other paraneoplastic syndromes that affect neuromuscular function.

   b.   Avoiding N_2O or administering intravenous droperidol on emergence can help reduce postoperative nausea and vomiting. Intraoperative placement of a gastric tube may decrease gastric distention to help reduce postoperative nausea and vomiting.

   c.   Patients who had ileus or were nauseated preoperatively should not be extubated until they are in full control of their airways.

VI. POSTOPERATIVE CARE

  A. Invasive lines should be removed as soon as possible because of the immunocompromised state of most patients with neoplastic disease.

  B. Postoperative analgesia may be best accomplished with a patient-controlled analgesia device in those who have been on opiates preoperatively, as these patients often require larger doses than are prescribed routinely. This same population of patients usually requires a larger dose of epidural opiate.

  C. Any prophylactic measures initiated preoperatively to prevent DVT are continued, especially for those patients who are immobilized postoperatively.

VII. SUMMARY OF ANESTHETIC CONSIDERATIONS

Patients with active malignancies are usually malnourished and immunosuppressed. Their clinical course is often complicated by paraneoplastic problems such as Cushing's syndrome, hypoglycemia, metabolic acidosis, SIADH, electrolyte imbalance, anemia, coagulopathy, neuromuscular abnormalities, pericardial effusion, obstructive uropathy, superior vena caval obstruction, brain metastases, and spinal cord compression. Further complicating patient management is chemotherapy and radiation therapy, both of which are potentially toxic to the bone marrow, heart, lungs, liver, and kidneys. Abnormalities in fluid and electrolyte balance and in metabolic, endocrine, and immunologic function are also found. These problems must be addressed before surgery.

Generally, patients with malignancies will benefit from hydration and nutrition. All procedures should be carried out in aseptic fashion. Preoperative medication will need to be reduced in the very malnourished patient or increased in patients who are receiving large amounts of analgesics or sedatives.

Regional anesthesia should be avoided in patients with brain metastases, possible increased intracranial pressure, spinal metastases, and coagulopathy. Inhaled anesthetics can be used safely, but the potential for myocardial depression in patients treated with doxorubicin and for pulmonary failure in those given bleomycin should be kept in mind. Intravenous anesthetics need to be carefully titrated because the decreased serum protein allows more free drug to be available, causing an increase in immediate potency. The action of muscle relaxants can be prolonged in patients who have paraneoplastic syndromes that affect the neuromuscular junction. The use of a nerve stimulator will help with the dosage of muscle relaxants. Postoperatively, most patients will have the same problems as before surgery, and all precautions and treatment used preoperatively should be carried out postoperatively.

Recommended Reading

Batist G, Andrews JL. Pulmonary toxicity of antineoplastic drugs. JAMA 1981;246:1449.

Beutler B, Cerami A. Cachectin: more than a tumor necrosis factor. N Engl J Med 1987;316:379.

Calabresi P, Parks RE Jr. Antiproliferative agents and drugs used for immunosuppression. In: Gilman AG, Goodman LS, Rall TW, Murad F, eds. The pharmacological basis of therapeutics. 7th ed. New York: Macmillan, 1985:1247.

Calabresi P, Parks RE Jr. Chemotherapy of neoplastic diseases. In: Gilman AG, Goodman LS, Rall TW, Murad F, eds. The pharmacological basis of therapeutics. 7th ed. New York: Macmillan, 1985:1240.

Chung F. Cancer, chemotherapy and anesthesia. Can Anaesth Soc J 1982;29:364.

Dillman JB. Safe use of succinylcholine during repeated anesthetics in a patent treated with cyclophosphamide. Anesth Analg 1987; 66:351.

Goldiner PL, Rooney SM. In defense of restricting oxygen in bleomycin-treated surgical patients. Anesthesiology 1984; 61:225.

Goldiner PL, Schweizer O. The hazards of anesthesia and surgery in bleomycin-treated patients. Semin Oncol 1979;6:121.

Kaplan BS, Klassen J, Gault MH. Glomerular injury in patients with neoplasia. Annu Rev Med 1976;27:117.

Kopec IC, Groeger JS. Life-threatening fluid and electrolyte abnormalities associated with cancer. Crit Care Clin 1988;4:81.

LaMantia KR, Glick JH, Marshall BE. In reply [letter]. Anesthesiology 1984;61:225.

Lewis KP. Anesthetic implications in the patient receiving cancer chemotherapy I. Anesth Rev 1988;15(2):35.

Lewis KP. Anesthetic implications in the patient receiving cancer chemotherapy II. Anesth Rev 1988;15(3):45.

McCammon RL. Cancer. In: Stoelting RK, Dierdorf SF, eds. Anesthesia and co-existing disease. New York: Churchill Livingstone, 1983:631.

McClay EF, Bellet RE. Preoperative evaluation of the oncology patient. Med Clin North Am 1987;71:529.

Mundy GR. Ectopic hormonal syndromes in neoplastic disease. Hosp Pract 1987;April:179.

Selvin BL. Cancer chemotherapy: implications for the anesthesiologist. Anesth Analg 1981;60:425.

Wise RP. A myasthenic syndrome complicating bronchial carcinoma. Anaesthesia 1962;17:488.

Young RC, Ozols RF, Myers CE. The anthracycline antineoplastic drugs. N Engl J Med 1981;305:139.

CHAPTER 10

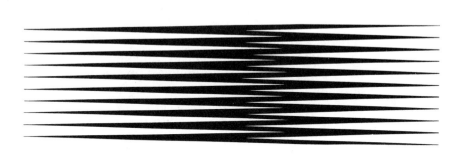

Infection

Brian J. McGrath

Pneumonia

I. COMPLICATIONS AND RISK FACTORS

   A. Immunosuppression

      Immunocompromised states are present in patients with malignancies or AIDS and in those receiving cancer chemotherapy or other immunosuppressive treatments.

   B. Chronic Obstructive Lung Disease

      Patients with chronic obstructive lung disease frequently suffer postoperative pulmonary complications. Atelectasis, retained secretions, impaired mucociliary clearance, and reduced cough are common postoperatively.

   C. Mechanical Ventilation

      Patients already on mechanical ventilation have altered bacterial flora, reduced mucociliary clearance, and bypass of the normal glottic defense mechanisms.

   D. Mechanical Obstruction

      Processes obstructing the airways, such as tumor, foreign body, or tenacious secretions, predispose to infection distal to the obstruction.

   E. Altered Neurologic Function

      Patients having reduced ability to protect the airway (e.g., drug overdose, alcoholics, stroke victims) are at increased risk for aspiration.

   F. Sepsis

      Bacteremia can lead to seeding of the lung with organisms.

   G. Smoking

      Cigarette smoking causes increased carboxyhemoglobin levels, leftward shift of the oxyhemoglobin disassociation curve, copious secretions, and reduced mucociliary clearance.

II. PREOPERATIVE EVALUATION

   A. History

      1. Patients with pneumonia usually present with productive cough, fever, chills, hemoptysis, dyspnea, or mental status changes. Elderly, debilitated, or neutropenic patients may have minimal clinical manifestation of pulmonary infection.

      2. Evidence of prior lung disease should be sought, because the effects of acute infection will be compounded by further alterations in the work of breathing, secretion clearance, and gas exchange.

      3. Patients with significant heart disease tolerate poorly the hypoxemia and increased work of breathing secondary to pneumonia or sepsis.

B. Physical Examination

    1. Tachypnea, rales, rhonchi, bronchial breath sounds, and wheezing may be present.

    2. Hypovolemia secondary to infection or poor fluid intake should be sought and corrected prior to surgery.

C. Laboratory Assessment

    1. Gram stain and cultures with sensitivity studies should be checked to see if patients are receiving proper antibiotics.

    2. An elevated leukocyte count with an increase of immature polymorphonuclear cells indicates active infection.

    3. Chest radiography

    Lobar, segmental, or a more diffuse interstitial pattern may be present. Hypovolemic patients may have minimal infiltrate until they are rehydrated. In some patients, the chest radiograph provides the only evidence of pneumonia.

    4. Arterial blood gas measurement

    There is often hypoxemia and concomitant respiratory alkalosis. Hypercarbia may imply severe acute lung impairment or prior lung disease. Concomitant metabolic acidosis signifies poor tissue oxygenation.

    5. Pulmonary function tests

    Spirometry is of little value in acute lung disease. However, evidence of chronic lung disease from previous tests can be helpful in predicting difficulty in weaning the patient from mechanical ventilation.

    6. Electrocardiogram

    Dysrhythmias and myocardial ischemia can occur in the setting of hypoxemia, hypercarbia, or acidosis. Chronic cor pulmonale from emphysema will typically produce right-axis deviation, right ventricular hypertrophy, prominent P waves in II, III, and aVF (P-pulmonale pattern), and low-voltage QRS complexes, especially over the left precordium.

III. ANESTHETIC CONSIDERATIONS

A. Preoperative Preparation

    1. Appropriate antibiotics should be instituted prior to surgery, guided by Gram stain and culture.

    2. Mobilization of secretions via suctioning, chest physiotherapy, and incentive spirometry will improve lung mechanics and ventilation-perfusion ($\dot{V}/\dot{Q}$) matching.

   3. Any bronchospasm should be controlled with bronchodilators.

B. Anesthetic Choice

   1. A patient needing general anesthesia who has pneumonia and a tenuous hemodynamic state is best managed by carefully titrated doses of benzodiazepines, opiates, and muscle relaxants during induction and maintenance.

   2. Intravenous agents will allow the use of high concentrations of oxygen intraoperatively and a smooth transition to the ICU.

   3. Because of the adverse effects of general anesthesia on pulmonary function, regional anesthesia should be used whenever possible. Experience with spinal and epidural anesthetics and analgesics supports their utility in reducing postoperative pulmonary dysfunction.

C. Induction Agents

An induction agent is chosen on the basis of cardiovascular status as well as the potential for bronchospasm.

   1. Sodium thiopental

   Although controversial for patients with bronchospasm, a thiopental induction in a hemodynamically stable patient is still favored by many. Hypovolemic patients or patients with multisystem organ failure may not tolerate sodium thiopental because of its tendency to produce hemodynamic depression. If sodium thiopental is titrated slowly, minimal hemodynamic depression will occur, even in these patients.

   2. Ketamine

   Ketamine may be useful because it produces rapid anesthesia combined with bronchodilation and hemodynamic stability. It has a direct myocardial depressant effect, however, and may cause hypotension with larger doses.

   3. Opiates

   The absence of adverse hemodynamic effects of narcotics must be weighed against their tendency to prolong respiratory depression.

   4. Etomidate

   Caution should be used when considering etomidate

in a patient with adrenal insufficiency, as the drug has been associated with adrenal suppression. Even a single dose may cause adrenal suppression for as long as 24 hours.

D. Effects of Inhaled Anesthesia

    1. Functional residual capacity (FRC)

General anesthesia leads to a fall in FRC, causing reduced compliance and increased $\dot{V}/\dot{Q}$ inequality. High inspired oxygen concentrations and PEEP may be necessary to maintain an adequate Ca_{O_2}. PEEP will help restore FRC by alveolar recruitment. This will improve compliance, decrease the work of breathing, and decrease $\dot{V}/\dot{Q}$ inequalities (Figure 10-1). An acceptable Ca_{O_2} for most patients will be achieved with a hemoglobin arterial saturation exceeding 90% or an arterial pO_2 above 60 mmHg.

    2. Ventilation

Halothane, enflurane, and isoflurane reduce the normal ventilatory responses to hypercarbia and hypoxemia. Residual anesthetic gas can reduce respiratory drive after a long procedure, which may

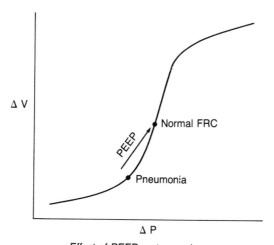

Effect of PEEP on transpulmonary
pressure gradient and lung compliance

Figure 10-1 Normalizing functional residual capacity with PEEP will improve lung compliance, reducing the work needed to move a given lung volume.

impair weaning from mechanical ventilation. For intubated patients who require high inflation pressures to deliver adequate volumes and large minute ventilation, the usual anesthesia machine ventilator often is inadequate: a ventilator similar to that used in the ICU may be required.

3. Hypoxic pulmonary vasoconstriction
Inhalation anesthetics interfere with the normal pulmonary vasoconstrictive response to alveolar hypoxia. Patients with pneumonia thus may develop worsening hypoxemia during anesthesia.

4. Respiratory work
The ventilatory response to increased mechanical loading from pneumonia is impaired by certain inhalational anesthetics. Therefore, mechanical ventilation may be preferable to spontaneous ventilation during general anesthesia.

5. Mucociliary function
General anesthesia interferes with mucociliary clearance (an important respiratory defense mechanism) via direct anesthetic action, dry inspired gas delivery, high F_{IO_2} and the presence of an endotracheal tube. If the underlying lung pathology is not known, suctioning the trachea after intubation and sending sputum for appropriate tests would be helpful. Meticulous attention to secretion clearance with frequent suctioning should be maintained throughout the case to prevent plugging of small airways.

IV. POSTOPERATIVE CARE

A. A major issue is deciding when to remove the patient from mechanical ventilation. Prior pulmonary impairment often precludes early weaning and extubation. The questions to be answered are: "Is the patient able to perform the work of breathing?" "Can the patient oxygenate adequately?" and "Is the patient able to protect the airway?" Residual anesthesia or muscle relaxation, hypothermia, hemodynamic instability, or inadequate analgesia are of immediate concern postoperatively.

B. In patients with marginal pulmonary function, it usually is best to maintain intubation and mechanical ventilation. General guidelines for the ability to wean from mechanical ventilation are:

    1. Vital capacity greater than 15 ml/kg
    2. Alveolar–arterial O_2 gradient below 350 mmHg
    3. PaO_2 exceeding 60 mmHg with FI_{O_2} below 0.50
    4. Negative inspiratory force greater than -25 cmH$_2$O
    5. Respiratory rate below 30/minute.

  C. Postoperative Pulmonary Function
After thoracic and upper abdominal incisions, pain, chest-wall splinting, and diaphragmatic dysfunction lead to atelectasis and reductions in lung volume. This problem reaches a peak 48 to 72 hours after surgery and may persist for a week.

V. SUMMARY OF ANESTHETIC CONSIDERATIONS
Pneumonia will increase ventilation–perfusion mismatching and shunt. Preoperative treatment with appropriate antibiotics and vigorous pulmonary maneuvers to clear secretions will help with perioperative oxygenation and decrease postoperative pulmonary morbidity.

Whenever possible, regional anesthesia should be used, as inhaled anesthetics will worsen $\dot{V}/\dot{Q}$ matching, decrease normal ventilatory responses to hypercarbia and hypoxemia, and inhibit mucociliary function and hypoxic pulmonary vasoconstriction. After a general anesthetic, prior to extubation, the patient must have good recovery of respiratory muscle strength. The patient must be able to clear secretions as well as cope with the increased minute ventilation required during an active pulmonary infection for oxygenation and CO_2 elimination.

Septic Shock

I. CLINICAL CHARACTERISTICS
  A. Gram-negative bacteremia is the most common cause of septic shock. However, almost all microorganisms, including gram-positive bacteria, fungi, and rickettsiae, can produce the same clinical picture.
  B. Sepsis has become an increasingly common cause of death among the critically ill. Aggregate mortality rates in septic shock are 40% to 60%, with rates exceeding 90% in some high-risk groups. Survival rates are better in patients having a surgically treatable focus of infection. Therefore, when the probability of surgical control of

sepsis is high, it is best to proceed with the operation rather than wait for long periods to achieve greater hemodynamic stability.

II.   PATHOPHYSIOLOGY

A.   Once infection is established, the organism produces widespread effects via direct actions of the microbe and its toxins on the body's immune system. Immunologic interactions lead to production of various humoral mediators, which are thought to cause most of the physiologic derangement in sepsis. The implicated mediators include complement components, prostaglandins, leukotrienes, chemotactic factors, oxygen free radicals, tumor necrosis factor (cachectin), platelet-activating factor, histamine, and endorphins.

B.   The concept of a progression from a hyperdynamic state to a hypodynamic one is based on old data. In the era of vigorous volume resuscitation and inotropic support, there is little evidence to support the concept of a progression of phases. Hyperdynamic septic patients often die in a hyperdynamic state. It is true that a small subgroup of septic patients exhibit a hypodynamic circulation; these tend to be the patients with underlying cardiac disease.

III.   PREOPERATIVE ASSESSMENT

The wide-ranging physiologic effects of septic shock mandate careful preoperative evaluation. In assessing such patients, a systematic approach to each organ system will avoid overlooking significant problems.

A.   Cardiovascular

1.   Existing function

The presence of coronary artery disease, abnormal ventricular function and dysrhythmias should be sought. Cardiac disease indicates a limited physiologic reserve and less ability to tolerate hemodynamic stress.

2.   Cardiac output

Cardiac output is abnormally increased in most patients secondary to a low systemic resistance. Despite elevated output, there often is substantial depression of contractility such that the heart may be unable to meet the circulatory demands of further vasodilatation caused by anesthetic agents. A low cardiac output state implies pre-existing cardiac disease or inadequate volume resuscitation. Low cardiac output does not necessarily imply a progression to end-stage sepsis, but it is a poor prognostic factor.

3. Vasodilatation

Inappropriate vasodilatation occurs in the muscle and other peripheral tissues, often compromising flow to critical organ systems.

4. Hypovolemia

Vasodilatation, fever, and diffuse capillary leakage lead to reductions in intravascular volume.

5. Defective oxygen consumption

There is inefficient utilization of oxygen as well as abnormal dependence on increased oxygen delivery. Mixed venous oxygen saturation is often normal or elevated despite the presence of tissue ischemia and lactic acidosis.

B. Respiratory

1. Adult respiratory distress syndrome (ARDS)

Sepsis is the most common cause of the ARDS. Pulmonary capillary leakage results in noncardiogenic pulmonary edema, reduced pulmonary compliance, and hypoxemia.

2. Pneumonia

Pulmonary infection may be the primary source of sepsis. Pneumonias will increase $\dot{V}/\dot{Q}$ mismatching, decrease pulmonary compliance, and increase the risk of hypoxemia.

C. Hematologic

Coagulation abnormalities occur, the most common being an isolated thrombocytopenia. Clotting factor deficiencies also are possible. Disseminated intravascular coagulation (DIC) occurs in a minority of patients. The overall effect is to increase the risk of bleeding, especially from the gastrointestinal tract. Usually, DIC will resolve with treatment of underlying disorder. Treatment with heparin or epsilon-aminocaproic acid is seldom effective.

D. Renal

Hypotension, hypovolemia, DIC, endotoxemia, and the use of nephrotoxic drugs contribute to the development of acute renal failure. Acute renal failure is associated with a poor prognosis.

E. Hepatic

Sepsis may result in hepatocellular injury and cholestasis. A frequent problem in these patients is acalculus cholecystitis.

IV. PHARMACOLOGIC THERAPY

A. Vasoactive Drugs

Sympathomimetic drugs are often needed in the septic patient to maintain adequate tissue perfusion pressure. These adrenergic agents may produce arrhythmias, elevations in myocardial oxygen consumption, and diffuse vasoconstriction. Drugs such as pancuronium or halothane, when used in conjunction with sympathomimetics, can increase the risk of arrhythmias. Any anesthetic drugs require careful titration because of their tendency to reduce sympathetic tone and myocardial contractility.

B. Antibiotics

Renal and hepatic damage and alterations in hematologic function can occur with many antibiotics. Aminoglycosides, polymyxin, and clindamycin can interfere with neuromuscular function and prolong paralysis with the use of neuromuscular blockers.

C. Corticosteroids

Previously, high-dose steroids were used in the treatment of septic shock, but their use has been shown in multicenter studies not to be beneficial. Recommendations would be to avoid their use unless adrenal suppression is highly suspected or documented. If steroids are used, serum glucose levels should be closely monitored, because hyperglycemia is a common complication.

D. Naloxone

Although high-dose naloxone has been advocated for the treatment of septic shock, recent human data do not support its utility. Potential adverse effects include hypertension, dysrhythmias, pulmonary edema, and myocardial ischemia.

V. PREOPERATIVE DIAGNOSTIC TESTS

A. ECG

An electrocardiogram may detect myocardial ischemia, conduction defects, or dysrhythmias.

B. Chest Radiograph

Chest radiography is indicated to document baseline pulmonary status and to search for problems that can be reversed preoperatively. Common pulmonary complications include aspiration, pneumothorax, pulmonary edema, pneumonia, and ARDS.

C. Hematology

A complete blood count and coagulation studies are needed because of the potential for coagulopathy, bleeding, and anemia.

D. Blood Chemistry

Electrolytes, creatinine, and BUN will be helpful in evaluating the extent of renal dysfunction. Plasma phosphorus, magnesium, and ionized calcium should also be checked, because these ions are frequently decreased in the septic state. Electrolyte correction should be accomplished preoperatively to optimize myocardial, pulmonary, and neuromuscular function.

E. Liver Function

Hepatic dysfunction is assessed by liver enzymes and prothrombin time. Drug doses may have to be adjusted if there is hepatic dysfunction. Vitamin K or fresh frozen plasma should be considered if there is evidence of coagulopathy.

F. Arterial Blood Gases

Metabolic acidosis is frequent in sepsis. Correction guided by blood gas measurements should be done expeditiously. Respiratory alkalosis is also seen and may complicate electrolyte balance.

VI. ANESTHETIC MANAGEMENT

A. Premedication

Because septic patients are often obtunded and hemodynamically unstable, premedication usually is not warranted.

B. Transport

Adequate hemodynamic monitoring and ventilation must be assured. The transport of the patient with multisystem organ failure over even short distances may be very difficult because of the numerous automatic infusion devices and the need for the maintenance of extraordinary ventilatory support. A reasonable checklist should include the four Ps:

1. Precordial (or esophageal) stethoscope

2. Proper transport monitors (pulse oximeter, portable ECG and pressure monitor)

3. Pressurized breathing device or PEEP Ambu bag with supplemental oxygen

4. Pairs of hands to help with IV lines and monitors.

C. Intraoperative Monitoring

1. In addition to routine noninvasive monitoring

(ECG, blood pressure, temperature, pulse oximetry), invasive techniques are usually helpful. Whenever possible, monitoring lines should be placed before induction to obtain baseline hemodynamic measurements.

2. Arterial catheter placement
Rapid changes in blood pressure make beat-to-beat monitoring important. Frequent arterial blood gas analysis is expedited by an arterial catheter.

3. Pulmonary artery catheter
It is rare for physical and laboratory evaluations to define hemodynamic abnormalities clearly in the anesthetized septic patient. Central venous pressure measurement is frequently an unreliable indicator of left ventricular preload. Therefore, a pulmonary artery catheter is often the best indicator of intravascular volume. In addition, an estimation of cardiac performance may be obtained by thermodilution cardiac output measurement.

D. Regional Technique
Regional anesthesia is appropriate for peripheral procedures; however, there is a high risk of complications in patients with coagulopathy or infection at the needle site. Sympathectomy produced by a spinal or epidural anesthetic may produce unacceptable hypotension. Regional techniques should be avoided in patients with recently documented bacteremia.

E. Induction Agents
Induction is hazardous because of the existing vasodilation, hypovolemia, and myocardial depression. Appropriate monitoring and fluid resuscitation prior to induction provides a smoother hemodynamic course. The following are the potential problems and advantages of commonly used induction agents.

1. Thiopental
Myocardial depressant and vasodilating properties limit its usefulness.

2. Ketamine
The central catecholamine-releasing properties of this drug are desirable, but when catecholamine reserves are limited, the direct myocardial depressant effects may predominate.

3. Etomidate
This is a useful agent in maintaining hemodynamic

stability. Because of its corticosteroid-inhibiting properties, etomidate should not be used unless the patient is already committed to steroid support.

4. Opiates

The synthetic opiates fentanyl, sufentanil, and alfentanil have minimal hemodynamic effects while providing analgesia when carefully titrated. Amnesia is not always assured.

5. Benzodiazepines

These are useful agents for amnesia and usually do not cause hemodynamic instability when used alone. When they are used with other anesthetic agents, hypotension may occur more frequently than if each agent was used alone.

F. Maintenance of General Anesthesia

1. Anesthetics

Inhalation agents should, in most cases, be avoided because of their myocardial depressant and vasodilating properties. Opioids such as fentanyl and sufentanil may offer the greatest hemodynamic stability.

2. Muscle relaxants

Relaxants should be chosen on the basis of hemodynamic effect and route of elimination. For example, *d*-tubocurarine should be avoided because of its histamine-releasing potential. Atracurium is useful in patients with hepatic and renal dysfunction. Histamine release is associated with rapid injection of atracurium and is minimized with slow infusion using doses less than 0.5 mg/kg. Vecuronium has the least effect on blood pressure and pulse rate compared with other nondepolarizing muscle relaxants and is rapidly metabolized by the liver.

VII. POTENTIAL INTRAOPERATIVE PROBLEMS

A. Respiration

1. Airway control should be established in patients with a tendency toward hypoventilation and respiratory acidosis. Hypoxemia will occur more quickly when acute lung injury is present. Many patients will be intubated before transport to the operating room. High inspired oxygen concentrations are required if there is severe pulmonary dysfunction. PEEP is helpful in improving oxygenation and lung mechanics.

2. Because of hypermetabolism with increased CO_2 production and increased dead space, controlled breathing with high minute ventilation may be needed. Operating room ventilators may not be able to provide the high minute ventilation, PEEP, and inspiratory pressure needed to ventilate patients with low compliance. Arterial blood gas analysis is needed to determine optimal support.

B. Hemodynamics

1. Hypotension should be treated according to the physiologic abnormalities present. Information derived from the pulmonary artery catheter is helpful in guiding therapy (Table 10-1).

2. Inadequate preload

    a. Hypovolemia is worsened by surgical bleeding and the increased capillary permeability of sepsis. Reductions in preload, as determined by pulmonary artery occlusion pressure (PAOP) measurement, should be corrected with fluid challenges to optimize cardiac output and mean arterial pressure (MAP).

    b. Given the myocardial depression associated with sepsis as well as the frequent use of PEEP, there will be reductions in left ventricular com-

Table 10–1. Treatment of Hypotension in Sepsis

Causes	Treatment
Decreased preload	Volume Maintain PAOP >15 mmHg
Decreased contractility	Inotropes Maintain cardiac output >10 L/min before using vasoconstrictors
Reduced heart rate	Atropine Isoproterenol Pacemaker Maintain rate above 60/min
Decreased SVR	Vasoconstrictors to be used after cardiac output and preload are optimized Use only enough vasoconstrictors to maintain minimal blood pressure needed for organ perfusion

pliance. A PAOP of at least 15 mmHg provides better assurance of an adequate preload.

3. Inadequate contractility

Inotropic drugs are required when there is significant myocardial depression and hypotension after intravascular volume has been optimized. There is no clear evidence to support the use of any particular agent. Pharmacologic effects will differ with dosage range (Table 10-2). These drugs should be titrated to maximize oxygen transport (cardiac output $\times$ Ca_{O_2}).

4. Low systemic vascular resistance

Even when cardiac output has been maximized

Table 10–2. Uses of Inotropes and Vasopressors

Drug	Dose per Kg per Min	Effect
Dopamine	0.5–3 µg	Dopaminergic receptor stimulation increases renal and splanchnic blood flow
	3–10 µg	β-Agonist stimulatory effect. At the higher range, α-receptor stimulation occurs
	>10 µg	α-Agonist stimulatory effect will predominate, which will increase vasoconstriction
Dobutamine	2–20 µg	β_1-Receptor stimulation will increase contractility. It may cause decrease in blood pressure because of β_2 effects at higher doses
Epinephrine	0.04–0.1 µg	β effects predominate
	≥0.15 µg	α effects predominate, which usually will increase blood pressure of peripheral vasoconstriction
Norepinephrine	0.005–0.03 µg	At low doses, both β_1 and α_1 effects will be seen
	>0.03 µg	At higher doses, main effects from α_1-receptor stimulation will predominate. This dose is usually used when all other drugs fail to increase SVR and blood pressure
Phenylephrine	20–200 µg/min	Generalized vasoconstriction from α_1-receptor stimulation

with volume therapy and inotropic drugs, perfusion pressure may be inadequate. A vasoconstrictor should then be used to elevate the blood pressure to the minimum necessary for organ function. The danger in using high doses of these agents is generalized vasoconstriction, especially in the kidney, gut, and digits, leading to ischemic damage.

C. Renal

1. Oliguria should trigger a search for reversible causes of renal dysfunction. Frequent intraoperative causes are renal hypoperfusion from reductions in cardiac output or intravascular volume or obstruction of urine outflow.

2. If oliguria persists after correction or exclusion of reversible causes, low-dose dopamine may be helpful in increasing urine output. Diuretics may also increase urine output; however, they may cause further volume depletion from a brisk diuresis, with subsequent worsening of renal perfusion. If the patient is at high risk for oliguria, preload must be optimized prior to anesthetic induction.

VIII. POSTOPERATIVE CARE

Postoperative management is a continuation of cardiovascular and respiratory resuscitation. Mechanical ventilation should be maintained for most patients until they clearly meet extubation criteria (see previous section). During transport, provisions must be made for continuous monitoring of hemodynamics and for ventilatory support.

IX. SUMMARY OF ANESTHETIC CONSIDERATIONS

Septic patients usually have multisystem organ failure. The decision whether to monitor these patients invasively is usually already made. Most will be intubated, on high levels of oxygen supplementation and PEEP, and receiving inotropic drugs and high infusion rates of fluids.

Preoperative sedation is usually not needed. During transport, it is critical to maintain PEEP and a constant infusion of vasoactive drugs, as even short interruptions can cause hypoxemia and hypotension that is difficult to treat. Regional techniques are rarely used because of the prevalence of coagulopathy and bacteremia. A balanced anesthetic technique is probably the best. High oxygen concentrations can be provided, and the vasodilation and cardiac depression of inhalational agents are avoided. The risk of intraoperative renal insult is high. Therefore, propylactic measures to preserve renal function, such as optimizing preload and dopamine infusion at "renal" levels, are recommended. Postoperative transfer entails the same problems encountered before surgery. Ensuring continuous high-level respiratory and cardiac support is essential.

Viral Hepatitis

I. ETIOLOGY
Acute inflammation of the liver (hepatitis) can result from infection, toxins, circulatory derangements, and metabolic abnormalities. Hepatitis A, B, and non-A, non-B are responsible for most acute cases of infectious hepatitis, the only type to be discussed.

II. TYPES OF VIRAL HEPATITIS
    A. Hepatitis A
    Hepatitis A is highly infectious. It is transmitted by the fecal–oral route and is often seen in endemic outbreaks originating with a single infected person in nursing homes, military camps, and other closed environments. There is a 2- to 3-week incubation period, with infectivity potentially lasting 3 weeks before and after the onset of symptoms. Jaundice is usually mild, and fulminant hepatic failure is rare. There is no progression to a carrier state or to chronic hepatitis. Acute infection is marked by an elevation in serum IgM. The later production of IgG can persist for years.

    B. Hepatitis B
        1. Infection with hepatitis B is transmitted primarily by the parenteral route but may also occur by contact with saliva, semen, vaginal secretions, and feces. High-risk groups include intravenous drug users, hemophiliac and hemodialysis patients, health care workers, and homosexual men with multiple partners. There is an incubation period of 4 to 24 weeks, with an average of 50 days. Approximately one quarter of those infected develop clinical hepatitis. Thus, most of those infected never realize that they have contracted the virus. One per cent of those with clinical hepatitis develop fulminant hepatic failure, and 5% become chronic carriers or develop chronic hepatitis. Hepatocellular carcinoma is 200-

fold more likely to occur in chronic carriers of the virus.

2. The immune response to the virus can be helpful in determining the course of hepatitis B infection. Hepatitis B surface antigen (HBsAg) appears 2 weeks to 2 months prior to the onset of symptoms and persists for about 6 weeks in most patients. The presence of HBsAg or HBeAg, an antigen derived from the core particle, implies infectivity. Antibody to the core antigen (Anti-HBc) appears around the time of clinical onset and can be present for years after the infection. Antibody to the surface antigen (Anti-HBs) appears during the convalescent phase in about 90% of patients. This means the patient is no longer infectious and has active immunity against reinfection. Persistence of HBsAg for more than 6 months in the absence of antibody implies a chronic carrier state, with the potential for infectivity and chronic liver disease. HBsAg is present in 10% to 20% of patients with chronic liver disease.

C. Non-A, Non-B Hepatitis

A third type of viral infection, termed non-A, non-B, has become the principal cause of transfusion-related hepatitis. Transmission occurs in a manner similar to hepatitis B, but there have been reports of outbreaks similar to those of type A. The incubation period is from 2 to 20 weeks, with an average of 8 weeks. Fulminant hepatic failure and chronic liver disease occur with about the same frequency as in hepatitis B. A promising test for diagnosing non-A, non-B hepatitis is measuring for anti-HCV. Currently, there is no commercial serologic test available for this disease.

III. CLINICAL COURSE

A. The clinical course is similar with all three types of infection.

1. There is a prodromal phase that may include nausea, vomiting, anorexia, malaise, arthralgia, and abdominal pain.

2. This is followed by the icteric phase characterized by bilirubinuria, jaundice, light-colored stools, scleral icterus, and an enlarged, tender liver. Various laboratory abnormalities coincide with the onset of symptoms. Elevations in serum transaminases (ALT [SGPT] more than AST [SGOT]), alkaline phospha-

tase, bilirubin, and serum globulins routinely occur. In more severe cases, prothrombin time is prolonged, and hypoglycemia may become a problem.

3. The convalescent phase brings a gradual resolution of symptoms and laboratory abnormalities.

B. Complications

1. Fulminant hepatic failure (or widespread necrosis of the liver) has a mortality rate approaching 80%. The protein-synthesizing function of the liver is markedly impaired, as reflected by the elevation of prothrombin time and reduction of serum albumin.

2. Chronic persistent hepatitis is characterized by moderate elevation of ALT and AST (40–200 IU/L) for at least 6 months. These patients may be infectious, but liver function is usually stable, and cirrhosis and liver failure are rare.

3. Chronic active hepatitis is a variably progressive disease that ultimately results in cirrhosis and hepatic failure. Serum aminotransferase concentrations are usually greater than 400 IU/L.

4. Aplastic anemia occurs rarely but carries a poor prognosis.

5. Hepatitis B infection can be associated with immune complex deposition, producing arthritis, urticaria, glomerulonephritis, and vasculitis. Pancreatitis occurs occasionally.

IV. PREVENTION

A. There is currently no treatment for viral hepatitis. Therefore, prevention of the disease becomes all the more important.

B. Hepatitis A

1. The principal step is limitation of contact with infectious individuals, including their food, utensils, and clothing.

2. Passive immunization with immunoglobulin of anyone who has been infected by hepatitis A can prevent infection.

C. Hepatitis B and Hepatitis non-A, non-B

1. Hepatitis B and non-A, non-B are of particular concern to anesthesiologists because of the modes of virus transmission. Serologic markers for Type B infection have been found in more than 20% of anesthesia personnel, compared with less than 5% of the general population.

2.   Recognition of those infected with the virus and those at high risk can be difficult. Therefore, adoption of certain isolation precautions for *all* patients, as outlined in the section on AIDS, is the best way to avoid exposure.

3.   There is a safe, effective vaccine now available against the Type B virus. Given the risk of infection for anesthesia personnel, vaccination is recommended.

4.   If an exposure occurs, such as a needle stick from an infectious patient, treatment with immunoglobulin enriched with anti-HBs (HBIG) is recommended.

5.   The virus survives on contaminated surfaces for as long as 6 months at room temperature. Therefore, good sterilization technique for potentially contaminated surfaces and safe handling of high-risk items such as needles is crucial.

V.   SUMMARY OF ANESTHETIC CONSIDERATIONS

The patient with acute hepatitis should be anesthetized only for a truly emergency procedure, as anesthesia and surgery can worsen hepatic function or precipitate acute hepatic failure. This risk probably relates to decreases in blood flow to an already-compromised liver.

Preoperative medication should be carefully titrated because of its unpredictable effect on mental status and potential prolongation of postoperative recovery secondary to decreased metabolism. Intraoperative factors such as hypotension, hypercarbia, positive pressure ventilation, anesthetic agents, and, particularly, surgical stimulation lead to a reduction in blood flow to the liver with possible ischemia. If an inhaled anesthetic is to be used, isoflurane causes less reduction in hepatic blood flow than halothane or enflurane. Drugs and dosages should be chosen in light of the fact that metabolism by the liver will be reduced. For this reason, many have advocated the use of the inhalational anesthetics for these patients.

Coagulopathy and anemia should be corrected as much as possible prior to the operation. Care should be taken with the rate of blood transfusion, as citrate toxicity is more likely with rapid transfusions. Metabolic derangements such as hypoglycemia and acidosis must be looked for and corrected.

Emergence from anesthesia may be prolonged because of the variable effect of the anesthetics on mental status in the setting of liver disease. Patients with significant liver disease often hyperventilate and appear to have an adequate respiratory status. This may be misleading, as mental status could still be impaired and the risk of aspiration high. Therefore, it is necessary to keep the patient intubated until protective airway reflexes have returned.

Tuberculosis

I. PRIMARY INFECTION
    A. Tuberculosis (TB), a chronic granulomatous disease caused by *Mycobacterium tuberculosis*, was once a significant health problem throughout society. Tuberculosis is now largely confined to overcrowded urban areas and to the debilitated, malnourished, and immunosuppressed.
    B. The infection is spread primarily through aerosol transmission, although there are occasional cases of parenteral exposure among health care workers. The risk of transmission is greatest from patients with cavitary or laryngeal TB and is related to the concentration of organisms in the sputum, the closeness and duration of contact, and the cough frequency.
    C. Once in the body, the organism spreads by local extension, intrabronchial spread, and hematogenous or lymphatic dissemination. The hallmark of TB is the production of caseating granulomas in response to the mycobacterium.
    D. Signs and Symptoms
        1. Infection begins with the primary stage, when there are few or no symptoms. Occasionally, there are pleural effusions, meningitis, bone and joint disease, or cavitation in the lung.
        2. The lung parenchyma usually develops an inflammatory pneumonic process with enlarged hilar nodes, but lesions often are not apparent on the chest radiograph.
        3. Primary disease is usually confirmed by positive skin testing with PPD. However, 5% to 20% of newly identified patients initially have negative skin tests.
        4. The primary stage will then heal, with some calcified scarring, after which the organism remains dormant.

II. REACTIVATION
    A. The reactivation phase accompanies decreased immunity such as in malnutrition, alcoholism or other drug abuse, emotional stress, infection, malignancies, hemodialysis, or steroid use.

    B. Reactivation usually appears in the posterior portion of the upper lobes of the lung because of the higher oxygen concentration in that area. Occasionally, reactivation occurs in response to a repeat exposure to TB in a person already sensitized by the prior exposure.

    C. Reactivation can follow a variable course. Signs and symptoms include nonproductive cough, hemoptysis, or a flu-like syndrome with fever, cough, and myalgia.

    D. The diagnosis of reactivation may be suggested by chest radiographs, which can show a wide variety of lesions in addition to upper-lobe cavitation. The sputum will show acid-fast organisms on smear, and sputum cultures may grow the organism.

III. **EXTRAPULMONARY SITES**

    A. The pleura, chest wall, and pericardium can be involved via intrathoracic extension.

    B. Outside the thorax, lymphadenitis is the most common manifestation.

    C. The genitourinary tract is the next most common site.

        1. The kidney often develops abscesses followed by scarring and hydronephrosis.

        2. In males, prostate, seminal vesicle, and epididymal involvement can occur.

    D. Skeletal disease usually manifests as thoracic or lumbar spondylitis. Arthritis and tenosynovitis may also be found.

    E. In the gastrointestinal system, TB can cause peritonitis.

    F. Tubercular meningitis and cerebral abscesses are possible.

    G. Laryngeal, middle ear, and eye involvement are less likely to be seen. Rarely, vascular infection leads to mycotic aneurysm.

IV. **CHEMOTHERAPY**

    A. The incidence and mortality rate from tuberculosis have decreased dramatically since the discovery of effective chemotherapeutic agents. After 10 weeks of effective therapy, 75% of patients can be expected to have sputum that is free of the organism. In general, after 3 weeks of combined chemotherapy, patients may be considered noninfectious even though tubercle bacilli are still seen on smear. A full course of therapy ranges from 9 to 18 months.

    B. Drugs

        1. Isoniazid

        Isoniazid is the most widely used agent. Less common side effects are encephalopathy, memory loss, optic atrophy, seizures, hemolytic anemia, or lupus-like syndrome. Its most common side effect is a peripheral neuropathy, but its most serious side effect is hepatic toxicity, the risk of which is increased with heavy alcohol use and in the elderly. The hepatic metabolites of the drug may increase defluorination of volatile anesthetics, which can lead to increased fluoride levels and renal tubular toxicity.

2. Rifampin

Rifampin's most common toxicity is an allergic reaction consisting of rash and fever with nausea and vomiting. Acute renal failure, thrombocytopenia, hemolysis, and hepatitis are rare. The durations of action of many drugs may be shortened, because rifampin is a potent inducer of hepatic microsomal enzymes.

3. Ethambutol's principal side effect is optic neuritis.

V. SUMMARY OF ANESTHETIC CONSIDERATIONS

Any patient suspected of having pulmonary TB should be kept in strict respiratory isolation, with all those in proximity wearing masks. Care should be taken to minimize the spread of secretions during manipulations of the airway, and proper sterilization of all potentially contaminated equipment such as laryngoscopes and bronchoscopes is mandatory before their reuse. Disposable equipment and filters for the anesthetic circuit should be considered.

Patients with active TB should have elective operations postponed until treatment has been initiated. Three weeks of chemotherapy is usually sufficient to eliminate the risk of infectivity; however, sputum must be documented to be negative for the organism before this can be assured.

Anesthesia for the patient with tuberculosis will be complicated by the type and severity of organ dysfunction present either as a result of the disease itself or of its treatment. The most common organ involved is the lung, giving rise to the same problems present in patients with other forms of pneumonia.

Acquired Immunodeficiency Syndrome

I. DIAGNOSIS

A. The acquired immunodeficiency syndrome (AIDS) has become a significant health threat throughout the world.

Since its identification in 1981, there have been more than 90,000 cases reported in the United States. The number of persons who either carry the virus or who are at high risk for becoming infected is rising.

B.   Clinical diagnosis of AIDS requires the presence of Kaposi's sarcoma or certain opportunistic infections associated with defective cell-mediated immunity in a person without another defined cause. An ever-broadening range of infections and malignancies in association with a positive test for the human immunodeficiency virus (HIV) are being included in the definition of the disease.

C.   Although there are less severe categories of HIV infections, such as AIDS-related complex (ARC), recent data suggest that infection with the virus is equivalent to having the disease eventually. The latency period for expression of the virus can be quite long, 6 years or more. Detection is by an enzyme-linked immunosorbent assay (ELISA) of antibody to disrupted virus or by assay of antibody to specific viral antigens (Western blot technique).

D.   Risk Groups

    1.   Homosexual and bisexual men make up approximately 70% of patients with AIDS.

    2.   Intravenous drug abusers are the second largest group (15%) with AIDS in the US. Sharing of needles is the principal mode of transmission of the virus in this group.

    3.   Transfusion recipients (especially those receiving pooled blood products such as hemophiliacs), sexual partners of infected individuals, and newborn children of infected mothers are small but growing risk groups.

II.   PREOPERATIVE EVALUATION

    A.   Pulmonary

        1.   For many patients, secondary respiratory infections represent the most severe manifestation of AIDS.

        2.   Infections caused by *Pneumocystis carinii* (most common), cytomegalovirus (CMV), *Mycobacterium tuberculosis, Mycobacterium avium-intracellulare, Legionella, Cryptococcus, Candida,* Herpes, *Toxoplasma,* and various other organisms produce severe acute lung disease.

        3.   Noninfectious pneumonitis, which is less common, may produce significant pulmonary compromise.

4. Pleural disease manifested by effusions and pleural thickening can limit lung compliance.

5. Kaposi's sarcoma of the airways can produce significant hemoptysis.

B. Cardiovascular

The AIDS virus itself has been reported to cause cardiomyopathy, endocarditis, and pericardial disease.

C. Neurologic

The most common central nervous system (CNS) manifestation is a progressive encephalitis produced by direct HIV infection of neural tissue. Myelopathy, encephalitis, meningitis, brain abscess, progressive multifocal leukoencephalopathy, and peripheral neuropathy may occur via secondary infection. Lymphoma and Kaposi's sarcoma of the CNS are rare.

D. Renal

Proteinuria, nephrotic syndrome, and glomerulosclerosis have all been described, but their etiology is unknown. The most significant risk is the development of acute renal failure, usually in association with sepsis and treatment of infection with nephrotoxic drugs.

E. Hematologic

Anemia, lymphopenia, thrombocytopenia, or neutropenia can be secondary to HIV infection of the bone marrow or can result from drug therapy, secondary malignancy, or autoimmune mechanisms.

F. Gastrointestinal

Enteric involvement is common and occurs via opportunistic infection, lymphoma, or Kaposi's sarcoma. These have the potential to produce malabsorption, hypovolemia, and bleeding.

G. Ophthalmic

Not infrequently, AIDS-related chorioretinitis and conjunctivitis leads to progressive blindness.

III. SUMMARY OF ANESTHETIC CONSIDERATIONS

Monitoring, anesthetic technique, and choice of agents should be determined by the type of organ dysfunction present. The principal problems usually involve pulmonary disease or cardiovascular instability.

A significant concern for anesthesiologists is the risk of viral transmission. According to Centers for Disease Control (CDC) statistics, a small number of health workers appear to have developed AIDS as a result of occupational exposure. The majority of these cases involved needle sticks, although some may have been caused by open skin or mucous membrane contact with infected material. The virus has been identified in blood, semen, saliva, cerebrospinal fluid, urine, stool, tears, and breast milk. The CDC guidelines for health care workers recommend that all patients, regardless of HIV status, be treated with proper precautions as follows:

Wear gloves when performing patient procedures.

Use appropriate barrier precautions when exposure to aerosolization or splashes is likely (gowns, masks, eye covering). This includes endotracheal intubations and tracheal suctioning.

Do not recap needles. Dispose of all sharp implements in designated containers.

Avoid performing invasive procedures or handling potentially infected material if you have open skin lesions.

Use respiratory isolation precautions for patients with pneumonia.

Keep equipment for artificial ventilation readily available to avoid mouth-to-mouth resuscitation.

HIV survives drying and storage at 25°C and remains viable in dried material at room temperature for 3 days. Hospital sterilization techniques utilizing disinfectants such as dilute sodium hypochlorite (bleach) will remove the virus from contaminated surfaces such as the anesthesia machine. Instruments such as laryngoscopes and anesthetic circuits should be safe to use after appropriate treatment, although many institutions have adopted the use of disposable equipment for patients with AIDS.

Soft Tissue Infections

I.   SIGNIFICANT TYPES

     A.   Soft tissue infections such as clostridial myonecrosis and necrotizing fasciitis are life-threatening emergencies. Surgical debridement, often involving extensive, disfiguring resection, is the mainstay of treatment.

     B.   Gas Gangrene

         Infection and necrosis of muscle by gas-producing bacteria is called gas gangrene. *Clostridium perfringens* is most often responsible. The bacterium is usually introduced by penetrating trauma such as a gunshot wound or motor vehicle accident, but infection can follow surgery. After implantation into anoxic, devascularized tissue, the organism multiplies rapidly and releases toxins leading to necrosis, sepsis, and death.

C. Necrotizing Fasciitis

Infection of the deep subcutaneous tissues without myonecrosis can follow minor trauma. Streptococci and staphylococci are often implicated. After introduction, the organisms multiply, invade deep tissues, and produce necrosis of blood vessels and lymphatics.

II. PREOPERATIVE EVALUATION

A. Unsuspected renal failure may be caused by myoglobin released from tissue necrosis or free hemoglobin and red cell stroma from intravascular hemolysis.

B. Electrolyte abnormalities such as hyperkalemia and hypocalcemia, if uncorrected, are associated with cardiac dysrhythmias and muscular irritability, respectively.

C. Cardiac function needs to be closely evaluated. Myocardial depression from endotoxin, myocardial depressant factors from sepsis, and valvular dysfunction from vegetations are frequent complications.

III. SUMMARY OF ANESTHETIC CONSIDERATIONS

Extensive surgical dissection should be anticipated, along with a need to infuse large amounts of blood and crystalloid. Meticulous attention to maintaining intravascular volume is essential to prevent hypovolemia and possible hypoperfusion of vital organs. For frequent debridement procedures, the anesthetic technique should provide good analgesia and amnesia for short periods with minimal residue effect.

Intraoperative antibiotic administration is frequently required of the anesthesiologist. The most commonly used antibiotics and their potential side effects may affect anesthetic management (Table 10-3). Special consideration should be paid to antibiotic hypersensitivity, because anesthesia may mask the initial signs or symptoms of reactions. Almost all antimicrobials can cause hypersensitivity reactions, which can range from minor skin rashes to fatal anaphylactic shock. The penicillins are the most frequent cause. The overall incidence of penicillin hypersensitivity is between 0.5% and 10%. IgE-related anaphylaxis accounts for 0.02% of allergic reactions.

A common perioperative question is whether to administer a cephalosporin to a patient with a history of penicillin allergy. The incidence of cross-reactivity to the cephalosporins

Table 10–3. Adverse Reactions to Antibiotics

Antibiotic	Reaction
Penicillins	Nephritis (pcn G); bone marrow depression (nafcillin and methicillin); platelet dysfunction (carbenicillin and ticarcillin); hepatitis and seizures
Vancomycin	Hypotension (direct myocardial depression, histamine release); nephrotoxicity; ototoxicity
Cephalosporins	Hemolytic anemia; nephrotoxicity (especially in combination with aminoglycosides); thrombocytopenia; granulocytopenia
Aminoglycosides	Nephrotoxicity; ototoxicity; skeletal muscle weakness; potentiation of neuromuscular blockade
Erythromycin	Cholestatic jaundice; thrombophlebitis; fever; eosinophilia; deafness
Tetracyclines	Hepatic dysfunction; thrombophlebitis
Trimethoprim–sulfamethoxazole	Renal toxicity; rash; jaundice; megaloblastic anemia
Pentamidine	Hypotension (IV); hypoglycemia; leukopenia; thrombocytopenia
Amphotericin B	Hypotension, hypoxemia, fever, chills, headache, anorexia, renal dysfunction (80% of patients); hypokalemia, hypomagnesemia, thrombocytopenia, anemia
Isoniazid	Hepatitis; marrow depression; peripheral neuropathy
Chloramphenicol	Bone marrow toxicity

is low (5%–10%), and the reaction is not severe. In most cases, therefore, cephalosporins may be given. However, when a prior penicillin reaction has been serious, such as anaphylaxis or laryngeal edema, it is best to avoid the use of cephalosporins also.

Prophylaxis for Bacterial Endocarditis

There are certain cardiac lesions in which antibiotic prophylaxis is recommended to prevent the development of endocarditis when there is a risk of bacteremia. The following recommendations are taken from the American Heart Association's antibiotic prophylaxis guidelines (1986) for bacterial endocarditis.

I.   PATIENTS AT RISK

Prosthetic heart valves
Congenital malformations (most)
Surgical systemic-to-pulmonary shunts
Rheumatic and other acquired valve dysfunction
Idiopathic hypertrophic subaortic stenosis (IHSS)
History of endocarditis
Mitral valve prolapse with insufficiency.

II.   PATIENTS NOT AT RISK

Isolated secundum atrial septal defect (ASD)
Secundum ASD repair without patch more than 6 months ago
Ligation of patent ductus arteriosus more than 6 months ago.

III.   PROCEDURES REQUIRING PROPHYLAXIS FOR PATIENTS AT RISK

A.   Dental and Airway Procedures

Dental procedures likely to produce bleeding
Tonsillectomy and adenoidectomy
Surgery or biopsy of respiratory mucosa
Nasotracheal intubation
Incision and drainage of infected tissue.

B.   Gastrointestinal and Genitourinary Procedures (Prophylaxis Required for All Lesions)

Cystoscopy
Urethral catheterization
Prostate surgery
Urinary tract surgery
Colon surgery
Colonoscopy
Esophageal procedures
Vaginal hysterectomy
Cholecystectomy.

C.   Gastrointestinal and Genitourinary Procedures (Prophylaxis Required Only for Patients with Prosthetic Valves and Systemic–Pulmonary Shunts)

Percutaneous liver biopsy
Upper gastrointestinal endoscopy
Proctosigmoidoscopy without biopsy

Table 10–4. *Antibiotic Prophylaxis for Common Medical Procedures*

Procedure	Antibiotic Regimen
Dental; Surgery of the Upper Respiratory Tract	
Routine	Penicillin V, 2.0 g orally, 1 hour before, then 1.0 g 6 hours later
Maximal protection (e.g., prosthetic values)	Ampicillin 1.0–2.0 g IV/IM 30 min before *and* Gentamicin 1.5 mg/kg IV/IM 30 min before; penicillin V 1.0 g 6 hours later
Penicillin allergy	Erythromycin 1.0 g orally 1 hour before, then 500 mg 6 hours later
High risk with penicillin allergy	Vancomycin 1.0 g IV over 60 min started 1 hour before; no repeat dose is needed
Gastrointestinal and Genitourinary Procedures	
All lesions	Ampicillin 2.0 g IV/IM 30 min before and 8 hours later *and* Gentamicin 1.5 mg/kg IV/IM 30 min before and 8 hours later
Penicillin allergy	Vancomycin 1.0 g IV 1 hour preoperatively; may be repeated 8 hours later *and* Gentamicin 1.5 mg/kg IV/IM 1 hour before and 8 hours later
Cardiac Surgery	
	Cefazolin 1 g IV/IM 1 hour prior to and every 6 hours for 48 hours after surgery

        Vaginal delivery (uncomplicated)
        Bladder catheterization (sterile urine).

    D. All Cardiac Operations

IV. Standard antibiotic regimens have been established for common medical procedures (Table 10-4).

Recommended Reading

Benumof JL. General respiratory physiology and respiratory function during anesthesia. In: Benumof JL, ed. Anesthesia for thoracic surgery. Philadelphia: WB Saunders, 1987:39.

Berry AJ, Isaacson IJ, Hunt D, Kane MA. The prevalence of hepatitis B viral markers in anesthesia personnel. Anesthesiology 1984;60:6.

Centers for Disease Control. Classification system for human T-lymphotropic virus type III/lymphadenopathy-associated virus infections. JAMA 1986;256:20.

Centers for Disease Control. Recommendations for preventing transmission of infection with human T-lymphotropic virus type III/lymphadenopathy-associated virus during invasive procedures. Ann Intern Med 1986;104:824.

Gelman SL. Disturbances in hepatic blood flow during anesthesia and surgery. Arch Surg 1976;111:661.

Gilbert EM, Haupt MT, Mandanas RY, et al. The effect of fluid loading, blood transfusion, and cathecholamine infusion on oxygen delivery and consumption in patients with sepsis. Am Rev Respir Dis 1986;134:873.

Hess ML, Hastillo A, Greenfield LJ. Spectrum of cardiovascular function during gram-negative sepsis. Prog Cardiovasc Dis 1981;23:279.

Jacobson MA, Young LS. New developments in the treatment of bacteremia. West J Med 1986;144:185.

Kaiser AB. Antimicrobial prophylaxis in surgery. N Engl J Med 1986;315:1129.

Kaye D. Prophylaxis for infective endocarditis: an update. Ann Intern Med 1986;104:419.

Kunkel SE, Warner MA. Human T-cell lymphotropic virus type III (HTLV-III) infection: how it can affect you, your patients and your anesthesia practice. Anesthesiology 1987;66:195.

Masur H. Antimicrobials. In: Chernow B, Lake CR, eds. The pharmacologic approach to the critically ill patient. Baltimore: Williams & Wilkins, 1983:607.

Pavlin EG. Respiratory pharmacology of inhaled anesthetic agents. In: Miller RD, ed. Anesthesia, vol 1. 2nd ed. New York: Churchill Livingstone, 1986;667.

Rawal N, Sjostrand U, Christoffersson E, et al. Comparison of intramuscular and epidural morphine for postoperative analgesia in the grossly obese: influence on postoperative ambulation and pulmonary function. Anesth Analg 1984;63:583.

Rosenthal MH. Physiologic approach to the management of shock. Semin Anesth 1982;1:285.

Selwyn PA. AIDS: what is now known III: clinical aspects. Hosp Pract 1986;Sep 15:119.

Shulman ST, Amren DP, Bisno AL, et al. Prevention of bacterial endocarditis: a statement for health professionals by the Committee on Rheumatic Fever and Infective Endocarditis of the Council on Cardiovascular Disease in the Young. Circulation 1984;70:1123A.

Stover DE, White DA, Romano PA, et al. Spectrum of pulmonary diseases associated with the acquired immunodeficiency syndrome. Am J Med 1985;78:429.

West JB. Respiratory physiology: the essentials. 2nd ed. Baltimore: Williams & Wilkins, 1984.

Zaritsky AL, Chernow B. Catecholamines, sympathomimetics. In: Chernow B, Lake CR, eds. The pharmacologic approach to the critcally ill patient. Baltimore: Williams & Wilkins, 1983:481.

CHAPTER 11

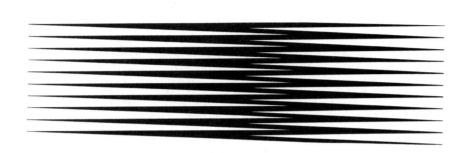

Immunologic Disorders

John F. Williams

The function of the immune system has important implications for the anesthesiologist. The primary immunodeficiency diseases usually are seen in children and present as recurrent bacterial infections. However, with the success of antibiotic therapy, the anesthesiologist is now presented with patients who survive to adulthood and are on multiple drug regimens that can increase the likelihood of allergic and autoimmune reactions.

Because the lungs serve as a filter of both blood and air, many substances enter the lung, where they can be trapped and set off a series of potentially detrimental responses. Anesthetic drugs may alter the immune response to infection or malignancy. As a result of this alteration, the lungs can be involved in many immunologic disorders, including allergic asthma, anaphylaxis, sarcoidosis, and systemic lupus erythematosus (Table 11-1). A knowledge of the immune system and its interaction with anesthetic drugs thus is essential for the safe conduct of anesthesia.

Immune System

I. BASIC CONCEPTS
   A. Mechanisms of Immunologically Mediated Inflammation
   The immune system has been described as a surveillance mechanism that distinguishes "self" from "nonself." When something is recognized as nonself, such as neoplastic cells or microorganisms, there is recruitment of both cellular and humoral elements to defend the host. This response is usually beneficial, but there are situations in which it can be detrimental. Such adverse responses may occur in the lungs or kidneys, where blood or air can become trapped and recognized as "nonself," initiating a cellular or humoral response directed at normal (self) host tissue that can cause inflammation, fibrous deposition, granuloma formation, and bronchospasm.

   The classification system that has been useful in understanding the pathogenesis of immunologically mediated disorders was developed in 1968 by Coombs and Gell (Table 11-2).
   B. Mechanisms of Immunologically Mediated Inflammation
      1. Type I
      The Type I sensitivity reaction is mediated by IgE. This reaction leads to edema and smooth-muscle

Table 11–1.　Lung Diseases Known or Suspected to be Immunologically Mediated

Known to be immunologically mediated
　Allergic asthma
　Anaphylaxis
　Goodpasture's syndrome
　Hypersensitivity pneumonitis
Suspected of being immunologic reactions
　Pulmonary vasculitides (III, IV)
　　Classic Wegener's granulomatosis
　　Necrotizing sarcoid granulomatosis
　Systemic vasculitides in which lung may be involved (III)
　　Cryoglobulinemia
　　Polyarteritis nodosa
　Collagen vascular diseases complicated by pulmonary vasculitis (III)
　　Rheumatoid arthritis
　　Systemic lupus erythematosus
　　Sjögren's syndrome

(Adapted from Larkin AB, Compton CC, Irwin RS. Immunologic lung disease. In: Rippe JM, Irwin RS, Alpert JS, Dalen JE, eds. Intensive care medicine. Boston: Little, Brown, 1985:515.)

contraction, typically seen in anaphylactic or reagin-mediated reactions and allergic asthma. The reaction usually occurs within seconds to minutes, does not require complement activation, and does not cause cell lysis.

2. Type II
The Type II reaction is mediated by cytotoxic antibodies, which destroy cells or cell membranes. The reactions are caused by complement activation or phagocytosis by killer cells. The reaction typically is seen in Goodpasture's syndrome, transfusion reactions, and hemolytic anemia.

3. Type III
The Type III reaction is mediated by the deposition of circulating soluble complexes of antigen and antibody. Platelets and complement are activated, and IgM and IgG play a role in the reaction. This interaction causes the inflammatory response typically seen in diseases such as systemic lupus erythematosus, polyarteritis nodosa, and post-streptococcal glomerulonephritis.

Table 11–2. Mechanisms of Immunologically Mediated Inflammation

Type	Characteristics of Response	Clinical Disease Type
Allergic (IgE-mediated)	Basophil and mast cell products leading to immediate flare and wheal	Atopy, anaphylaxis
Cytotoxic or tissue-specific antibody (IgM- or IgG-mediated)	Acute inflammation via phagocytic cells and deposition of complement in tissues; lysis or phagocytosis of target cells	Goodpasture's syndrome; anti-red cell antibodies in transfusion reactions
Immune complex (IgG-, IgM-, IgA-mediated)	Accumulation of neutrophils, macrophages, and complement components	Systemic necrotizing vasculitis, systemic lupus erythematosus, serum sickness syndromes
Delayed hypersensitivity	T-cell-induced mononuclear cell accumulation of regulatory and effector T cells and macrophages. Lymphokines and monokines released. Often, granuloma formation	Tuberculosis, sarcoidosis, rheumatoid arthritis, Wegener's granulomatosis

(Adapted from Austen KF. Diseases of immediate type hypersensitivity. In: Braunwald E, Isselbacher KJ, Petersdorf RG, et al, eds. Harrison's principles of internal medicine. 11th ed. New York: McGraw-Hill, 1987:1407.)

4. **Type IV**

The Type IV, or delayed hypersensitivity, reaction is mediated by T lymphocytes that cause mononuclear cellular inflammation without complement or antibody activation. This reaction is characteristically delayed 24 to 48 hours. The Type IV reaction is typically seen in the granulomatous diseases such as tuberculosis and sarcoidosis.

II. **MEDIATORS OF IMMUNOLOGIC RESPONSES**

A. Lymphocytes are the most important cells in the immune response. There are two distinct types, which are derived from a common bone-marrow stem cell: T (thymus-dependent) and B (bursa-dependent) lymphocytes. T lymphocytes are programmed to distinguish self from nonself and are responsible for cell-mediated immunity. B lymphocytes, when activated by contact with an antigen, become plasma cells and produce antibodies.

B. A molecule's ability to act as an antigen is known as immunogenicity. Antigens are large molecules that stimulate an immune response on their own or when bound to proteins (haptens). These antigens are capable of interacting with B lymphocytes to create plasma cells that secrete antibodies.

C. Drugs as Antigens
1. Drugs such as succinylcholine may be able to act as antigens without first binding to protein because they have two antigenic groups an appropriate distance apart for bridging cell-bound IgE molecules and therefore initiating an allergic reaction.
2. Metabolic breakdown products of the parent molecule can also be the antigenic component, altering the host tissue and stimulating autoantibodies; for example, hydralazine and procainamide can chemically alter nuclear material, stimulate formation of antibodies, and, occasionally, cause systemic lupus erythematosus.
3. Drugs such as antibiotics (penicillin being the classic model) are small molecules (called haptens) that combine with protein to stimulate antibody formation. This contact leads to a series of biochemical events within the mast cell resulting in the release of mediators that may produce urticaria, wheezing, rhinorrhea, and, occasionally, hypotension.

D. Antibodies
1. Antibodies are formed when antigens stimulate B lymphocytes to become plasma cells. The plasma cells also secrete protein macromolecules with the ability to bind the antigen that stimulated their production.
2. In general, these antigen–antibody complexes are phagocytized and destroyed by macrophages of the reticuloendothelial system. Occasionally, however, these complexes are deposited in tissues (lung, kidney), causing inflammation and tissue damage.
3. Antibodies are largely responsible for the protective immunity so critical for the survival of the human

host. Any dysfunction or alteration in the antibody system can lead to death. Antibodies produced by the B lymphocytes are called immunoglobins (Ig). Five classes of immunoglobins are recognized on the basis of their structure and function: IgA, IgG, IgD, IgE, and IgM (Table 11-3).

a. Immunoglobin A

IgA appears in serum and some seromucous secretions such as saliva, tears, nasal fluids, sweat, and pulmonary and nasogastric fluids. It is secreted by plasma cells and is the first line of defense against bacteria. It has the ability to inhibit the binding of bacteria to mucosal cells and to activate complement. IgA-deficient patients may develop severe pulmonary edema when given blood products.

b. Immunoglobin G

IgG is the principal antibody produced by the body to fight infection; it is also the most abundant immunoglobin in the serum. Also called gamma-globulin and complement-

Table 11–3. Properties of Human Immunoglobins

	Location	$T_{1/2}$ in the Serum (days)	Serum Concentration (mg/dl)	Function
IgA	Serum, saliva, tears	6	60–333	Topical defense against infection
IgG	Serum, amniotic fluid	23	550–1900	Immunity and defense against systemic infection
IgD	Serum	3	0.3–30	Not known
IgE	Serum	2.5	Trace	Immune-mediated hypersensitivity (anaphylaxis)
IgM	Serum	5	45–145	Lysis of bacterial cell walls

(Adapted from Roesch RP. The immune system. In: Stoelting RK, Dierdorf SF, eds. Anesthesia and co-existing disease. 2nd ed. New York: Churchill Livingstone, 1988.)

fixing gamma-globulin, it has been isolated from patients' sera during reactions to protamine and local anesthetics.

    c. Immunoglobin D

IgD appears to be a membrane receptor for lymphocytes, but its specific role has not been confirmed.

    d. Immunoglobin E

IgE exists in very small concentrations in serum and is the primary cause of anaphylaxis. Most IgE is bound to mast cells, and elevated levels are found in patients with a history of allergy, atopy, or asthma.

    e. Immunoglobin M

IgM binds to and activates complement and is responsible for cell wall lysis.

E. The Complement System

    1. The complement system consists of a group of plasma proteins that are activated via two sequences: the "classic" and "alternate" pathways. Human disease related to complement may present as defective resistance to infection secondary to impaired activation of the system or as hypersensitivity states caused by excessive complement activation.

    2. Activation of the complement system generally requires an antigen–antibody complex, which initiates a cascade of enzymes, proteins, and lytic factors (Figure 11-1). The common final pathway leads to generation of anaphylatoxins, which have direct effects on target organs and cause mediator release. The complement system consists of 18 proteins found in plasma.

        a. The classic pathway for complement system activation consists of proteins designated C_1 through C_9, with the cascade initiated by the activation of the normally inactive C_1 protein (Figure 11-2). An enzyme in human serum, C_1 inhibitor, regulates the progression of the complement cascade. Any decrease in this protein will lead to an excess of the components of the complement system (Table 11-4). An excess of complement components can lead to increased vascular permeability and release of histamine

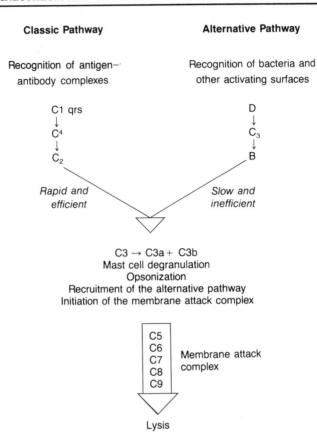

Figure 11-1 Classic and alternative pathways of complement activation. *(Adapted from Braunwald E, Isselbacher KJ, Petersdorf RG, et al, eds. Harrison's principles of internal medicine. 11th ed. New York: McGraw-Hill, 1987:1407.)*

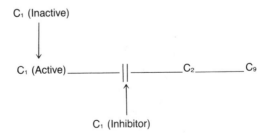

Figure 11-2 C_1 of the complement cascade normally is inactive in the serum. C_1 inactive is converted to C_1 active by an antibody–antigen reaction. C_1 active then initiates the complement cascade. *(Adapted from Roesch RP. The immune system. In: Stoelting RK, Dierdorf SF, eds. Anesthesia and co-existing disease. 2nd ed. New York: Churchill Livingstone, 1988.)*

Table 11–4. Biologic Activities of Principal Complement Components

Component	Activity
C_4, C_2 kinin	Increases vascular permeability
C_{3a}	Anaphylatoxin; evokes release of histamine from basophils and of serotonin from platelets
C_{5a}	Anaphylatoxin; evokes histamine release from basophils; potent chemoattractant for monocytes and neutrophils
C_{3b}	Enhancement of phagocytosis by neutrophils and monocytes. Promotes immune-complex binding to cells within monocyte–macrophage system, as well as neutrophils. With Bb, forms alternate pathway. Promotes solubilization of immune complexes
C_5–C_9	Membrane attack complex; forms transmembrane channels leading to cell destruction

(Adapted from Austen KF. Diseases of immediate type hypersensitivity. In: Braunwald E, Isselbacher KJ, Petersdorf RG, et al, eds. Harrison's principles of internal medicine. 11th ed. New York: McGraw-Hill, 1987:1407.)

and bradykinin, causing vasodilatation and hypotension mimicking a full-blown acute anaphylactic reaction.

b. The alternate pathway can be activated by contrast media, many classes of drugs, and bacteria, causing reactions ranging from mild vasodilation and hypotension to acute anaphylaxis. The alternate pathway is more complex than the classic pathway, as two C_3-converting enzymes are formed. Patients who develop clinical anaphylaxis via the alternate pathway may react to structurally different drugs and may not react on every occasion despite having underlying immunopathology. Patients who have had an anaphylactic reaction without a clear precipitating agent or an agent that does not usually cause anaphylaxis should have complement measured by assaying the function of its components.

c. Treatment of hypotension caused by activation of the complement system consists of stopping any anesthetic agents, increasing FIO_2 to 1.0, and initiating fluid therapy. These patients usually respond quickly to fluid therapy, obviating pharmacologic intervention. A decrease in complement proteins renders the patient much more susceptible to pyogenic infections, glomerulonephritis, and Raynaud's syndrome.

III. ALLERGIC REACTIONS
  A. Anaphylaxis or Immune-Mediated Hypersensitivity
    1. Definition

Anaphylaxis is a syndrome in which cardiovascular collapse is the predominant feature (Table 11-5). Airway swelling, bronchospasm, and pulmonary edema are life-threatening manifestations. Cutaneous manifestations are characterized by urticaria and pruritus with or without angioedema. The life-threatening anaphylactic reaction seen in a sensitized person appears within minutes after the administration of the inciting antigen. Patients under general anesthesia may not manifest any cutaneous warning symptoms, and the anesthesiologist will be presented with cardiovascular collapse as the only symptom.

    2. Incidence

A number of studies have reported an in-hospital incidence of anaphylactic reactions of 3 per 10,000 patients. The incidence of anaphylaxis for anesthetic drugs is 1 in 20,000 patients; for blood volume replacement solutions, 1 in 400; and for intravenous contrast media, 1 in 1000. Mediators of anaphylaxis range from histamine and serotonin to prostaglandins and leukotrienes (Table 11-6). Death occurs in 3% to 9% of patients.

Table 11–5.   Clinical Features of Anaphylaxis

Minor	Major
Urticaria	Cardiovascular collapse
Rash	Bronchospasm
Pruritus	Laryngeal edema
Flush	Angioneurotic edema
Rhinitis	Generalized edema
Lacrimation	Coma
Cough	Gastrointestinal (vomiting, diarrhea)

Table 11–6. Mediators of Anaphylaxis

Mediator	Source	Function
Histamine	Preformed in mast cell/ basophil	Elevates AMP levels Feedback regulation Increases vascular permeability Smooth muscle constriction Generates prostaglandins Pulmonary vasoconstriction Increases gastric secretion Stimulates suppressor lymphocytes Cardiac effects
Serotonin	Preformed in mast cells	Increases vascular permeability
Eosinophil chemotactic factors	Preformed in mast cells	Attracts and activates eosinophils Increases eosinophil complement receptors
Platelet-activating factor	Generated in mast cells, ?macrophages, neutrophils, eosinophils	Aggregates platelets Releases amines and thromboxane Increases vascular permeability Bronchoconstriction Myocardial depression Vasoconstriction Sequesters platelets
Prostaglandins	Generated in mast cells	Increases cAMP Smooth muscle constriction Increases vascular permeability
Leukotrienes	Generated in mast cells, macrophages, neutrophils, eosinophils	Smooth muscle constriction Increases vascular permeability Decreases peripheral blood flow Generates prostaglandins Cardiac depression Coronary vasoconstriction Decreases lymphocyte response
Neutrophil chemotactic factor	Preformed in mast cells	Attracts and activates lymphocytes

3. Etiology

   a. Anesthetic drugs

      The muscle relaxant drugs produce the majority of reactions, usually in patients without previous exposure. Cross-sensitivity between muscle relaxants is more common than with other groups of drugs. These reactions are IgE mediated. The thiobarbiturates and methohexital have all been reported to cause anaphylaxis or immune-mediated hypersensitivity responses. Unfortunately, even a history of prior safe barbiturate exposure does not guarantee the safety of repeated exposure.

b. Colloid solutions
Dextrans and hydroxyethyl starch solutions can produce severe anaphylaxis. These reactions rarely occur when the solutions are used to resuscitate patients in shock but rather primarily in hemodynamically stable patients who require volume repletion.

c. Osmotic solutions
Mannitol and 50% glucose can both produce anaphylaxis through osmotic-induced histamine release. Adverse reactions are less likely if these solutions are infused slowly.

d. Antibiotics
Penicillin is the most common cause of drug-induced hypersensitivity reactions. Approximately 30% of patients who have an anaphylactic reaction to penicillin will have a significant cross-sensitivity to cephalosporins. Cephalosporins, trimethoprim–sulfamethoxazole, and vancomycin are all known to produce drug-induced anaphylaxis. Although these drugs are the most common antibiotics to cause reactions, virtually all antibiotics have caused anaphylaxis.

e. Other drugs
The cardiac drugs, particularly digoxin, quinidine, procainamide, and beta-blockers, may produce allergic reactions. As many as 10% of asthmatics may be allergic to nonsteroidal anti-inflammatory agents.

4. Predisposing factors
a. More common in women than men.
b. More common in people with a history of allergy, atopy, or asthma.
c. Allergy to seafoods is associated with increased reactions to contrast media.

d. More common in well patients than in patients in shock.

5. Natural history

The majority of reactions (>90%) to intravenous drugs occur within seconds to minutes after the introduction of the antigen. There is a slower onset when the antigen is ingested or given subcutaneously. Most patients who die from anaphylaxis do so within an hour of the onset of symptoms.

6. Clinical features

The onset and clinical manifestations of anaphylaxis vary (see Table 11-5), depending on the route of administration of the antigen. There is no universal human response pattern or particular "shock" organ that is involved. There is, however, a characteristic pattern of response in individuals exposed to antigens capable of initiating a reaction.

a. Cutaneous reactions

The most common manifestations of systemic reactions are cutaneous. The characteristic features are generalized erythema giving a cherry red or tomato appearance or eruptions that are well-circumscribed wheals with erythematous blanched centers. A generalized raised red rash, frequently on the legs and lower trunk, is also common.

b. Respiratory reactions

There are two patterns of respiratory failure. The first is upper airway obstruction caused by edema of the larynx or epiglottis, which can cause acute distress and death by suffocation. The second involves diffuse lower-airway bronchoconstriction similar to the respiratory abnormalities observed in status asthmaticus. Such airflow compromise is not relieved by endotracheal intubation and may lead to hypoxemia and hypercarbia.

c. Cardiovascular reactions

Perhaps the most severe clinical manifestation of anaphylaxis is cardiovascular collapse, which can develop with or without other symptoms. It is caused by peripheral pooling of blood secondary to direct vasodilatation, which then reduces venous return and cardiac output. Increased capillary permeability with loss of intravascular blood volume into the interstitial spaces is thought to be a contributing factor. Electrocardiographic abnormalities, including arrhythmias, conduction disturbances, and ischemic and infarction patterns, have been observed. These changes may reflect myocardial ischemia caused by decreased coronary perfusion and increased oxygen demand.

d. Metabolic changes
Metabolic abnormalities include increased blood histamine levels, which correlate with the duration and severity of shock.

e. Coagulation reactions
There is depletion of clotting factors V, VIII, and fibrinogen. The utilization of these coagulation factors is consistent with disseminated intravascular coagulation and may account for the clotting defects observed in clinical anaphylactic syndromes.

f. Angioneurotic edema
Angioneurotic edema consists of urticaria involving large vessels in the deeper skin layers. This occurs in a significant number of patients, with involvement of the head, neck, and upper airway. Clinically, angioedema progresses slowly and mandates close observation of the patient who has been resuscitated for at least 12 hours.

7. Differential diagnosis

    a. Cardiac causes

       1) Acute myocardial infarction

       2) Arrhythmias

       3) Drug-induced vasodilation

       4) Preoperative volume deficit.

    b. Respiratory causes

       1) Upper airway obstruction

       2) Tension pneumothorax

       3) Asthmatic bronchospasm.

8. Treatment

The primary goals of treatment are similar to those in other forms of shock (Table 11-7). Sympathomimetic drugs are the primary pharmacologic antagonist of anaphylactic shock.

    a. The underlying cause is treated by inhibiting further release of vasoactive substances with epinephrine. Epinephrine will also antagonize mediator effects on the end organs and support blood pressure.

    b. Fluid replacement with a balanced salt solution, colloid, or both should be undertaken immediately.

    c. The patient should be intubated and given a high oxygen concentration.

    d. Clinical features are treated with appropriate pharmacologic therapy (i.e., bronchodilators for bronchospasm).

    e. Antihistamines have no clear role. By the time anaphylaxis is diagnosed, their effects are unlikely to be of value. There are those who argue, however, that antihistamines may help by counteracting any circulating histamine that remains.

    f. There is no evidence to support the use of steroids in anaphylactic shock.

B. Anaphylactoid Reactions

    1. The anaphylactoid mechanism of action is indistinguishable from the immune-mediated hypersensitivity reaction. This reaction is caused by the release of histamine from mast cells after the ad-

Table 11–7. Treatment of Anaphylaxis

Intubation and mechanical ventilation with 100% O_2

Epinephrine 0.03–0.3 µg/kg IV or small boluses of 5–10 µg IV

Intravascular fluid replacement with normal saline, lactated Ringer's solution, and/or colloid

Antagonization of circulating histamine with intravenous diphenhydramine (0.5–1 mg/kg)

Treatment of the clinical features of shock. Increase of perfusion pressure with sympathomimetic drugs if necessary

ministration of a particular drug. Several important features distinguish this reaction from the Type I reaction.

    a.   Histamine release is independent of an antigen–antibody reaction.

    b.   Previous sensitization is not necessary for the reaction; it may occur with the first exposure to the drug.

    c.   The magnitude of histamine release is reduced by decreasing the rate of infusion or the dose of the drug.

    d.   Prophylaxis can be provided preoperatively.

2.   Drugs commonly causing anaphylactoid reactions include radiocontrast media, protamine sulfate, dextran, hydroxyethyl starch, and muscle relaxants. With the exception of contrast material, these agents are commonly administered by the anesthesiologist.

3.   Prophylaxis for the anaphylactoid reaction
Prophylaxis with an H_1 antagonist needs to be started 16 to 24 hours before exposure to a suspected antigen, as H_1-receptor antagonists seem to require this much time to act. Treatment 8 to 12 hours prior to antigen exposure with promethazine, cimetidine, or ranitidine has been reported to prevent or ameliorate anaphylactoid reactions secondary to intravenous contrast material. Volume status should be optimized prior to exposure to a suspected allergen. Although some authors have recommended large-dose steroid therapy (1–2 g of methylprednisolone) to prevent an anaphylactoid reaction, the efficacy of such therapy has not been confirmed.

4.   The treatment is the same as for anaphylactic shock (see Table 11-7).

C. Allergic Reactions to Local Anesthetics
Although often cited, allergic reactions to local anesthetics are extremely rare: less than 1% of reactions to local anesthetics have a true allergic mechanism. Frequently, these "allergic" reactions can be attributed to excessive blood levels of a local anesthetic, producing ringing in the ears, hypotension, and seizures. A true allergic response will manifest itself as a classic Type I reaction with erythema, rash, wheezing, etc. A reaction

that goes away without treatment is not an anaphylactic reaction. Ester local anesthetics, because of their structural similarity to paraminobenzoic acid (ester anesthetics have a benzoic acid ring), are more likely than amide local anesthetics to produce an allergic reaction. If a patient has had a reaction to an ester anesthetic, this does not preclude the use of an amide anesthetic.

IV. **SUMMARY OF ANESTHETIC CONSIDERATIONS**
Allergic reactions occasionally occur during anesthesia. Local anesthetics, especially the ester derivatives, succinylcholine, hydralazine, procainamide, and antibiotics have been associated with perioperative allergic reactions. Most often, patients have only minor reactions, which are characterized by generalized erythema or rash with urticaria and wheezing. Often, it is difficult to isolate the offending drug, but symptomatic treatment with H_1 blockers and bronchodilators is usually all that is needed. The rare occurrence of anaphylaxis is life threatening; anesthesia and surgery should be postponed until the patient has been stabilized and the etiology of anaphylaxis identified.

Immediate treatment includes controlling the airway and ventilating with 100% oxygen, fluid administration, bolus injection or continuous infusion of epinephrine to support blood pressure and inhibit further release of anaphylactic mediators, and bronchodilators.

Immunoglobin Disorders

I. **X-LINKED (BRUTON'S) AGAMMAGLOBULINEMIA**
  A. This genetic disorder predisposes patients to infections caused by pneumococci, streptococci, and *Haemophilus influenzae*. The most common infections are sinusitis, pneumonia, otitis, meningitis, and septicemia. The diagnosis is suspected if serum concentrations of IgG, IgA, and IgM are below 95% confidence levels. The disease is characterized by a serum concentration of IgG of less than 100 mg/dl. These patients tend to have little difficulty with fungi, gram-negative organisms, and viruses, with the exception of enteroviruses and hepatitides.
  B. Management
    1. Preoperatively, these patients should be receiving appropriate antibiotics.

      2. When signs of bacterial infection occur, signs of sinusitis, otitis, meningitis, and pneumonia should be sought. Diagnostic tests should always include complete blood count, chest radiograph, and Gram stain and culture of the suspected primary site of infection.

      3. Patients with bacterial infection should be given gamma-globulin so that the IgG level is above 200 mg/dl.

II. SELECTIVE IgA DEFICIENCY

  A. Selective IgA deficiency occurs in 1 of 700 persons and is manifested by repeated serious infections or connective tissue disorders. The infectious complications commonly involve the respiratory, gastrointestinal, and urogenital tracts. Associated connective tissue disorders include systemic lupus erythematosus, rheumatoid arthritis, and Sjögren's syndrome. These patients frequently have a history of diarrhea, a sprue-like malabsorption syndrome, or both.

  B. Management

      1. Preoperatively, intercurrent infection should be ruled out. One should maximize fluid status and check for electrolyte abnormalities.

      2. Intraoperatively, blood transfusion can cause anaphylaxis unless the blood is derived from an IgA-deficient donor. Type and cross-match orders should specifically state the need to look for IgA deficiency.

III. SELECTIVE IgM DEFICIENCY

  A. Patients with IgM deficiency develop septicemia caused by meningococci and other gram-negative organisms, recurrent staphylococcal pyoderma, respiratory infections, and pneumococcal meningitis.

  B. Preoperatively, management must include aggressive treatment with antibiotics to avoid fatal septicemia.

IV. MULTIPLE MYELOMA

  A. Multiple myeloma is a disseminated malignant disease in which transformed plasma cells proliferate in the bone marrow, invading adjacent bone and disrupting normal bone-marrow function.

      1. As a result of this marrow infiltration, the disease is frequently associated with extensive skeletal destruction, impaired renal function, hypercalcemia, anemia, thrombocytopenia, immunodeficiency, and increased susceptibility to infection.

2. Multiple myeloma is most frequently observed in the middle aged and elderly, with the incidence increasing with age.

3. These patients usually have severely depressed serum levels of normal immunoglobins and a decreased ability to manifest a normal humoral response. Consequently, they are particularly susceptible to pneumococcal pneumonias and herpes zoster, including generalized varicella infections.

4. Presenting signs and symptoms of multiple myeloma include bone pain (frequently associated with pathologic fractures of the ribs or spine), recurrent infection, symptoms of hypercalcemia (e.g., constipation, polyuria, calculus formation, confusion, stupor or coma), and, occasionally, bleeding disorders.

B. Management

1. Preoperatively, serum Ca^{2+} levels and electrolytes should be checked. Existing hypercalcemia is best treated initially with hydration. Bedrest and inactivity will increase Ca^{2+} and predispose to renal calculi and symptoms of hypercalcemia. Hyperviscosity from myeloma (Bence-Jones) protein should be treated with plasmapheresis before any surgical procedure. Renal function must be carefully checked. If renal insufficiency is present, preoperative hydration will help decrease the incidence of postoperative renal failure.

2. Intraoperative positioning for intubation or surgical procedure must be gentle, because the bones may be extremely fragile secondary to plasmacytomas.

3. Postoperatively, inadvertent fractures of vertebral bodies or ribs could cause cord compression or a decrease in respiratory function, respectively.

V. CRYOGLOBULINEMIA

A. In cryoglobulinemia, abnormal circulating immunoglobins precipitate in response to lowered body temperature. Renal dysfunction occurs in approximately 20% of these patients, sometimes in the face of a normal body temperature, probably because of deposition of IgM–IgG complexes in the kidney.

B. Management

1. Intraoperative maintenance of body temperature above 35°C is desirable. The best way is by increas-

ing the ambient temperature. Using warm humidified anesthetic gases and warmed intravenous fluids also is helpful.

2. Postoperative maintenance of body temperature above 35°C is as important as intraoperative temperature balance.

VI. MACROGLOBULINEMIA

A. Waldenström's or primary macroglobulinemia is characterized by the accumulation and proliferation of malignant cells that secrete IgM.

1. The neoplastic proliferation of these cells results in large quantities of monoclonal IgM, which produces a variable clinical pattern associated with increasing weakness, fatigue, bleeding manifestations, and anemia. Recurrent infection, weight loss, neurologic symptoms, and visual disturbances are frequent.

2. As the disease progresses, lymphadenopathy, splenomegaly, and hepatomegaly develop, producing a clinical pattern that resembles leukemia or lymphoma. Serum viscosity is usually elevated, and these patients may have severe hyperviscosity syndromes.

3. Preoperative plasmapheresis for hyperviscosity will help resolve neurologic symptoms (e.g., paresis or impending coma) and bleeding disorders. These patients are frequently treated with steroids and will need supplemental coverage perioperatively.

B. "Amyloidosis" is an inclusive term applied to a variety of conditions associated with tissue infiltrates of insoluble proteins, protein–polysaccharide complexes, or both.

1. Involvement of the kidney, spleen, heart, skin, peripheral nerves, skin, and small intestine is common.

2. Preoperative evaluation of the kidneys and heart will help determine the extent of organ damage. Macroglossia from amyloid invasion of the tongue may compromise the airway on induction.

VII. COMPLEMENT SYSTEM DISORDERS

A. Hereditary Angioneurotic Edema

1. This autosomal dominant genetic disorder causes a functional abnormality or deficiency of the C_1 inhibitor protein.

a. The condition is characterized by episodic edema involving the face, limbs, and respiratory tract.

    b. Patients frequently present with abdominal pain, but the most serious and life-threatening manifestation is laryngeal edema.

  2. Management

    a. Preoperatively, treatment may include:

      1) Danazol, an androgen derivative that induces an increase in the level of C_1 inhibitor protein.

      2) Fresh frozen plasma, two units 24 hours prior to surgery (contains C_1 inhibitor protein).

      3) Epsilon-aminocaproic acid or tanexamic acid (plasminogen inhibitor) needs to be given 2 to 3 days before surgery for any patient requiring an endotracheal tube.

    b. Regional anesthesia should be used whenever possible. Also, the anesthesiologist must be prepared for emergency endotracheal intubation. Traumatizing of the patient during intubation and preoperative positioning must be avoided.

B. Complement Deficiency Disorders

Deficiencies of C_3, C_5, C_6, C_7, and C_8 render patients more susceptible to infection. Deficiency of C_3, in particular, carries an increased risk of life-threatening bacterial infections. Any preoperative infections should be treated vigorously.

VIII. SUMMARY OF ANESTHETIC CONSIDERATIONS

There is a wide variety of immunologic disorders. Many of these patients are at increased risk of infections because of specific defects in immunologic functions. Not breaking aseptic technique is important. Perioperative antibiotics are also important in preventing significant postoperative morbidity from infections.

Several immunologic disease states have unique features that must be considered. Patients with selective IgA deficiency must be given only blood from an IgA-deficient donor; otherwise, anaphylaxis may occur. Multiple myeloma with hypercalcemia and increased plasma protein increases the risk of perioperative renal failure. Preoperative fluid loading and measures to increase intraoperative urine output should be considered. Maintaining body temperature above 35°C is essential in patients with cryoglobinemia, as lower temperatures will cause the precipitation of abnormal immunoglobulins and increase the risk of renal failure. Macroglobulinemia causes hyperviscosity syndrome. Patients with this disease state should receive plasmapheresis before surgery. Patients with hereditary angioneurotic edema develop extensive swelling with even minimal trauma, and there is an increased risk of laryngeal obstruction from edema after intubation. Regional anesthesia should be used in these patients whenever possible.

Recommended Reading

Austen KF. Diseases of immediate type hypersensitivity. In: Braunswald E, Isselbacher KJ, Petersdorf RG, et al, eds. Harrison's principles of internal medicine. 11th ed. New York: McGraw-Hill, 1987:1407.

Buckly RH. Immunodeficiency disease. JAMA 1987;258:2841.

Coombs RRA, Gell PGH. Classification of allergic reactions responsible for clinical hypersensitivity and disease. In: Gell PGH, Coombs RRA, Lachmann PJ, eds. Clinical aspects of immunology. 3rd ed. Oxford: Blackwell Scientific Publications, 1975:761.

Fisher M. Anaphylaxis [review]. Dis Mon 1987;33:433.

Larkin AB, Compton CC, Irwin RS. Immunologic lung disease. In: Rippe JM, Irwin RS, Alpert JS, Dalen JE, eds. Intensive care medicine. Boston: Little, Brown, 1985:515.

Lasser EC, Berry CC, Talner LB, et al. Pretreatment with corticosteroids to alleviate reactions to intravenous contrast material. N Engl J Med 1987;317:845.

Lichtenstein LM. Anaphylaxis. In: Wyngaarden JB, Smith LH Jr, eds. Cecil's textbook of medicine. 18th ed. Philadelphia: WB Saunders, 1988:420.

Moudgil GC. Anesthesia and allergic drug reactions. Can Anaesth Soc J 1986;33:400.

Patten B. Immunohematologic disease. JAMA 1987;258:2945.

Roesch RP. The immune system. In: Stoelting RK, Dierdorf SF, eds. Anesthesia and co-existing disease. New York: Churchill Livingstone, 1983:645.

Sage DJ. Management of acute anaphylactoid reactions. Int Anesthesiol Clin 1985;23(3):175.

Stoelting RK. Allergic reactions during anesthesia. Anesth Analg 1983;62:341.

Walton B. Anesthesia, surgery and immunology. Anesthesiology 1978;33:322.

Wood AJJ, Oates JA. Adverse reactions to drugs. In: Braunswald E, Isselbacher KJ, Petersdorf RG, et al, eds. Harrison's principles of internal medicine. 11th ed. New York: McGraw-Hill, 1987:352.

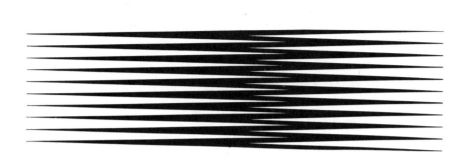

Muscular Connective Tissue Diseases and Malignant Hyperthermia

John Morley

Collagen–vascular and muscular disease states affect many organ systems that will influence anesthetic management. A comprehensive preoperative evaluation and preparation will be required to reduce the risk of intraoperative and postoperative complications. The organ compromise may be directly related to either the progress of the disease or its therapy (e.g., steroids and immunosuppressants).

Muscular Dystrophy

I. DEFINITION
   A. "Muscular dystrophy" refers to a group of inherited primary muscle diseases. Each form of the disease involves degeneration of muscle fibers and an increase in fibrofatty tissue. The patient becomes progressively weaker as the muscle cells are replaced by fatty tissue. The process is painless. Although there have been several theories on the etiology of the muscular dystrophies, it is clear now that there is a defect in one of the genes coding for a protein found on the muscle cell membrane.
   B. There are three forms of muscular dystrophy, each with its own pattern of inheritance, age of onset, severity, and presence or absence of cardiac involvement. The fact that there are multiple names for each form indicates that there are various degrees of penetration of the genetic defect.

II. DUCHENNE TYPE
   A. Duchenne muscular dystrophy (DMD; pseudohypertrophic dystrophy; Becker's dystrophy) occurs in 1 of 3000 live births by X-linked recessive inheritance, making it the most common form of dystrophy. The disease presents in early childhood, but victims are usually asymptomatic up to 6 to 7 years of age.
   B. Clinical Course
      1. These patients have a high incidence of cardiac involvement, affecting both the conducting system and contractility. Dysrhythmias are common, and conduction abnormalities are seen in about 50% of patients. Patients are also predisposed to mitral valve prolapse.
      2. Respiratory muscle weakness leads to restrictive lung disease, which is frequently compounded by the development of scoliosis. Because of the de-

creased muscle strength, seen as poor vital capacity and negative inspiratory force, many patients with DMD are unable to cough adequately to clear secretions. This leads to chronic respiratory infections.

3. Pharyngeal muscle involvement causes difficulty with swallowing and an increased risk of aspiration.

4. Gastrointestinal smooth-muscle involvement predisposes to postoperative gastric dilation that increases the potential for regurgitation and aspiration.

III. OTHER FORMS

A. Facioscapulohumeral muscular dystrophy is an autosomal dominant form. Its onset is in adolescence and begins with the muscles of the face and shoulder. The disease gradually progresses to involve the hips and legs.

B. Limb-girdle dystrophy is an autosomal recessive form presenting in early adulthood.

C. Neither of these forms involves the muscles of breathing or swallowing, and cardiac involvement is rare. Neither condition shortens the life expectancy. Depolarizing muscle relaxants are best avoided, but no special anesthetic modification is necessary.

IV. PREOPERATIVE EVALUATION

A. Pulmonary

1. The majority of patients with DMD presenting for surgery will be children. Particular attention should be paid to the extent of weakness. Patients unable to stand by themselves frequently have a diminished vital capacity and respiratory infections. Forced vital capacity (FVC) should be measured preoperatively. An FVC less than 20 ml/kg or less than 50% of predicted indicates a significant risk of postoperative pulmonary complications.

2. Froese and associates recommend measurement of inspiratory capacity (IC) or "usable VC." An IC of less than 15 ml/kg indicates inability to clear secretions without assistance.

3. Arterial blood gas measurement and a chest roentgenogram are required. Carbon dioxide retention in restrictive lung disease occurs in the end stage, and the patient may require prolonged postoperative mechanical ventilation.

4. Prior to elective surgery, the patient should be in the best possible medical condition. Respiratory infec-

tion must be treated with a full course of antibiotics and chest physiotherapy given to help clear secretions.

B. Cardiac

1. Cardiac function must be evaluated for signs of failure. Tachycardia may be present at rest. Patients with severe cardiac dysfunction may not complain of cardiac symptoms because skeletal muscle atrophy restricts their activity. The same may be true for respiratory symptoms.

2. Typical ECG changes include sinus tachycardia, shortened P-R interval, Q waves in V_{5-6}, and tall R waves in V_1.

3. A radionuclide or sonographic evaluation of cardiac function is helpful in determining the extent of the disease process in patients suspected of having myocardial dysfunction.

V. ANESTHETIC MANAGEMENT

A. Premedication

Premedication should be used cautiously in patients with DMD, because their compromised pulmonary and cardiac status may easily be worsened by sedatives or opioids. Metoclopramide may not accelerate gastric emptying. H_2 blockers will help reduce acidity and, potentially, gastric volume.

B. Induction

1. These patients usually have a delayed gastric emptying time and so must have nothing by mouth for at least 6 hours preoperatively. If any doubt exists as to the volume of gastric contents, either an awake intubation under light sedation and topical anesthesia or a rapid-sequence induction should be performed.

2. Patients with DMD are more susceptible to the cardiac and respiratory depressant effects of induction agents, and careful titration is necessary. Arrhythmias, including ventricular fibrillation and asystole, have occurred during induction.

3. Depolarizing muscle relaxants should be avoided. There have been reports of K^+ release and increased serum levels after use of succinylcholine in DMD patients. For a rapid-sequence induction, nondepolarizing agents are best. However, one must remember that use of a priming dose (1/10th the

intubating dose) may, in advanced disease, compromise the airway and breathing.

C. Maintenance

Just as DMD patients are more sensitive to benzodiazepines, narcotics, and barbiturates, they are more sensitive to potent inhalation agents. Patients have a diminished cardiac reserve and may develop cardiac failure intraoperatively. Tachycardia when the patient is under adequate anesthesia may be an early sign of heart failure.

D. Monitoring

1. Monitoring of the neuromuscular junction is suggested for all patients but is of special concern in DMD patients, as they are very sensitive to nondepolarizing muscle relaxants. Train-of-four (T_1/T_4) should be followed as the muscle relaxant is titrated. The newer short-acting agents are recommended if a muscle relaxant is needed. Ideally, the agent can be timed to terminate its activity with the end of surgery. Buzello and colleagues point out that reversal with anticholinesterase agents in patients with muscle disease is unpredictable and therefore best avoided if possible.

2. Arterial catheterization and a pulmonary artery catheter are often necessary in these patients, who frequently have underlying cardiopulmonary disease.

E. Postoperative Management

1. Owing to their sensitivity to anesthetic drugs, these patients are at increased risk for cardiorespiratory depression postoperatively. First and foremost is the maintenance of an airway and adequate breathing. Prior to terminating mechanical ventilation and to extubation, tidal volume (≥ 5 ml/kg), vital capacity (FVC ≥ 15 ml/kg), and negative inspiratory force (NIF ≥ -25 cmH$_2$O) must be checked for minimal acceptable values. Also, before extubation, the patient should demonstrate an ability to breathe spontaneously through the endotracheal tube without CO_2 retention or hypoxemia on supplemental O_2 (FIo$_2$ ≤ 0.5). In addition, consideration should be given to placement of a nasogastric tube to empty a distended stomach, which could compromise diaphragmatic movement. Wislicki and coworkers have suggested leaving a nasogastric tube in place for all patients nursed in the supine position because of the risk of gastric dilation as late as 48 hours after surgery.

2.   Patients with DMD are not candidates for outpatient surgery. Even those having minor procedures under general anesthesia without muscle relaxants or under regional anesthesia should be admitted overnight. Patients undergoing a long general anesthetic and receiving muscle relaxants should be monitored in an ICU. Particular attention should be paid to postoperative chest physiotherapy, including suctioning and incentive spirometry to assist in the clearance of secretions.

3.   Bush has described a delayed reaction in six patients after general anesthesia consisting of muscle weakness and respiratory failure after an apparent recovery from general anesthesia. Five of the six died. Use of a nondepolarizing muscle relaxant appears to be the only common factor in the anesthesia of these patients.

4.   Patients should be out of bed and walking as soon as possible. This disease progresses more quickly with prolonged bed rest or febrile illness.

VI.   SUMMARY OF ANESTHETIC CONSIDERATIONS

Patients with Duchenne muscular dystrophy often have respiratory trouble from restrictive lung disease and muscular weakness. There is also a high incidence of cardiomyopathy and arrhythmia. Preoperative evaluations should include pulmonary function tests and an echocardiogram or radionuclide scan of the heart.

Preoperative medication should be kept to a minimum because of the underlying cardiopulmonary dysfunction. H_2 agonists will help reduce acidity and gastric volume. Regional anesthesia can be used where appropriate. There is an increased sensitivity to intravenous and inhaled anesthetics, so both groups of drugs must be titrated carefully. Hyperkalemia has been associated with succinylcholine. Short-acting nondepolarizing muscle relaxants should be used in conjunction with a nerve stimulator. Reversal of muscle paralysis with anticholinesterase is unpredictable, and patients must be monitored closely.

Prior to extubation, these patients must exhibit good respiratory muscle strength, tested by measuring FVC and NIF as well as systemic strength. Because of the increased sensitivity to anesthetic drugs, careful observation of the cardiopulmonary status is necessary for the first 24 hours after extubation.

The Myotonias

I.   DEFINITION

Myotonias are a group of hereditary conditions passed on in an autosomal dominant pattern with varying penetration from generation to generation. The three forms are myotonia dystrophica, myotonia congenita, and paramyotonia. All forms are characterized by an inability of skeletal muscle to relax after chemical or physical stimulation. The forms are distinguishable by the age of onset, type of muscle affected, prognosis, and stimulus for contracture. The anesthetic implications are, for the most part, the same as for muscular dystrophy, with some additional considerations, which will be outlined below.

II.   MYOTONIA DYSTROPHICA

    A.   General Characteristics

        1.   Myotonia dystrophica usually presents in early adulthood (although there is a rare form presenting as hypotonia in infancy). The lesion is primarily an atrophy of Type I fibers and hypertrophy of Type II fibers in the early stages.

        2.   The muscle pathology creates both weakness and myotonia. Weakness is more prominent in the cranial and distal muscles.

        3.   The myotonic contractures are of particular concern to anesthesiologists. They can be brought on by acetylcholine, succinylcholine, physical stimulation (i.e., shivering, defasciculation), and cold.

        4.   Contractures in some patients are attenuated by warmth and repetitive movement. Some patients show improvement with quinine, quinidine, or procainamide.

        5.   Contracture will not respond to neural or neuromuscular junction blockade. In other words, regional anesthesia, increasing the concentration of potent inhalation anesthetics, dantrolene, and neuromuscular blockers are of no value in the treatment of myotonia.

B. Cardiopulmonary Involvement
  1. The muscles of breathing are affected, leading to restrictive lung disease. The involved muscle groups include the diaphragm, intercostals, and other accessory muscles.
  2. The sternocleidomastoid and facial muscles are affected earliest. This, along with pharyngeal muscle involvement, predisposes to aspiration and pneumonia.
  3. There is cardiac involvement (contractile fibers and conducting system) beginning early and insidiously.
C. Endocrine and Central Nervous System Function
  1. Male patients often have testicular atrophy.
  2. An abnormal insulin response to glucose is observed even in nondiabetic patients.
  3. Below-average IQ, including mental retardation, is noted in almost 25% of myotonics.
  4. Cataracts and cholelithiasis are more common in myotonics and are frequent indications for surgery.

III. PREOPERATIVE EVALUATION
  A. Cardiac
    1. Cardiac conduction abnormalities are assessed via the ECG. First-degree heart block is the most common finding.
    2. Contractility may be evaluated by assessing the ejection fraction (EF) by echocardiogram or radionuclide scan. Patients with a reduced EF (<40%) should be considered for intraoperative monitoring with a pulmonary artery catheter.
  B. Pulmonary
    Pulmonary function testing is done to look for significant restrictive lung disease: a proportional decrease in FVC and 1-second forced expiratory volume (FEV_1). If the FVC is less than 15 ml/kg or less than 50% of predicted, or the FEV_1/FVC is less than 50%, preparation should be made for long-term postoperative ventilation.

IV. ANESTHETIC CARE
  A. Preoperative Preparation
    1. Preoperative medication is best avoided because of the increased sensitivity to respiratory and cardiovascular depression in myotonia.
    2. Special attention should be given to keeping the patient warm to avoid cold-induced contracture.

The operating room should be warmed before the patient's arrival, and warm humidified anesthetic gases should be utilized.

B. Induction

    1. Titrating the drugs for a slow induction reduces the risk of acute hemodynamic changes.

    2. Depolarizing muscle relaxants must be avoided for several reasons: hyperkalemia, release of myoglobin, and contractures that may prevent adequate ventilation or intubation.

C. Maintenance Anesthesia

    1. Halothane is probably best avoided because of the increased risk of postoperative shivering. Other potent inhalational agents may be used.

    2. There may be an association between this syndrome and malignant hyperthermia (discussed later in this chapter).

    3. Nondepolarizing muscle relaxants may be used but must be monitored closely. Patients with severe myotonia dystrophica are very sensitive to these drugs. Short-acting nondepolarizing muscle relaxants are recommended to avoid use of anticholinesterases, which can induce contractures.

    4. The core temperatures must be maintained in a relatively narrow range, between 36° and 37.8°C.

    5. Myotonia developing intraoperatively is best treated with injection of local anesthetics directly into the abnormally contracted muscles.

V. EMERGENCE AND RECOVERY ROOM CARE

Aside from the special concern for maintaining temperature, the postoperative management is centered on evaluating the airway and breathing muscle strength prior to extubation, much as for DMD.

VI. OTHER MYOTONIAS

A. Myotonia congenita presents at birth with abnormal contractures brought on by sudden movement (intention myotonia), rest, and cold. Swallowing may be affected. Quinidine may be effective. No other organ systems are involved.

B. Paramyotonia is a rare form in which cold is the only stimulus to myotonus. No other organ system is affected. In both paramyotonia and myotonia congenita, anesthetic considerations are similar to those for myotonia dystrophica.

VII. SUMMARY OF ANESTHETIC CONSIDERATIONS
The myotonia of greatest concern is myotonia dystrophica, which is associated with both diffuse muscle weakness and the potential for clonic contractures. Preoperative evaluation is centered on the cardiopulmonary system. Conduction problems can be diagnosed by ECG and contractility by echocardiogram or radionuclide scan. Cardiac ejection fractions of less than 40% indicate limited cardiac reserve, and intraoperative monitoring should include an intra-arterial and pulmonary artery catheter. Pulmonary function tests showing severe restrictive disease suggest that postoperative mechanical ventilation will be needed.

Induction and maintenance anesthetic medications are directed at minimizing cardiac depression and preventing contractures. All anesthetics must be titrated slowly and blood pressure and pulse rate watched carefully. Depolarizing muscle relaxants must be avoided, as should situations that decrease the patient's temperature and cause shivering. If contractures are triggered by stress, pain, cold, or fasciculation, direct intramuscular injection of local anesthetics is the most effective treatment. Intravenous quinine is reported to decrease contractures. Postoperatively, patients must be kept warm and any shivering immediately treated. The patient is extubated only when fully awake and demonstrating good respiratory muscle strength.

Familial Periodic Paralysis

I. GENERAL CHARACTERISTICS
Familial periodic paralysis is an inherited disorder involving alterations in the ratio of extracellular to intracellular K^+. There are three forms, distinguished by an increased, decreased, or normal serum K^+ (hyperkalemic, hypokalemic, or normokalemic familial periodic paralysis). Each is passed on in an autosomal dominant pattern, but penetrance varies.

II. TYPES
    A. Hypokalemic
        1. Hypokalemic familial periodic paralysis was first described in 1882. It presents as attacks of muscle weakness, potentially quadriplegia, lasting from a few hours up to days. Rarely, attacks affect breathing and swallowing.

2. There are reports of patients dying from aspiration or respiratory or cardiac failure. These patients are especially sensitive to even very small changes in the serum K^+ level. They become weak at K^+ levels of 3.0 mEq/L and show ECG changes earlier than normal.

3. Anything that shifts K^+ intracellularly can potentiate an attack. This includes hyperventilation, glucose, insulin, beta-agonists, corticosteroids, and thyroxine. There is an association between thyrotoxicosis and hypokalemic periodic paralysis in Asians.

4. Acetazolamide is the treatment of choice, as it promotes acidosis, which reduces the hypokalemia.

B. Hyperkalemic

1. Attacks of weakness in hyperkalemic periodic paralysis are caused by a release of K^+ from muscle cells. Weakness frequently begins with the muscles of the back and spreads down to the thighs and calves and then to the arms and hands.

2. Attacks are most frequently brought on during a rest after strenuous exercise. They can be prevented by exercise and a gradual cool down period.

3. Unlike hypokalemic periodic paralysis, in which attacks can last for days, attacks of hyperkalemic periodic paralysis rarely extend longer than 1 hour.

4. Patients are especially sensitive to increases in K^+. A serum K^+ of 5.0 mEq/L can cause weakness, and above 7 mEq/L, paralysis develops. A high-Na^+, high-carbohydrate, and low-K^+ diet can help prevent attacks.

C. Normokalemic

1. Normokalemic paralysis is the rarest form of the syndrome. Attacks can occur in response to alcohol, cold, stress, or strenuous exercise. Whereas arrhythmias may occur in the other forms, they are common in the normokalemic form.

2. Suggested therapy includes a high Na^+ intake for paralysis, quinidine for arrhythmias, and acetazolamide to stabilize K^+ levels.

3. Anesthetic management, much as for the other types of familial periodic paralysis, involves prevention of cold and stress and avoiding neuromuscular blockers whenever possible. If muscle relaxants are

necessary, short-acting nondepolarizing agents should be used to monitor the effects on neuromuscular function.

III. SUMMARY OF ANESTHETIC CONSIDERATIONS

Muscle weakness is the principal characteristic of familial periodic paralysis. The weakness can cause failure of the myocardium and muscles of breathing.

Preoperatively, minimizing stress decreases attack rates. Also, manipulating intravenous sodium and glucose delivery can affect the attack rate. A high sodium intake helps prevent attacks of hyperkalemic and normokalemic periodic paralysis, whereas a low sodium intake decreases attacks of hypokalemic periodic paralysis. A high carbohydrate load will decrease attacks of hyperkalemic periodic paralysis but can increase attacks of the hypokalemic type. Acetazolamide is used in all three types of periodic paralysis to stabilize serum K^+ concentrations.

Perioperative laboratory assessment must include serial measurement of serum glucose and K^+. Intraoperatively, neuromuscular blockers should be avoided whenever possible. If muscle relaxants are used, a nerve stimulator is required to monitor neuromuscular function. If an attack does occur, airway control must be established. Other treatment includes acetazolamide, changing carbohydrate and Na^+ load, and quinidine for arrhythmias.

Glycogen Storage Diseases

I. GENERAL CHARACTERISTICS

Glycogen is a branched-chain polysaccharide stored in liver and muscle. The Cori classification is based on the missing enzyme and organ system(s) affected (Table 12-1). These hereditary disorders (autosomal recessive) are characterized by the absence or abnormality of a single enzyme in the metabolic pathway of glycogen breakdown. The disorders of primary concern affect cardiac and skeletal muscle function.

II. CORI CLASSIFICATION

    A. Cori II (Pompe's)

        Pompe's disease affects the skeletal and cardiac muscle. Two forms are known: infantile and adult. The infantile form presents with hypotonia and cardiomyopathy and is rapidly progressive: patients often do not survive beyond

Table 12–1. Cori Classification of Glycogen Storage Diseases

Type		Enzymatic Defect	Organs Affected
II	(Pompe's)	α-1,4-glucosidase	Skeletal and cardiac muscle
III	(Cori's, Forbes')	Amylo-1,6-glucosidase	Liver, skeletal, and cardiac muscle and blood cells
IV	(Andersen's)	Branching enzyme	Liver, skeletal, and cardiac muscle and blood cells
V	(McArdle's)	Muscle phosphorylase	Muscle
VII	(Thompson's)	Phosphofructokinase	Muscle
VIII	(Tarin's)	Hepatic phosphorylase kinase	Muscle and red blood cells

age 2. The chest radiograph shows cardiomyopathy with a globular heart. Left-axis deviation on ECG is frequent in early infancy. The heart is often three to four times normal size. The adult form follows a more benign course with long-term survival. No therapy is available for either form.

B. Cori III (Forbes')

Mild hypotonia and weakness is seen in Forbes' disease because of the limited glycogen deposition. Cardiac involvement is rarely clinically significant. The primary problems are hepatomegaly, retarded growth, and fasting hypoglycemia.

C. Cori IV (Andersen's)

Muscle involvement in Andersen's disease is mild. However, the liver becomes cirrhotic at an early age, with large amounts of unmetabolizable glycogen in storage.

D. Cori V (McArdle's)

The Cori V type primarily involves skeletal muscle, in which changes are severe. There is a single case report, by Ratinov et al., describing a patient with McArdle's disease and ECG changes. The disease presents in childhood with muscle pain and weakness. Exercise may induce contractures that are relieved by rest. Progressive deterioration eventually leads to muscle atrophy in the fifth decade. Depolarizing muscle relaxants should be avoided because of the risk of myoglobinuria, which may be manifested as a decrease in urine output and burgundy discoloration or be diagnosed only by direct testing of urine. Mannitol or other diuretics may be necessary to maintain a urine output of at least 1.5 ml/kg (if preload and cardiac output are adequate) to clear the myoglobin and minimize renal tubular toxicity.

E.   Cori VII (Thompson's)
The Cori VII type consists of mild myopathy with episodic contracture of the calf muscles. No special anesthetic care is indicated.

F.   Cori VIII (Tarin's)
There is involvement of both skeletal muscle and erythrocytes in Tarin's disease. It is similar in presentation and prognosis to Cori V.

III.   SUMMARY OF ANESTHETIC CONSIDERATIONS
Each specific disorder affects different organs to a different extent. Generally, careful workup of the cardiac, renal, and hepatobiliary systems is needed preoperatively.

There are no special anesthetic considerations for these diseases, but attention to two important factors will decrease perioperative morbidity. First, any stimulus that can increase serum myoglobin, such as depolarizing muscle relaxants, must be avoided to reduce the incidence of postoperative renal failure. Second, a glucose infusion must be used to provide a constant energy substrate, because glycogen metabolism is abnormal.

Malignant Hyperthermia

I.   GENERAL CHARACTERISTICS
A.   Malignant hyperthermia (MH) is a hypermetabolic state that develops in susceptible individuals in response to a triggering event (such as physical or emotional stress or a specific drug). Susceptibility is genetically determined and inherited in what is probably an autosomal dominant pattern with variable penetrance.
B.   The specific defect involves the Ca^{2+} stored in sarcoplasmic reticulum, which is used to link excitation of the muscle membrane to contraction. The normal reuptake of Ca^{2+} that terminates contraction does not occur, and the sustained muscle contracture results in the hypermetabolic state manifested as increased O_2 consump-

tion, increased CO_2 production, rapidly rising temperature, and respiratory and metabolic acidosis. Ventricular arrhythmias are common. The earliest indicator, resulting from the increased CO_2 production, is either an increase in end-tidal CO_2 in patients paralyzed and on a set minute ventilation (MV) or a large increase in MV in a spontaneously breathing patient.

C. The most frequent triggering agents are potent inhalation anesthetics and depolarizing neuromuscular blockers. Other triggering agents include the amide local anesthetics in large volumes. Use of small volumes of lidocaine for muscle biopsy or dental procedures is accepted as safe.

D. Masseter muscle rigidity (MMR) may occur during induction. Although this has been associated with MH, it is very nonspecific. MMR can develop in patients with myotonia (a condition frequently undiagnosed before age 25), muscular dystrophy, polymyositis, and amyotrophic lateral sclerosis. It has also occurred in some patients without apparent muscle pathology when succinylcholine is given in the presence of halothane. Distinguishing MMR from MH may be difficult initially, but when doubt exists, the reaction should be treated as MH.

II. RISK FACTORS AND PROPHYLAXIS

A. Patients at risk for MH include those with central core disease, muscular dystrophy, myotonia dystrophica, scoliosis, strabismus, musculoskeletal abnormalities, or creatine phosphokinase (CPK) values above 20,000 IU. MH is most common in males aged 3 to 30 years.

B. High-risk patients are given prophylactic dantrolene preoperatively.

    1. Oral administration is no longer recommended because of unreliable absorption.

    2. Dantrolene (1–2 mg/kg) is best given IV prior to surgery under direct observation.

    3. Patients with primary muscle disorders and decreased muscular function have been reported to be especially sensitive to the muscle relaxant effects of dantrolene, and respiratory failure has been reported after as little as 2 mg/kg.

    4. The half-life of dantrolene is approximately 6 to 8 hours. Patients receiving prophylaxis should receive a second dose intravenously in cases lasting more than 6 hours. Patients who develop MH should be maintained on dantrolene for three or four doses of 1 to 2 mg/kg each after all symptoms have subsided.

III.   TREATMENT

A.   When suspicion of MH arises, as when MMR occurs, all potential triggering agents (i.e., volatile anesthetics) should be discontinued and the patient given 100% O_2. A period of close observation follows to see if any more signs develop, such as increasing end-tidal CO_2 and temperature. Arterial blood gases should be followed for signs of acidosis.

B.   If the temperature and end-tidal CO_2 remain normal or stabilize after a small increase for 15 to 20 minutes, it is possible to continue surgery, but a high degree of suspicion for MH should be maintained throughout the case. On the other hand, if it is still not clear in 15 to 20 minutes, elective cases should be stopped and drug therapy initiated.

C.   Patients in whom the temperature rises 1°C in 15 minutes or with a rapid increase in end tidal CO_2 above 60 mmHg, leaving little doubt of the diagnosis, are immediately started on dantrolene at 2 mg/kg IV. The dose is repeated every 5 minutes until either the trend reverses or a maximum dose of 10 mg/kg is reached.

D.   Additional treatment includes benzodiazepines and muscle relaxants. Benzodiazepines are used to sedate the patient and reduce anxiety-induced stress; paralysis improves ventilatory control over the patient and helps reduce O_2 consumption. Vecuronium can provide complete neuromuscular blockage without the tachycardia seen with pancuronium or the hypotension associated with the histamine released in response to curare-like drugs.

E.   Patients should be ventilated to maintain the PCO_2 below 40 mmHg and given bicarbonate to treat a base excess below -5 mEq/L.

F.   Although dantrolene is the definitive treatment and should be given early, fever is also a significant concern. Intravenous fluids should be iced, the external body surface cooled, and body cavities (bladder, stomach, peritoneum and, perhaps, even pleura) lavaged with iced sterile fluids. Shivering in response to attempts at cooling can be a severe problem but is prevented by paralyzing the patient.

G. Ventricular ectopy is common and should be controlled with procainamide.

IV. MONITORING

A. Continuous hemodynamic monitoring during therapy is required, because large shifts in fluid, with changes in blood pressure, occur rapidly.

B. Urinary output should be maintained above 1 ml/kg per hour to hasten excretion of potential nephrotoxins such as myoglobin, free hemoglobin, or hemoglobin stroma.

    1. If urine output drops, ventricular filling pressures should be optimized.

    2. Thereafter, a diuretic such as mannitol (0.25–1.0 g/kg) may be needed to maintain urine output).

C. Electrolytes, glucose, liver enzymes, partial thromboplastin time, prothrombin time, fibrinogen, fibrin split products, hemoglobin, and platelets need to be followed and abnormalities corrected.

D. If MH develops during an emergency case, the anesthetic technique must be modified. The most important concerns are the total avoidance of the potent inhalation anesthetics (ideally, there is an anesthetic machine available for MH cases that never had a volatile anesthetic running through it) and of other triggering agents (depolarizing muscle relaxants) and the administration of dantrolene with 100% oxygen. Narcotics with a benzodiazepine will provide analgesia and amnesia without triggering or sustaining MH.

V. SUMMARY OF ANESTHETIC CONSIDERATIONS

Patients with documented malignant hyperthermia or at high risk should receive IV dantrolene 1 to 2 mg/kg prior to surgery. If the anesthetic is long, subsequent doses should be given at 6-hour intervals until the end of surgery. Oral prophylaxis is not recommended because of unreliable absorption.

Intraoperatively, oxygenation and ventilation should be done with an anesthetic machine that has not been exposed to inhalation anesthetics. Succinylcholine must also be avoided. General anesthetic can be provided safely with benzodiazepines, opiates, and nondepolarizing muscle relaxants. Regional anesthesia may be performed with ester-type local anesthetic or small amounts of amide-type local anesthetics.

Despite all precautions, malignant hyperthermia may occur. Intravenous dantrolene should be given immediately in 2-mg/kg boluses every 5 minutes until the hyperthermia or acidosis reverses or a maximum dose of 10 mg/kg has been reached. Cooling measures include infusion of cooled IV fluids and body cavity lavage with iced sterile fluids. Ventricular ectopy is common, and procainamide is the effective treatment. Because of the hemodynamic lability and the need for frequent blood gas analysis and fluid challenges, arterial and central venous catheter placement is necessary. Patients who develop malignant hyperthermia should be maintained on dantrolene for three or four doses of 1 to 2 mg/kg after all symptoms have subsided.

Rheumatoid Arthritis

I.   GENERAL ASPECTS
Rheumatoid arthritis (RA) is a systemic disease originating from a defect in the immune system. The onset is usually between ages 20 and 40 years. It occurs in women three times more frequently than in men. Rheumatoid factor is neither 100% sensitive nor specific diagnostically. Diagnosis is based on a constellation of signs and symptoms and is difficult because classic adult RA probably is not a single disease and almost certainly does not have a single etiology.

II.   SYSTEMIC MANIFESTATONS
    A. Musculoskeletal
Classically, the hands and wrists are involved. Carpal (or tarsal) tunnel syndrome is frequently seen. It is the frequent cervical spine involvement that is of most concern, as it may be associated with neurologic complications. Atlantoaxial subluxation can create a separation of the atlas from the odontoid process. This separation, which can be 3 mm or greater, may allow the odontoid process to protrude through the foramen magnum, compressing the vertebral arteries, the medulla, or both. This potential problem usually is easy to see on a lateral roentgenogram during flexion. Erosion of the dens often develops and reduces the risk of compression of neurovascular structures.
    B. Cardiac
        1. Granulomas, inflammation of the myocardium or endocardium, or fibrosis of the valves are not infrequent. Evidence of inflammation and rheumatoid granulomas may be seen on the ECG as intra-

ventricular conduction delay or heart block. Amyloidosis, one of the many potential complications of RA, can affect the conducting system as well as myocardial contractility.

2. Pericardial involvement (inflammation, effusion, thickening) is a major concern. Tamponade or constriction can result in presentation to the OR for pericardiectomy.

C. Pulmonary

The lungs are commonly affected in patients with severe RA. Pleural effusions may even be the presenting manifestation of rheumatoid disease. Rheumatoid nodules can invade both parenchyma and pleura. Radiographs commonly show abnormalities, but pulmonary symptoms often develop much later or not at all. In rare cases, the patient has severe symptoms of restrictive lung disease.

D. Vascular

1. Patients with severe disease and high rheumatoid factor levels are prone to develop vasculitis, which, in turn, can affect all organ systems (myocardial, cerebral or bowel infarction, skin ulcerations, mononeuritis multiplex).

2. Vasculitis of the vessels supplying nerves can cause severe and irreversible damage. Both sensory and motor loss occurs. Weakness at affected joints without sensory loss is common but generally secondary to primary muscle involvement.

E. Hematologic

1. Hematologic abnormalities include anemia, leukopenia (when associated with splenomegaly, it is known as Felty's syndrome), and thrombocytopenia (rarely severe).

2. The leukopenia–neutropenia predisposes to infection, especially when skin ulceration is present. Rheumatoid joints are a potential source of sepsis because the signs of infective arthritis are masked by the chronic inflammation of RA.

III. DRUG THERAPY

A. Anti-inflammatory Drugs

The initial treatment utilizes anti-inflammatory drugs (salicylates and nonsteroidal anti-inflammatory agents, which reduce both inflammation and pain). Unfortunately, in the doses usually required, gastric irritation or even ulceration is not uncommon, which can exacerbate the anemia of RA.

B. Immunosuppressants

  1. Steroids are generally the next step. The potent immunosuppression they cause often provides great relief to severely arthritic patients. However, the side effects may be significant enough to necessitate withdrawal of the drug. Problems include predisposition to infection (especially fungal), hypertension, hyperglycemia, osteoporosis and aseptic necrosis of the femoral head, thinning of the skin, and gastric ulceration.

  2. More potent immunosuppressants, such as methotrexate, cyclophosphamide, and azathioprine, are used in the most severely affected patients who have not responded to other treatments. Although patients often improve, side effects are common and potentially critical. Older patients and those with kidney or liver disease are most susceptible to side effects such as hepatic toxicity, anemia or pancytopenia (secondary to bone marrow suppression), and development of malignancy.

C. Treatment with gold salts can induce remission of symptoms. The response ranges from remission with minor side effects to no response but serious side effects. Toxicity includes bone marrow depression (leukopenia, thrombocytopenia, or pancytopenia) and skin rashes, which can be mild or exfoliative.

D. D-Penicillamine is another drug for the severely affected rheumatoid patient. Not only does it reduce inflammation throughout the body, but it reduces the noninflammatory components of the disease in other organ systems. However, side effects are particularly toxic and potentially worse than the primary disease. They include leukopenia, thrombocytopenia, pancytopenia, proteinuria, stomatitis, gastritis, and others. Penicillamine is also listed as a rare cause of a number of other syndromes such as systemic lupus erythematosus, polymyositis, and Goodpasture's syndrome.

IV. OTHER THERAPY

Other therapy not involving drugs has included surgery, plasmapheresis, and radiation of lymphoid tissue. Surgery can be useful in the initial stages. Synovectomy reduces pain and prevents or reduces the intensity of the advancing synovitis. In the later stages, patients present to the OR for prosthetic joint replacement. Plasmapheresis and radiation of lymphoid tissue have not been proved effective and are no longer being used.

V. PREOPERATIVE EVALUATION
  A. Airway
     1. Patients with advanced disease may be unable to open their mouths more than 1 to 2 cm because of temporomandibular joint involvement.
     2. The cervical spine can be involved in any of several ways, including subaxial subluxation, atlantoaxial instability, and vertical migration of the dens. The neck can become shortened and cause a scoliotic deformity of the larynx and trachea. The change in position of the larynx makes direct laryngoscopy and even fiberoptic laryngoscopy more difficult, if not impossible.
     3. Both atlantoaxial subluxation and subaxial subluxation cause an instability of the cervical spine, predisposing to spinal cord compression and paralysis.
     4. Involvement of the cricoarytenoid joint occurs in about 25% of severely rheumatoid patients and can cause glottic narrowing.
     5. All of these factors in any patient with rheumatoid disease creates a high risk of airway complications. With only a few exceptions, almost all patients with RA should have preoperative flexion and extension roentgenograms of the cervical spine.
  B. Pulmonary
       Additional preoperative evaluation of the rheumatoid patient, especially one with respiratory symptoms or an abnormal chest radiograph, includes pulmonary function testing and arterial blood gas analysis. Patients with abnormal test results are more susceptible to respiratory failure in the postoperative period and will require closer attention for an extended period of time. Rheumatoid patients are especially susceptible to interstitial pneumonia. Patients should be advised of the potential need for postoperative mechanical ventilation.
  C. Cardiac
       The ECG may show evidence of left ventricular hypertrophy or dysrhythmias. Patients with an abnormal ECG or symptoms potentially related to cardiac function should undergo echocardiographic studies. This will define wall thickness, diagnose hypertrophic cardiomyopathy or valvular dysfunction, and evaluate ejection fraction. Those with hypertrophic disease or ejection fraction of less than 40% should be considered for pulmonary artery catheter-

ization, especially for long anesthetics or when large fluid shifts are anticipated.

D. Hepatic and Renal

Both liver and renal function can be compromised by amyloidosis or drug therapy, and this should be taken into consideration when selecting anesthetic drugs.

E. Immunologic

These patients have severe compromise of the immune system from their primary disease state or therapy. Total white count; the proportion of neutrophils, lymphocytes, and immature polymorphonuclear cells in the total white count; and skin testing can provide information about the function of the immune system.

VI. SUMMARY OF ANESTHETIC CONSIDERATIONS

Prior to anesthesia and surgery on patients with RA, the airway and pulmonary and cardiac status must be evaluated thoroughly. Cervical neck instability, scoliotic deformity of the larynx and trachea, and limited mouth opening frequently complicate airway management. Excessive flexion and extension of the neck must be avoided. Direct laryngoscopy for intubation is difficult or impossible because of the anterior displacement of the larynx and the limited mouth opening. Awake fiberoptic intubation is a good method to secure the airway.

Evidence of pericardial disease from echocardiography or of significant pulmonary dysfunction from pulmonary function tests necessitates invasive arterial pressure monitoring. If intravascular volume assessment is needed, a pulmonary artery catheter should be used, because the central venous pressure will not be an accurate reflection of left-sided filling pressure.

Aseptic technique for any procedures is especially important because of the immune suppression from the primary disease state and many of the treatment medications.

If the intubation is difficult, extubation should not occur until the patient is fully awake and able to protect the airway.

Progressive Systemic Sclerosis

I. CLINICAL PRESENTATION

Progressive systemic sclerosis (PSS) is a true collagen disease in which excess fibrous connective tissue may be deposited in almost any organ system. Three forms occur, which are distinguished by the organs involved: scleroderma, involving just skin; CREST: calcinosis, Raynaud's phenomenon, esophageal hypomotility, scleroderma, and telangiectasis; and diffuse, with cardiac, pulmonary, or renal involvement alone or in combination. All three forms have anesthetic implications, but only when there is diffuse organ involvement is the prognosis uniformly poor.

II. COMPLICATIONS

    A. In scleroderma, the most obvious change is the fibrotic thickening of the face, fingers, and hands. Thickening of the facial skin can prevent jaw opening, making rigid laryngoscopy impossible.

    B. The CREST syndrome includes those changes in the skin plus calcinosis, telangiectasis, and vascular and esophageal involvement.

        1. Esophageal dysfunction with low esophageal sphincter tone and intestinal hypomotility increases the risk of regurgitation and aspiration. Also, intestinal involvement predisposes to dilation and obstruction and may reduce the absorption of fat-soluble vitamins. Inadequate amounts of vitamin K-dependent coagulation factors prevent adequate clotting.

        2. Narrowing of the arteries and arterioles and intermittent vasospasm with or without obvious Raynaud's phenomenon increases the risk of complications from invasive monitoring of blood pressure.

    C. Diffuse PSS has serious consequences, and, unfortunately, there is no therapy available.

        1. Arthritis, similar to rheumatoid but milder, can develop.

        2. Myopathy, similar to polymyositis, may occur; and skeletal muscle involvement is often associated with cardiac muscle involvement. When cardiac muscle is replaced by fibrous tissue, patients progress from conduction abnormalities to arrhythmias and, finally, intractable congestive heart failure. Small arterioles in the heart are often affected and may cause ischemia. Pericarditis and pericardial effusions have been reported.

        3. Pulmonary hypertension is common. Most often, pulmonary hypertension or interstitial fibrosis develops chronically, but it may be acute, fulminant, and rapidly fatal.

        4. Manifestation of renal involvement is usually limited to mild to moderate hypertension and proteinuria. Occasionally, the hypertension is malignant and does not respond well to pharmacologic therapy.

III. SUMMARY OF ANESTHETIC CONSIDERATIONS

Preoperatively, it should be established, whenever possible, which form of PSS the patient has and the degree of progression. Pulmonary function testing and baseline arterial blood gas data are required. Echocardiography is a noninvasive help in evaluating cardiac function. An inability to open the mouth at least 3.5 cm is an indication for awake (but sedated, topicalized, and breathing spontaneously) fiberoptic intubation.

Pulmonary artery catheterization provides specific and sensitive information on pulmonary pressures. This procedure should be done preoperatively in the hope of optimizing hemodynamics, especially of the pulmonary circulation, prior to anesthetic induction in patients with cor pulmonale or congestive cardiomyopathy. Intravenous nitroglycerin may help in reducing elevated pulmonary artery pressures. When arterial pressures are to be monitored, catheters should be placed in the central circulation; i.e. femoral or axillary arteries. Peripheral venous access is almost always difficult, and patients may require central vein cannulation.

Pregnancy deserves special consideration, as it exacerbates PSS in almost 50% of patients. Epidural anesthesia is contraindicated in patients with severe pulmonary hypertension, because a drop in peripheral resistance (sympathetic block) can reduce perfusion pressures to a critical level. Some of these patients may also have a coagulopathy, contraindicating any regional anesthetic. Normal spaces (and potential spaces) may be greatly reduced in PSS patients because of the dense excess collagen and taut overlying skin. (A case of acute ischemia has been reported after 5 ml of local anesthetic was injected into the wrist.) Regional analgesia (intrathecal and epidural narcotics) shows significant promise for reducing pain during labor (Stage I) but is of less value for delivery (Stage II). Patients with diffuse PSS have a very high perinatal mortality rate.

Systemic Lupus Erythematosus

I. GENERAL CHARACTERISTICS

Systemic lupus erythematosus (SLE) is a disease of the immune system and is regarded as one of the great masqueraders.

It affects all organ systems and can present as virtually any symptom or sign, including arthritis, fever, purpura, psychosis, seizure, chest pain, edema (nephrotic syndrome), infection (bacterial, viral, or fungal), and rash. Nine of ten patients are female. The course can be limited and benign or fulminant and fatal. Almost all patients have arthralgias, arthritis, and fever.

II. MULTISYSTEM ORGAN INVOLVEMENT
   A. Pulmonary
      Pulmonary involvement is common. The severity may range from an uncomplicated pleuritis to pulmonary infarction or pneumonia. Interstitial pneumonitis can develop chronically, causing restrictive lung disease.
   B. Cardiac
      The pericardium is the cardiac structure most commonly involved, either simple inflammation or with a small effusion (rarely tamponade unless there is a significant coagulopathy). Myocarditis can develop, manifesting as an arrhythmia or heart failure. Valvular involvement can include noninfectious endocarditis, subacute bacterial endocarditis, mitral stenosis and insufficiency, or aortic stenosis and insufficiency.
   C. Renal
      Patients characteristically have some degree of kidney disease, ranging from mild proteinuria and hematuria to nephrotic syndrome (membranous glomerulonephritis) to end-stage renal failure (diffuse proliferative nephritis).
   D. Neurologic
      Almost half of all patients manifest neurologic symptoms, most often depression and personality changes, although psychosis can be seen. Neurologic symptoms can be temporary and rapidly reversed when secondary to vasospasm, but when caused by cerebral hemorrhage are often permanent. Seizures, both focal and grand mal (including status epilepticus), can occur and may not respond to the usual antiseizure medications. Treatment of the underlying vasculitis will reverse most neurologic symptoms; however, the high doses of steroids that may be required also can induce psychosis.
   E. Hematologic
      Some of the more characteristic problems of SLE occur in coagulation. First is thrombocytopenia, which may be mild or severe but rarely causes problems if the platelet count is above 50,000 mm^3 unless there is another clotting defect. Antibodies can react with and lower clotting

proteins (especially factors VIII and IX). A particularly interesting antibody, known as lupus anticoagulant, reacts with a portion of the prothrombinase molecule, increasing the partial thromboplastin time (PTT). What makes the lupus anticoagulant interesting is the fact that although the PTT is altered (an in vitro phenomenon), the antibody does not create a bleeding diathesis in vivo. In fact, patients with the lupus anticoagulant have a predisposition to thrombosis.

F.   Other potential components to the SLE syndrome include Sjögren's sicca (dry mouth and eyes from lymphocytic infiltration of salivary and lacrimal glands) as well as a myopathy with CPK elevation and muscle degeneration very similar to polymyositis.

III.   SUMMARY OF ANESTHETIC CONSIDERATIONS

Patients whose only sign of SLE is a butterfly-shaped rash on the face offer no special problems to the anesthesiologist. In the asymptomatic patient, a physical examination, ECG, and chest radiograph may be all the workup necessary to exclude significant disease. However, any abnormality on the ECG or chest radiograph should be followed up with echocardiography to rule out endocarditis or valvular disease or with pulmonary function testing, respectively. In patients with end-stage renal failure, drugs such as pancuronium of which the majority is excreted by the kidney should be used with extra care or not at all when alternatives are available. When myopathy and elevated CPK are present, the following rules are suggested: avoid depolarizing muscle relaxants, reduce the dose of nondepolarizing muscle relaxants, and monitor the neuromuscular junction closely with a peripheral nerve stimulator. Coagulation must be checked and platelets transfused if the count is less than 50,000/mm^3. When the thrombocytopenia is a result of antibodies and platelet destruction, the transfusion should be given within 1 hour of surgery. Even with immediate preoperative platelet transfusion, it may not be possible to raise the platelet count significantly. Emergency or urgent (splenectomy) surgery should proceed despite refractory thrombocytopenia. Anemia should be treated with transfusion up to a hematocrit of at least 30%. Abnormalities of the prothrombin times and partial thromboplastin times (lupus anticoagulant) should be discussed with the rheumatologist or hematologist involved in the patient's care. Patients with both restrictive lung disease and myopathy are at very high risk for postoperative mechanical ventilation, and they should be forewarned.

Recommended Reading

Aldridge LM. Anaesthetic problems in myotonic dystrophy: a case report and review of the Aberdeen experience comprising 48 general anaesthetics in a further 16 patients. Br J Anaesth 1985;57:1119.

Azar I. The response of patients with neuromuscular disorders to muscle relaxants: a review. Anesthesiology 1984;61:173.

Bernstein RL, Rosenberg AD. Anesthesia for orthopedic surgery. Semin Anesth 1987;6(1):36.

Berry FA. Clinical update in pediatric anesthesia. IRS Rev Course 1987:69.

Boheimer N, Harris JW, Ward S. Neuromuscular blockade in dystrophia myotonica with atracurium besylate. Anaesthesia 1985;40:872.

Buzello W, Krieg N, Schlickewei A. Hazards of neostigmine in patients with neuromuscular disorders: report of two cases. Br J Anaesth 1982;54:529.

Coaldrake LA, Livingstone P. Myasthenia gravis in pregnancy. Anesth Intens Care 1983;11:254.

Ellis FR. Inherited muscle disease. Br J Anaesth 1980;52:153.

Graham DH. Monitoring neuromuscular block may be unreliable in patients with upper-motor-neuron lesions. Anesthesiology 1980;52:74.

Grossman A, Martin JR, Root HS. Rheumatoid arthritis of the cricoarytenoid joint. Laryngoscope 1961;71:530.

Hodgkinson R. Anesthetic management of a parturient with severe juvenile rheumatoid arthritis. Anesth Analg 1981;60:611.

Johns RA, Finholt DA, Stirt JA. Anaesthetic management of a child with dermatomyositis. Can Anaeth Soc J 1986;33:71.

Kaufman J, Friedman JM, Sadowsky D, et al. Myotonic dystrophy: surgical and anesthetic considerations during orthognathic surgery. J Oral Maxillofac Surg 1983;41:667.

Keenan MA, Stiles CM, Kaufman RL. Acquired laryngeal deviation associated with cervical spine disease in erosive polyarticular arthritis: use of the fiberoptic bronchoscope in rheumatoid disease. Anesthesiology 1983;58:441.

McLeod ME, Creighton RE. Anesthesia for pediatric neurological and neuromuscular diseases. J Child Neurol 1986;1:189.

Melnick B, Chang JL, Larson CE, et al. Hypokalemic familial periodic paralysis. Anesthesiology 1983;58:263.

Milne B, Rosales JK. Anaesthetic considerations in patients with muscular dystrophy undergoing spinal fusion and Harrington rod insertion. Can Anaesth Soc J 1982;29:250.

Mora CT, Eisenkraft JB, Papatestas AE. Intravenous dantrolene in a patient with myasthenia gravis. Anesthesiology 1986;64:371.

Mudge BJ, Taylor PB, Vanderspek AFL. Perioperative hazards in myotonic dystrophy. Anaesthesia 1980;35:492.

Neill RS. Progressive systemic sclerosis: prolonged sensory blockade following regional anaesthesia in association with a reduced response to systemic analgesics. Br J Anaesth 1980;52:623.

Oka S, Igaraski Y, Takagi A, et al. Malignant hyperpyrexia and Duchenne muscular dystrophy: a case report. Can Anaesth Soc J 1982;29:627.

Perloff JK, Roberts WC, DeLeon AC Jr, et al. The distinctive electrocardiogram in Duchenne's progressive muscular dystrophy. Am J Med 1967;42:179.

Person DA. Juvenile rheumatoid arthritis: anesthetic and surgical considerations. AORN J 1986;44:439.

Phelps JA. Laryngeal obstruction due to cricoarytenoid arthritis. Anesthesiology 1966;27:518.

Phillips DC, Ellis FR, Exley A, et al. Dantrolene sodium and dystrophia myotonica. Anaesthesia 1984;39:568.

Ravin M, Newmark Z, Saviello G. Myotonia dystrophica—an anesthetic hazard: two case reports. Anesth Analg Curr Res 1974;54:216.

Roelofse JA, Shipton EA. Anaesthesia in connective tissue disorders. S Afr Med Times 1985;67:336.

Sethna NF, Rockoff MA. Cardiac arrest following inhalation induction of anaesthesia in a child with Duchenne's muscular dystrophy. Can Anaesth Soc J 1986;33:799.

Sinclair JR, Mason RA. Ankylosing spondylitis: the case for awake intubation. Anaesthesia 1984;39:3.

Smith CL, Bush GH. Anaesthesia and progressive muscular dystrophy. Br J Anaesth 1985;57:1113.

Thompson J, Conklin KA. Anesthetic management of a pregnant patient with scleroderma. Anesthesiology 1983;59:69.

Wang JM, Stanley TH. Duchenne muscular dystrophy and malignant hyperthermia: two case reports. Can Anaesth Soc J 1986;33:492.

Weber S. Caudal anesthesia complicated by intraosseous injection in a patient with ankylosing spondylitis. Anesthesiology 1985;63:716.

Younker D, Harrison B. Scleroderma and pregnancy: anaesthetic considerations. Br J Anaesth 1985;57:1136.

CHAPTER 13

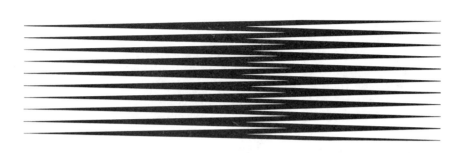

Psychiatric Problems

≡ Psychiatric Disorders and Their Treatment

J. David Haddox

Psychiatric disorders are common in the general surgical population, although the severity and type may vary widely. Important anesthetic considerations are the effect of anesthetics on existing psychiatric disorders, their interactions with drugs used in psychiatric treatment, and their ability to elicit psychiatric signs and symptoms even in patients with no psychiatric history. Psychiatric problems may manifest in a wide range of ways, from acute (e.g., the intoxicated patient with a metacarpal fracture) to chronic (e.g., the institutionalized schizophrenic taking chlorpromazine and benztropine who presents with a bowel obstruction). The objectives of this chapter are to review the salient features of some of the more common mental and behavioral disorders and to provide practical information on how they affect anesthetic management.

Disorders

I. GENERAL CONSIDERATIONS
    Several fundamental principles are noteworthy in the anesthetic care of patients with psychiatric disease.
    A. Extent of Medical Disease
        1. Between one-third and two-thirds of psychiatric patients have significant medical disease.
        2. Medical disease is underdiagnosed and undertreated in this population. Unrecognized (by the patient or the primary physician) medical disease is present in 6% to 15% of psychiatric patients. As many as two-thirds of psychiatrists do not perform physical examinations of their patients.
        3. Five to forty per cent of psychiatric syndromes are caused by medical disease.
    B. Informed Consent
        1. The presence of a psychiatric diagnosis does not, in itself, imply that a patient is unable to give informed consent for anesthesia. Competency to give consent is a legal decision, not a medical one. Although usually based on medical/psychiatric opinion, the final decision rests with the courts.

2. The mere presence of a reference to "anesthesia" on a standard informed consent does not necessarily meet statutory requirements. The anesthesiologist must:
   a. Explain the risks and benefits of each option to the patient and guardian (if applicable).
   b. Be reasonably certain that the patient (or guardian) understands the risk and benefit issues.
3. If an informed consent document for anesthesiology services is unavailable, writing the above information in the chart and having the patient (or guardian) cosign the note is an acceptable alternative.
4. When one must obtain a competency ruling immediately before surgery, consent for the anesthetic management plan must also be addressed.
5. In a true surgical emergency involving a psychiatric patient, it is customary to assume that the doctrine of implied consent is in force if the guardian cannot be found.
6. Informing a patient's relatives of anesthetic risks and options, although generally a good policy, does not supplant a court-appointed guardianship in the case of the incompetent patient.

C. Plasma Cholinesterase
A higher than normal frequency of genetic varieties of plasma cholinesterase deficiency has been reported in patients with various psychiatric diagnoses. This abnormality will affect the pharmacokinetics of depolarizing muscle relaxants. Patients undergoing electroconvulsive therapy have been found to be sensitive to succinylcholine at a rate 20 times that of the general surgical population.

II. AFFECTIVE DISORDERS
The affective disorders are syndromes in which the predominant disturbance is one of mood. The spectrum ranges from depression to mania.

A. Depression
1. Depression (unipolar affective disease) may be endogenous or associated with numerous medical conditions of anesthetic importance.
2. Hypothyroidism can be a cause of depression, especially the treatment-resistant forms. Its incidence in psychiatric populations is as high as 14%. Hypo-

thyroidism will decrease cardiac output and can alter drug metabolism. For example, barbiturates will have a much longer duration of action. Hypothyroidism can also complicate weaning from mechanical ventilation and cause intraoperative hypotension.

3. Other endocrine disorders can present as depression, notably Cushing's disease, Addison's disease, and parathyroid adenomas.

4. Various neoplastic and paraneoplastic conditions, such as pancreatic carcinoma and lymphomas, are often associated with depression.

5. Depression can also be drug induced, notably from:
    a. Neurotransmitter-depleting agents (reserpine, guanethidine)
    b. Beta-blockers (especially lipophilic drugs such as propranolol)
    c. Methyldopa
    d. Chronic use of CNS depressants (barbiturates, alcohol, benzodiazepines, glutethimide)
    e. Steroids.

6. Depression and other psychiatric conditions can be associated with an imbalance in electrolytes such as sodium, potassium, magnesium, and calcium.

B. Bipolar Affective Disorder

1. Bipolar affective disorder (formerly called manic depression) is classically characterized by cycling between periods of extreme elation and euphoria (mania) and periods of profound depression. Extended periods of relatively normal mood may be interspersed.

2. Lithium carbonate is the standard drug for the treatment of bipolar disorders and may be used with recurrent unipolar depression, cluster headaches, and a variety of other disorders of a paroxysmal nature.

3. Acutely manic patients may be difficult to sedate preoperatively. These patients will respond in the usual fashion to sedative-hypnotics such as benzodiazepines, although doses will need to be higher than is customary. Neuroleptics are the drugs of choice in most institutions to calm the manic patient.

4. The new onset of mania (especially in a previously

well patient with no depressive history) should initiate the search for an organic cause.

a. Hyperthyroidism, from thyroiditis or Graves' disease, can mimic mania. Hypertension, tachycardia, and hyperthermia may also be present.

b. Intoxication, especially with sympathomimetic agents such as decongestants, amphetamines, cocaine, or diet pills, may create a manic state accompanied by a hyperdynamic cardiovascular picture.

III. PSYCHOSES

The *sine qua non* of psychosis is a breakdown in reality testing, which may be manifested by hallucinations, illusions, and delusions. Psychosis can be thought of as organic (where a causative agent or condition is implicated) and nonorganic (functional).

A. Organic Psychosis

Many of the previously listed organic factors that can cause depressive and manic symptoms may also give rise to psychotic conditions. An organic cause should be vigorously sought in any acutely psychotic patient with no prior history.

B. Nonorganic Psychosis

Patients with nonorganic psychosis may be outpatients or institutionalized, depending on their degree of impairment.

C. Neuroleptics are frequently used to control the symptoms of psychoses from organic or nonorganic causes.

1. A neuroleptic dopamine blocker, droperidol, should be considered as premedication in this group of patients, because in addition to its well-known antiemetic properties, it generally will decrease the psychiatric symptoms.

a. If the patient is already receiving a neuroleptic drug, the dose should be 1 to 1.5 times the patient's usual morning dose of that drug or 50 to 100 mg of chlorpromazine orally 1 to 1.5 hours prior to surgery.

b. Low-potency neuroleptics (chlorpromazine, thioridazine) are preferable to high-potency drugs (haloperidol, fluphenazine) because of the former's increased sedative effects and higher anticholinergic profile.

   2. In the paranoid individual, premedications are best avoided, because the resulting decrease in sensory input may exacerbate the paranoia.

   3. Patients receiving chronic neuroleptic maintenance may not be as responsive to dopamine infusions because of dopamine-receptor blockade peripherally as well as centrally.

IV. MENTAL RETARDATION

Mentally retarded individuals may present for a variety of surgical procedures. Management of preoperative anxiety is similar to that for the pediatric population.

   A. Short-lived sedative agents are preferred for premedication so that emergence will not be complicated by central disinhibition.

   B. Adequate analgesia is of paramount importance in the treatment of these patients.

   1. Like the pediatric population, these patients are frequently undermedicated for pain.

   2. Mentally retarded patients may have difficulty expressing pain. The use of "smiley face" visual analog scales or pictures of people in various degrees of pain can provide a means for the patient to convey pain nonverbally.

   3. Behavioral observations are important in assessing pain.

   a. Classic signs such as guarding or splinting should be watched for.

   b. Nontypical signs, such as becoming noncommunicative or uncooperative or making repetitive vocalizations, may be clues to inadequate analgesia in this population.

   c. As in other patients, scheduled (not "prn") analgesics with breakthrough "rescue" doses provides the best pain management in the early postoperative period.

   C. Associated disease should be diagnosed and its treatment optimized preoperatively. Mental retardation occurs from myriad causes, but certain syndromes, such as Down's (trisomy 21) are associated with:

   1. Congenital cardiac defects

   2. Pulmonary hypertension

   3. Subglottic stenosis

   4. Excessive ligamentous laxity, predisposing to atlanto-occipital dislocation

5. Obesity

6. Seizure disorders.

D. The retarded aggressive patient who is unresponsive to verbal reassurance and behavioral control may be managed in the following manner:

   1. The patient is placed in a confined space with no more people present than are necessary to restrain him or her manually.

   2. Ketamine 1 to 2 mg/kg is given IM, and the patient is released, taking care not to allow harm to come to either the patient or the health care team.

   3. When the ketamine becomes effective, IV access can be obtained.

   4. The above procedure should be done in the operating suite or where full resuscitation measures are available.

E. The NPO status of the mentally retarded patient should always be suspect, and precautions for full stomach are reasonable.

V. DEMENTIA

Dementia is defined as a decrease in cognitive function below the level at which the individual functioned previously. The sensorium is usually clear. An organic cause is presumed (multiple cerebral infarcts, slow virus, heavy metal toxicity, metabolic), although in many cases, the pathophysiology is not known (Alzheimer's disease).

A. Symptoms can be made transiently worse by:

   1. Long-acting benzodiazepines

   The half-life of many of these drugs increases with age, such that the long-acting metabolite of diazepam, for example, may persist for well over a week after a single dose.

   2. Anticholinergics

   Even in normal doses, anticholinergics that readily cross the blood–brain barrier (atropine, scopolamine) can worsen the dementia without giving rise to a clinical anticholinergic toxicity syndrome.

B. The dental condition of the demented patient is notoriously poor. Tooth removal is a frequent indication for general anesthetics in this population.

   1. Periodontal disease predisposes to foreign body aspiration from accidental tooth extraction during intubation.

> **2.** Rampant caries predispose to fracture of the teeth during intubation, as well as to lip lacerations.
>
> **3.** Dentures may be left in to provide lip support for masking provided they fit reasonably well.

C. As with the mentally retarded patient, it is probably safest to consider the demented patient to have a full stomach at all times.

Psychiatric Medications

Various drugs are used to help control the symptoms of psychiatric disease. Some of these have significant implications for anesthetic management.

I. CYCLIC ANTIDEPRESSANTS

Cyclic antidepressants are generally referred to as tricyclic antidepressants, because the original drugs of this class did possess three-ring structures. However, newer members may be tetracyclic (maprotiline) or noncyclic (trazodone), and some dicyclic compounds are being readied for marketing.

A. These compounds are generally prescribed for depression but also may be used for anxiety or panic disorders, chronic pain, and several other disorders.

B. All of the cyclic antidepressants have the following characteristics to a greater or lesser degree:

1. Act by blocking reuptake of neurotransmitter that has been released into the synaptic cleft.

2. Sedation (except desipramine, fluoxitine, and bupropion).

3. Anticholinergic activity (especially amitriptyline and doxepin), causing tachycardia, urinary retention, and decreased gastrointestinal motility.

4. Antihistaminic properties (both H_1 and H_2 receptors).

5. Peripheral alpha$_1$-adrenergic blockade, producing orthostatic hypotension.

C. Arrhythmogenic Potential of Cyclic Antidepressants

1. Usual therapeutic doses rarely cause clinically significant arrhythmias.

2. The cardiac effects of these drugs can be thought of as similar to those of quinidine.

3. Pancuronium may cause arrhythmias during halothane anesthesia in people chronically taking antidepressants (specifically imipramine).

4. These drugs may cause tachycardia, supraventricular and ventricular dysrhythmias; T-wave and ST segment abnormalities, and prolongation of the QT interval at high serum levels.

D. Anesthetic management ideally involves discontinuance of antidepressants 2 weeks before surgery, but this is not always possible (emergencies) or desirable (from a psychiatric perspective). In general, drugs can be continued perioperatively without problem.

E. If anesthesia is provided to someone receiving chronic antidepressant therapy, one may encounter prolongation of sleeping time, increased effects of vasopressors, and ineffectiveness of some antihypertensives (guanethidine).

F. Acute Management of Cyclic Antidepressant Overdose

1. Airway and ventilatory support is often necessary, because many patients are obtunded with either decreased respiratory drive or acute upper airway obstruction.

2. Because of the enterohepatic circulation of the drugs, the patient's state of consciousness may wax and wane, making the decision to extubate difficult. A long period of alertness should be seen prior to extubation. Nasogastric suction and activated charcoal decrease the drug effect from enterohepatic circulation.

3. Management of arrhythmias
Rhythm disturbances are usually tachyarrhythmias and generally respond to the judicious use of physostigmine. Because this drug crosses the blood–brain barrier, it also may clear the sensorium for 30 to 40 minutes. Multiple doses of physostigmine are not recommended, because cholinergic crises may be initiated. Most arrhythmias will respond appropriately to the usual antiarrhythmics.

II. MONOAMINE OXIDASE (MAO) INHIBITORS
First synthesized in the search for antitubercular agents, MAO inhibitors have long been used to treat depression. The well-publicized dietary restrictions (avoiding high-tyramine sources), coupled with litigation fears, caused these drugs to fall from favor in the 1970s. Now, with the realization that some patients are responsive only to MAO inhibitors, the drugs are being used more frequently. One MAO inhibitor, pargyline (Eutonyl), has even been used to treat hypertension, although rarely.

A. Mechanism of Action
1. Monoamine oxidase is a mitochondrial enzyme that catalyzes the breakdown of certain biogenic amines, notably norepinephrine and dopamine. The MAO inhibitors bind in an irreversible fashion to this enzyme and render it inactive.
2. Termination of the effect of the drugs is by generation of new enzyme, a process that may require 2 weeks.

B. In all but absolute emergencies, surgery should be delayed for a 2-week drug-washout period in a patient taking MAO inhibitors.

C. If anesthesia must be provided for a patient receiving MAO inhibitors:
1. Postural hypotension is a common effect, and subarachnoid anesthesia and intravenous anesthetics should be administered cautiously to prevent hypotension.
2. Use of vasopressors can cause hypertensive emergencies. This applies to vasopressors used systemically or in conjunction with agents for conduction anesthesia.
3. There are anecdotal reports that local anesthetic duration is shortened.
4. The MAO inhibitors increase the sleep time after methohexital and, presumably, other barbiturates.
5. Prolonged respiratory depression is seen after general anesthesia.
6. A short-duration direct-acting vasopressor such as epinephrine has been recommended for controlling intraoperative hypotension.
7. Intraoperative hypertension can be managed with phentolamine or sodium nitroprusside.
8. Phenelzine has been reported to potentiate succinylcholine.

D. MAO Inhibitors and Narcotics
1. The concomitant use of MAO inhibitors and narcotic analgesics has been reported to cause a syndrome characterized by hypertension, tachycardia, hyperpyrexia, convulsions, and apnea.
2. The drug most frequently implicated in this interaction is meperidine, but it has been seen with other narcotics.
3. Morphine, given cautiously, is the narcotic recommended most often for use in these patients.

    E.   Overdoses of MAO inhibitors are generally characterized by hypertension to a life-threatening degree.

        1.   Cerebral hemorrhages are common.

        2.   Muscle rigidity and an increase in temperature are seen.

        3.   Rapid-acting intravenous vasodilators are indicated to treat hypertensive emergencies.

        4.   Dantrolene has been reported to be useful for management of overdose when rigidity is the predominant feature.

III. NEUROLEPTICS

Phenothiazines, butyrophenones, and similar compounds are useful in controlling psychotic processes in patients suffering from schizophrenia and related disorders. These drugs are also useful in anesthetic practice as preoperative sedatives and antiemetics. Historically, chlorpromazine (Thorazine) was used intravenously to provide induced or controlled hypotensive anesthesia. Droperidol and metoclopramide are the only other agents in this class approved for IV use.

    A.   All neuroleptics appear to work by blockade of limbic system dopamine receptors (the "dopamine hypothesis" of schizophrenia). Unfortunately, they also affect other areas of dopaminergic transmission such as the nigrostriatal areas and peripheral sites.

    B.   The neuroleptics share several properties, which include antidopaminergic, antihistaminic, antimuscarinic, and anti-alpha$_1$-adrenergic effects.

    C.   Chronic administration of these drugs in large doses (such as in the institutionalized patient) may result in megacolon and an increased risk of bowel obstruction. Precautions against pulmonary aspiration should be used in this population.

    D.   Extrapyramidal reactions of cogwheel rigidity, akinesia, tremor, and akathisia (a syndrome of profound restlessness in which relief is sought by moving the extremities) to these drugs are generally managed with anticholinergic agents.

    E.   Generally, neuroleptics should be given as scheduled up until surgery in a patient chronically treated with them. An increased dose may be given as premedication with or without narcotics.

    F.   Neuroleptic malignant syndrome (NMS) is associated with the use of these drugs on an acute or chronic basis. It is more common in patients with organic brain disease, persons treated with depot injection drugs, and young men.

1. The syndrome is characterized by muscle rigidity, hyperpyrexia, delirium, and autonomic instability.
2. Elevated creatine phosphokinase (CPK), lactic dehydrogenase (LDH), alkaline phosphatase, and transaminases and leukocytosis are frequently seen.
3. Rhabdomyolysis and, subsequently, acute renal failure may ensue.
4. There is a possibility that patients with NMS are more likely to experience malignant hyperthermia than is the general population. Therefore, it is probably safest to avoid drugs that are known to trigger malignant hyperthermia in patients with known NMS.
5. NMS has been treated with dantrolene (the current agent of choice), bromocriptine, amantadine, and pancuronium.

G. Tardive Dyskinesia
1. Tardive dyskinesia (TD) is believed to be secondary to a supersensitivity of dopamine receptors that have been blocked for long periods of time. It is a late and frequently irreversible complication of neuroleptic use.
2. TD is characterized by involuntary choreoathetoid movements of any muscle group, most commonly the orofacial musculature.
3. Although temporarily masked, it is probably made worse by continued administration of neuroleptics.
4. The anesthesiologist should avoid any elective use of neuroleptic drugs in patients with TD.

IV. ANTICHOLINERGICS
Anticholinergic drugs are frequently employed to counteract the extrapyramidal side effects of neuroleptics. They work to restore a central equilibrium between dopaminergic and cholinergic activity.
A. The drugs used are benztropine (Cogentin), trihexyphenidyl (Artane), and diphenhydramine (Benadryl).
B. Any of these may be used, although diphenhydramine in doses of 25 to 50 mg orally, IM, or IV, is generally the drug most available to the anesthesiologist. When given IV, diphenhydramine may cause hypotension.
C. Additional anticholinergics should be used with caution in people taking these drugs regularly.
D. The reduction of lacrimation by these drugs makes ocular protection under general anesthesia a prime concern.

E. Xerostomia produced by this class, although aiding intubation, increases the risk of mucosal trauma on extubation secondary to adherence of the dry mucosa to the endotracheal tube.

V. LITHIUM SALTS

A. Lithium is used for a variety of cyclic or periodic disorders, most commonly bipolar affective disorder. It is handled by the cells in a manner similar to the sodium ion, but how this translates into clinical usefulness is unclear. The carbonate salt is the most frequently used form.

B. Lithium has a narrow therapeutic index. Patients on chronic lithium therapy may develop hypothyroidism, and nephrogenic diabetes insipidus is fairly common.

C. Lithium carbonate is commonly thought to potentiate the neuromuscular blockade produced by several agents, both depolarizing and nondepolarizing. Although there is some evidence to support that contention, the work most often cited employed toxic lithium levels. A review of the experience of the extrapyramidal side effects in a large hospital demonstrated no effect of lithium carbonate on succinylcholine duration.

D. Lithium levels can be elevated significantly by diuretics, especially thiazide derivatives.

V. BENZODIAZEPINES

A. The benzodiazepines are commonly, and many times improperly, used for the chronic treatment of anxiety. They are most useful in the management of panic disorders.

B. Patients taking benzodiazepines may undergo withdrawal if the drugs are discontinued. Common manifestations are restlessness, anxiety, insomnia, neuromuscular irritability, transient psychosis, and seizures.

C. Long-term treatment with these drugs will induce tolerance to them and cross-tolerance to barbiturates and general anesthetics, necessitating increased dosages.

Summary of Anesthetic Considerations

Psychiatric patients frequently have undiagnosed medical problems. Careful examination is needed to detect medical diseases that may need preoperative treatment.

Many patients who are receiving psychiatric care are mentally incompetent, and it is important to determine who is legally responsible for these patients. To avoid legal problems, anesthetic and surgical consent is required from the legal guardian, not from the patient.

Affective and psychotic disorders are often treated with medications. Potential side effects of cyclic antidepressants that can affect anesthetic management are their sedative effects, anticholinergic activity, peripheral α_1-adrenergic blocking action, and arrhythmogenic potential.

Monoamine oxidase inhibitors are occasionally used to treat depression. Several precautions should be taken when managing these patients. The use of opiates should be avoided, as hyperpyrexia occasionally occurs when narcotics, especially meperidine, are given. There is an increased sensitivity to vasodilating and vasoconstrictive drugs. If a vasopressor is needed, a direct-acting agent such as epinephrine is preferred to indirect-acting sympathomimetics. Nitroprusside or phentolamine can be used for hypertension. Prolonged respiratory suppression after general anesthesia is also associated with MAO inhibitors.

The antidopaminergic, antihistaminic, antimuscarinic, and alpha$_1$-blocking effects of neuroleptic drugs must be considered when administering anesthetic medications.

Patients receiving phenothiazines or butyrophenones may develop neuroleptic malignant syndrome. Its presentation is similar to that of malignant hyperthermia, and there is a possibility that patients who experience NMS are at higher risk of having malignant hyperthermia. Anesthetic agents that may trigger malignant hyperthermia should be avoided in these patients.

Intravascular volume status must be carefully assessed with patients receiving lithium, as long-term use can cause nephrogenic diabetes insipidus. There may be a mild potentiation of neuromuscular blockade.

≡ Psychiatric Side Effects of Anesthetic Drugs

J. David Haddox

Almost any anesthetic drug can cause some type of psychiatric side effect on occasion, but there are certain ones that do so with some regularity.

I. DROPERIDOL AND METOCLOPRAMIDE

    A. Droperidol alone or in combination with fentanyl (Innovar) was originally marketed as an ideal premedicant. Its use in this fashion was discontinued because of the unacceptable incidence of akathisia, especially in the younger patient, causing patients to refuse surgery. Akathisia may be treated with judicious intravenous diphenhydramine.

    B. Respiratory dyskinesia (an unusual extrapyramidal effect) has been reported with various neuroleptics and can complicate weaning from a ventilator.

    C. Any neuroleptic will worsen the symptoms and signs of Parkinson's disease, making the patient less comfortable and interfering with postoperative physical and respiratory therapy.

II. KETAMINE

    A. Ketamine, a phencyclidine ("angel dust") derivative, is noted for its psychotomimetic effects, although this may be less problematic in children.

    B. The hallucinatory quality can be used to advantage by:

        1. Telling patients in the preoperative visit that they will be getting a drug that enables them to dream.

        2. Asking them their preferred dream content.

        3. Repeating this content to them during the induction.

    C. The hallucinatory quality may be decreased by coadministration of small amounts of benzodiazepines or thiopental.

III. OPIATES

Although generally without psychiatric side effects and the mainstay of postoperative analgesia, opiates can cause untoward psychic reactions in some people.

    A. Sedation is common with methadone and morphine.

    B. Hallucinations can be seen with any narcotic but are more common with methadone and morphine.

    C. Derealization or depersonalization occurs occasionally.

    D. Myoclonic twitching occurs most frequently with meperidine.

    E. Excessive doses of opiates may cause life-threatening complications from respiratory depression with hypercarbia and hypoxemia.

IV. ANTICHOLINERGICS

    A. Certain patients are apt to develop an anticholinergic toxicity syndrome from premedication or intraoperative use of these drugs: the elderly, patients on any other drug with anticholinergic activity (antidepressants, neuroleptics, intestinal preparations, anti-Parkinson agents, antihistamines), and patients with dementia.

    B. The syndrome is characterized by tachycardia; hot, red, dry skin; dilated pupils; difficulty with visual accommodation; confusion or delirium; and hallucinations (especially visual).

V. BENZODIAZEPINES

The metabolism of the benzodiazepines is decreased in the elderly, causing exceedingly long half-lives. Also, with some drugs in this class (e.g. lorazepam), the brain half-life far exceeds the serum half-life, producing behavioral effects longer than would be expected. These drugs may cause:

    A. Respiratory depression postoperatively

    B. Postoperative confusion or sedation

    C. Anterograde amnesia

    D. Disinhibition, resulting in behavior similar to that caused by other intoxicants such as ethanol.

≡ Electroconvulsive Therapy

J. David Haddox

I. HISTORY

In 1934, on the basis of the observation that some schizophrenics who had seizures became less symptomatic after convulsions, Meduna used chemically induced seizures in patients to achieve therapeutic benefits. A few years later, Cerletti and Bini induced seizures by the application of transcranial electrical current. Today, electroconvulsive therapy (ECT) remains a potent option in the management of depression and, on occasion, other psychiatric diseases.

    In an attempt to control the anxiety, decrease the bony fracture or dislocation rate, mitigate the hemodynamic side effects, and minimize hypoxia from "unmodified" electroconvulsive therapy (i.e., application of electrical current to an unsedated patient spontaneously breathing room air), the services of anesthesiologists are employed. Such care has significantly reduced the morbidity and mortality rates of the procedure, as well as making it more acceptable to all concerned.

II. GENERAL CONSIDERATIONS

    A. The patient presenting for ECT is likely to carry the diagnosis of depression. Special attention must be given to:

1. Reevaluation for undiagnosed medical conditions
2. Known medical conditions
3. Concurrent drug use.

B. Electroconvulsive therapy is often used in the elderly, so problems of anesthetic concern attendant to that age group must be addressed:

1. Decreased cardiac output, with prolonged arm-brain circulation time.
2. Decreased muscle mass, necessitating lower doses of neuromuscular blockers.
3. Increased susceptibility to the deleterious effects of anticholinergic drugs.
4. Osteoporosis and degenerative skeletal diseases, increasing the likelihood of fracture or dislocation with convulsions that are not modified adequately with neuromuscular blockade.
5. Acquired macroglossia resulting from an edentulous state, which may make airway management difficult.
6. Periodontal disease with consequent loose teeth, which makes dislodging them into the airway more likely.
7. Atherosclerotic cardiovascular disease, which may enhance the likelihood of myocardial ischemia or stroke from the blood pressure changes during ECT.

III. ELEMENTS OF ANESTHETIC MANAGEMENT

A. Patients should receive nothing by mouth for at least 6 hours prior to anesthesia.

B. Premedication

1. Sedatives, hypnotics, and anxiolytics are generally avoided, because in a properly prepared patient, premedication is unnecessary.
2. Standard premedications, such as benzodiazepines, raise the seizure threshold, decreasing the chances of successful seizure induction or adequate seizure duration.
3. Anticholinergics can be useful in controlling secretions and reducing the bradycardia associated with ECT. In the patient taking antidepressants, one may wish to avoid anticholinergic agents (e.g., scopolamine, atropine) that cross the blood–brain barrier, because they could potentiate the anticholinergic syndrome. A quaternary amine anticholinergic, glycopyrrolate, will not cross the blood–

brain barrier. The usual dose is 0.2 mg IM or subcutaneously ½ to 1 hour before treatment.

4. Intravenous caffeine increases the likelihood of a successful seizure with ECT. If ordered, it should be given IV 10 minutes before anesthetic induction. If diluted in 250 to 500 ml of normal saline, it will cause less discomfort during infusion.

5. In patients at risk for regurgitation (esophageal reflux, hiatal hernia, obesity, etc.), a preinduction H₂ blocker and metoclopramide may be used. Metoclopramide may enhance the ECT by lowering the seizure threshold.

C. Preoxygenation is provided, as it would be for any general anesthetic.

D. Induction agents should be selected to provide rapid induction of anesthesia with short duration and rapid recovery.

1. Methohexital in a bolus of 0.75 to 1 mg/kg IV is the most frequently employed induction agent for ECT, as it causes the least EEG changes.

2. Thiopental may be used in doses of 3 to 4 mg/kg. It has a slightly longer duration and is associated with more EEG changes. It may produce less salivation during ECT than methohexital.

3. Neuromuscular blockade is an important part of modern anesthetic management of ECT. Succinylcholine is the agent of choice because of its rapid onset and metabolism. It is used primarily to decrease the motor activity that would accompany a seizure in order to reduce the risk of musculoskeletal injury.

a. Because intubation generally is not used for ECT, the dose of succinylcholine can be less than used for "routine" anesthetic cases. Approximately 0.5 mg/kg generally is adequate to attenuate the convulsion.

b. A pneumatic cuff is frequently inflated on an extremity to occlude arterial flow before succinylcholine administration. This creates a localized area of untempered tonic–clonic activity for observation by the treating psychiatrist.

c. Myalgia after ECT with succinylcholine appears to be less of a problem than in other populations so that it is generally not necessary to precede it with a nondepolarizing neuromuscular blocker.

E. A soft rubber mouth guard should be inserted to protect the patient from orodental trauma during the forceful mandibular movements that result from direct transcutaneous stimulation of the muscles of mastication during ECT.

F. The seizure threshold may be lowered by hyperventilation, thereby enhancing the efficacy of the treatment.

G. Ventilatory support should be provided until spontaneous breathing resumes.

H. A postictal state commonly follows ECT that may be characterized by confusion, sedation, uncooperative behavior, and emotional lability.

IV. MONITORING

A. Proper anesthetic management of ECT involves a general anesthetic and should be approached with monitors appropriate to the patient. A minimal scheme would include ECG, pulse oximeter, precordial stethoscope, and blood pressure cuff (preferably automated with recording ability for documentation).

B. Other monitoring may be used from the psychiatric viewpoint.

1. An EEG to monitor seizure activity and duration. Care must be taken to ensure that the electrodes are not placed so as to interfere with anesthetic management. Likewise, care should be exercised by the anesthesiologist to avoid disturbing the EEG electrodes, as artifacts can significantly decrease the utility of intraoperative EEGs.

2. Placement of a pneumatic cuff for assessing convulsions in an extremity depends on the placement of the stimulating electrodes. If a bilateral configuration is used, either arm can be used. If unilateral nondominant hemisphere stimulation is used, the occluding cuff must be placed on the arm ipsilateral to the electrode site, because convulsions in that arm will indicate successful propagation of seizure across the cerebral midline (secondary to crossing of the corticospinal tracts at the pyramidal decussation). This requires that intravenous access and blood pressure readings be obtained from the arm contralateral to the stimulus application. The above problems may be avoided by using the auxiliary cuff

to occlude a leg and watching for seizure activity in the foot.

V. COMPLICATIONS

A. Parasympathetic stimulation may be apparent immediately after ECT resulting in bradycardia (even asystole) and hypotension. This is generally prevented by premedication with anticholinergic drugs.

B. Sympathetic effects are seen more commonly and include:

  1. Hypertension, which is generally at its maximum 60 seconds after the seizure and lasts about 5 minutes. It can be treated if necessary with beta-blockers, hydralazine, sodium nitroprusside, or trimethophan. Two and a half inches of 2% nitroglycerin paste may prevent a hypertensive response.

  2. Tachycardia, which, like hypertension, is thought to be attributable to catecholamine release. It peaks at 30 seconds postseizure and generally subsides within minutes. Increases in heart rate can be lessened by preinduction administration of oral beta-blockers or use of intravenous esmolol.

  3. Hypertension and tachycardia from ECT can significantly increase myocardial oxygen consumption and compromise patients with coronary artery disease. Electroconvulsive therapy does not contribute to substantial elevation of CPK, LDH, or AST (SGOT) and should not confound serial enzyme testing if myocardial infarct is suspected.

  4. Arrhythmias, which occur in approximately half of the noncardiac population and even more of those with cardiac disease, frequently resolve spontaneously and, if not, will respond to traditional management such as lidocaine.

C. Electroconvulsive therapy causes a marked increase in cerebral blood flow, and this may be of concern in patients with increased intracranial pressure preoperatively, with vascular anomalies, or with a history of cerebrovascular accidents.

D. Certain drugs frequently influence ECT management.

  1. The MAO inhibitors may prolong the action of barbiturates and complicate the management of arrhythmias and hypotension.

  2. Cyclic antidepressants can prolong the action of barbiturate, enhance the activity of sympathomimetic drugs, and interact synergistically with other anti-cholinergics, producing post-treatment delirium.

3. Neuroleptics can lower the seizure threshold, cause hypotension via alpha$_1$-receptor blockade, and interact synergistically with other anticholinergics, producing post-treatment delirium.

E. Contraindications

It can be argued that there are no absolute contraindications for the administration of ECT, given the severity of morbidity that may present in a psychiatric population (e.g., the severely depressed psychotic patient who is pregnant and not accepting nourishment). A discussion between the anesthesiologist and the psychiatric care team is mandatory when ECT is contemplated in any of the following conditions:

1. Very high-risk conditions such as recent myocardial infarction or cerebrovascular accident, intracranial mass lesion, cerebral aneurysm, and MAO inhibitor therapy

2. Higher-than-usual risk conditions such as angina pectoris, congestive heart failure, serious pulmonary disease, severe osteoporosis, recent large-bone fracture, pregnancy, retinal detachment, glaucoma, and thrombophlebitis.

VI. SUMMARY OF ANESTHETIC CONSIDERATIONS

The patient must be properly premedicated for ECT. Usually, an anxiolytic agent is not needed and may change the seizure threshhold, decreasing successful seizure induction. Anticholinergic agents should be given to control secretions and reduce the incidence of bradycardia. Preinduction H$_2$ antagonists and metoclopramide should be given for aspiration prophylaxis, especially because many centers do not routinely intubate these patients.

Methohexital is the usual induction agent because it has the least effect on the EEG of the ultrashort-acting barbiturates. Succinylcholine is used to decrease the muscle activity that accompanies the induced generalized seizure.

Standard monitoring for a general anesthesia case should be used. Drugs must be readily available to treat hypertension, tachycardia, or bradycardia associated with ECT. Ventricular and supraventricular arrhythmias frequently follow ECT. Most resolve spontaneously after a short time. ECT should be postponed for patients suspected of having full stomachs or with increased intracranial pressure.

≡ Eating Disorders

Rebekah Wang-Cheng

I. INCIDENCE

Eating disorders cover a wide spectrum, ranging from anorexia nervosa and bulimia to morbid obesity. Although there are some overlapping manifestations, each entity has its own unique features. Reports differ as to whether the incidence of anorexia and bulimia has increased in the past few decades, but as many as 5% to 10% of adolescent girls and young women may be affected. Although eating disorders are much more common in young women, they have been diagnosed in all age groups and both genders. Often, patients are secretive about their eating habits, and the problem may go undetected by family members or physicians.

Obesity is prevalent in Western society, and it is not uncommon to encounter morbidly obese patients who present for surgical procedures specifically designed to reduce body weight, such as gastric bypass, gastric stapling, or liposuction, as well as for other operations.

II. ANOREXIA NERVOSA

A. Definition

The diagnostic criteria have been revised in the latest edition of the American Psychiatric Association *Diagnostic and Statistical Manual* (DSM-III-R).

1. Refusal to maintain body weight over a minimal normal weight for age and height, leading to body weight 15% below that expected.

2. Intense fear of gaining weight or becoming fat, even though underweight.

3. Disturbance in the way one's body weight, size, or shape is perceived.

4. In females, absence of at least three consecutive menstrual cycles when otherwise expected to occur.

B. Complications

Morbidity and mortality rates for anorexia nervosa are among the highest of any psychiatric disorder. Even though patients are usually teenagers or in their 20s, they can have multisystem organ problems (Table 13-1).

C. Preoperative Evaluation

1. The patient appears very thin, even cachetic. Body temperature may be below normal.

Table 13–1. Medical Abnormalities in Anorexia Nervosa

General	Cachexia
	Hypothermia
	Lanugo hair
	Edema
Cardiovascular	Hypotension
	Bradycardia
Renal	Decreased glomerular filtration rate
Gastrointestinal	Decreased gastric emptying
	Constipation
	Elevated transaminases
Hematologic	Anemia
	Leukopenia
	Thrombocytopenia
Endocrinologic	Amenorrhea
	Osteoporosis
	Euthyroid sick syndrome

2. These patients should always be considered to have a full stomach, no matter how long the period of fasting, as both delayed gastric emptying and decreased intestinal motility are common.
3. Cardiovascular considerations
   a. Although various arrhythmias, including sinus arrest, ectopic atrial rhythms, nodal escape beats, and ventricular ectopy, have been reported, patients usually are in normal sinus rhythm or sinus bradycardia. The resting heart rate may be as low as 30 to 40 beats/min.
   b. Resting ECG abnormalities such as nonspecific T-wave or ST changes and QT prolongation may be seen. Marked QT prolongation is associated with sudden death.
   c. Systolic blood pressures are usually below 100 mmHg. Hypotension is not infrequent (systolic pressure <90 mmHg).
   d. Myocardial mass and left ventricular function are both reduced. The response of the heart rate and blood pressure to exercise are blunted even though patients with anorexia are often physically hyperactive.

        e. Mitral valve prolapse appears to be slightly more common in patients with eating disorders.

D. Laboratory Abnormalities
1. Electrolytes are usually normal unless the patient has been vomiting or using diuretics.
2. Liver enzymes may be elevated, which probably reflects fatty infiltration.
3. Mild anemia, leukopenia, and thrombocytopenia are frequently seen, but no increase in the risk of infection or bleeding has been reported.
4. Thyroid function tests
A low triiodothyronine (T3) level reflects decreased peripheral conversion of thyroxine (T4) to T3. This "euthyroid sick" syndrome is probably an adaptive response to chronic starvation.

E. Perioperative Considerations
1. Cardiovascular abnormalities are of greatest concern. Electrolyte abnormalities, especially hypokalemia, may increase the risk of cardiac dysrhythmias unless corrected.
2. These patients do not tolerate excess fluid: pulmonary edema is a frequent complication of overly aggressive fluid management.
3. Decreased nutrition with hypoalbuminemia will alter the pharmacokinetics of protein-bound drugs. Dosages of most drugs will therefore need to be reduced because of increased free drug.
4. Invasive monitoring with arterial catheterization is often necessary because of limited cardiac reserve and existing hypotension.

III. BULIMIA NERVOSA
A. Definition
Formerly called bulimia or bulimarexia, bulimia nervosa is characterized by repeated binging and purging of food. The DSM-III-R criteria are:
1. Recurrent episodes of binge eating
2. A feeling of lack of control over eating behavior during the binges
3. Regularly engaging in either self-induced vomiting, use of laxatives or diuretics, strict dieting or fasting, or vigorous exercise in order to prevent weight gain
4. An average of at least two binge-eating episodes a week for at least 3 months
5. Persistent overconcern with body shape and weight.

B. Complications
   1. Most of the complications are directly related to the gastrointestinal system (Table 13-2). Because of the repeated binging, acute gastric dilatation and rupture have been reported. Hyperlipidemic pancreatitis is another complication.
   2. Purging may be accomplished by induced or spontaneous vomiting and may lead to benign parotid enlargement, dental enamel erosion, esophagitis, and Mallory-Weiss tears.
   3. Because bulimics may also abuse drugs or alcohol, vomiting that occurs during a lethargic state carries the risk of aspiration pneumonia.
   4. Chronic ipecac use may lead to myocardial damage.

C. Preoperative Evaluation
   1. Bulimic patients tend to be older than patients with anorexia, usually age 20 to 40 years. They often go unrecognized because they are secretive about their binging and purging behaviors.
   2. A reliable history may be difficult to obtain, but they should be specifically questioned about taking amphetamine derivatives, laxatives, or diuretics to lose weight.
   3. Many bulimic patients have problems with excessive drug and alcohol use. As many as 75% of patients are also clinically depressed.
   4. Patients are usually normal weight to moderately overweight. Bilateral painless parotid enlargement,

Table 13–2. *Medical Complications of Bulimia*

General	Volume depletion
	Dental enamel erosion
	Edema
Renal	Hypokalemia (diuretic induced)
	Hypochloremic metabolic alkalosis
Cardiovascular	Cardiomyopathy (chronic ipecac use)
	Orthostatic hypotension
Gastrointestinal	Gastric dilation, rupture
	Parotid enlargement
	Esophagitis
	Mallory-Weiss tears, esophageal rupture
	Pancreatitis
Pulmonary	Aspiration pneumonia

irritation of the pharyngeal mucosa, and dental enamel erosion with excessive caries suggest frequent vomiting. A callus on the dorsum of the index finger may be a clue to self-induced vomiting.

5. Because of frequent purging, patients often develop marked volume depletion and orthostatic hypotension.

6. Patients should be assumed to have a full stomach. Because of anxiety regarding the procedure, they may have had a recent exacerbation of binge eating or purging.

7. Laboratory abnormalities
Because bulimic patients abuse laxatives, emetics, and diuretics for weight control, electrolyte and acid–base abnormalities are common. Frequent abnormalities are hyponatremia, hypokalemia, hypomagnesemia, increased BUN, and hypokalemic hypochloremic metabolic alkalosis.

8. Electrocardiogram abnormalities may be present but are not as common as in anorexia. They are usually related to electrolyte aberrations.

D. Intraoperative Considerations
Severe hypokalemia poses the greatest risk of perioperative complications. Multifocal premature ventricular contractions and ventricular tachycardia intraoperatively have been reported in bulimics with hypokalemia.

E. Postoperative Concerns
Postoperatively, one must be concerned with continued electrolyte imbalance, limited cardiac reserve, and the potential for aspiration if reflex vomiting occurs before the patient is fully awake.

IV. MORBID OBESITY

A. Definition
Morbid obesity, which is defined as 100 or more pounds over or at least 100% over desirable body weight, should be considered a chronic illness and carries an increased risk of morbidity and mortality. The obese patient is probably at higher risk for postoperative complications, but there are few data to quantify the degree of risk for elective surgery.

B. Complications

1. Pulmonary
About one third of moderately or severely obese persons have impaired lung function with decreased

vital capacity, maximum voluntary ventilation, and total lung capacity. These abnormalities have led to lower postoperative arterial oxygenation compared with preoperative values. Pulmonary abnormalities are compounded if the obese patient is a smoker or has chronic obstructive lung disease.

2. Cardiovascular

Obesity is a dependent risk factor. Its effects on coronary artery disease are probably mediated through other risk factors such as hyperlipidemia, hypertension, and diabetes.

3. Obesity–hypoventilation syndrome

a. Approximately 10% of the morbidly obese have the obesity–hypoventilation syndrome. However, there is no direct relation between the degree of obesity and the presence of this syndrome, and about 20% of people affected are of normal weight.

b. The classic Pickwickian syndrome consists of marked obesity, somnolence, periodic breathing, hypoventilation, hypercarbia, hypoxia, polycythemia, and cor pulmonale. Symptoms differ greatly from patient to patient.

c. Obstructive sleep apnea is the result of occlusion of the upper airway leading to asphyxia. The apnea is terminated by arousal from sleep and resumption of airflow.

d. Functional residual capacity is frequently below closing volume. This leads to atelectasis and ventilation–perfusion abnormalities, resulting in shunting and hypoxemia. Chronic hypoxemia with metabolic acidosis probably is the mechanism for pulmonary hypertension or cor pulmonale in the patient with obesity–hypoventilation syndrome.

e. Of concern perioperatively are the cardiac arrhythmias. Severe sinus bradycardia, prolonged sinus pauses (up to 13 seconds), second-degree heart block, and tachyarrythmias have all been associated with arterial hypoxemia. Profound bradycardia is mediated by the vagus and related to the severity of hypoxemia and oxyhemoglobin desaturation.

f. Daytime somnolence is primarily secondary to

night-time hypoxemia and the consequent frequent interruption of sleep.

g.   Hypercarbia is present. The etiology may be related to a central decrease in sensitivity to CO_2 and impaired strength of the breathing muscles.

h.   Therapy includes weight loss, removal of obstructive tissue, and avoidance of sedatives and alcohol. If these fail, tracheostomy is effective in reversing symptoms.

C.   Preoperative Considerations

1.   Arterial blood gas measurement will show whether significant hypoxemia or hypercarbia is present.

2.   If the patient is a smoker or has chronic obstructive lung disease or coronary artery disease, pulmonary function tests should also be obtained. Abstinence from smoking for at least 4 weeks is necessary before a decrease in mucous production and a return of ciliary function is seen.

3.   If the patient is seen far in advance of elective surgery, weight loss should be strongly encouraged. Even a small loss may improve cardiopulmonary function and reduce glucose and catecholamine levels.

4.   Even after fasting, obese patients have significantly larger volumes of gastric contents than the non-obese. Because the pH of gastric contents is also lower, premedication with H_2 blockers or metoclopramide is particularly important to decrease the risk of aspiration pneumonitis, especially during induction.

D.   Anesthetic Management

1.   Because several problems may arise with intubation, it is preferable to perform awake intubation. A short thick neck, large tongue, and redundant soft tissue may cause supraglottic obstruction during induction.

2.   Maintaining adequate tidal volume and minute ventilation is of primary concern. Arterial blood gases should be measured frequently, because hypoxia and hypercarbia are not uncommon.

3.   Because routine sphygmomanometry is unreliable in very obese people, intra-arterial cannulation is preferred for blood pressure monitoring.

    4. Central vein catheterization is often necessary because of difficulty obtaining peripheral access.

    5. Increased doses of lipophilic anesthetic agents may be needed because of the increased volume of distribution.

E. Postoperative Complications

    1. Massively obese patients may have significant intraoperative depression of the cardiac index from anesthesia which will not return to the preoperative level in the immediate postoperative period.

    2. Patients should be fully responsive and in a semisitting position prior to extubation to help decrease the possibility of aspiration.

    3. Pulmonary complications may be more common with obesity, but there is very little documentation for this. Prolonged anesthesia with potent inhaled anesthetics may adversely affect the ventilatory response to hypoxia and hypercarbia until the fat stores are significantly diminished hours after the anesthetic is discontinued. Vertical laparotomies probably predispose to atelectasis and hypoxemia more than do horizontal laparotomies.

    4. Wound infections are more frequent in the obese and are the most common cause of postoperative morbidity in gastric bypass. Superficial wound disruption is probably also greater in the obese patient.

    5. There may be increased rates of venous thrombosis in the obese. Antithrombin III levels and fibrinolytic activity are both reduced in morbid obesity and return to normal with weight loss. Prophylactic subcutaneous heparin is recommended.

V. SUMMARY OF ANESTHETIC CONSIDERATIONS

Patients with anorexia nervosa and bulimia nervosa often have nutritional, electrolyte, and acid–base abnormalities. These problems can be associated with cardiac dysrhythmias. Cardiomyopathy, liver dysfunction, anemia, and euthyroid sick syndrome may also be noted in patients with anorexia nervosa. The bulimic patient may have problems with gastric dilatation, esophagitis, and chronic aspiration. Preoperative correction of fluid and electrolyte, acid–base, and volume status will minimize anesthetic problems.

    Caution should be used when giving intravenous anesthetics to anorexic patients because of the increased concentration of free drug from hypoalbuminia and possible cardiomyopathy. For bulimic patients, of special concern is the possibility of unexpected vomiting and markedly delayed gastric emptying.

The morbidly obese patient's primary problem is airway and pulmonary status. Careful preoperative evaluation of the airway is needed. Awake intubation is often preferred for these patients. Postoperative atelectasis is frequent. It is important for these patients to lose as much weight as possible before surgery and to be taught respiratory exercises to decrease atelectasis postoperatively. Prophylaxis for aspiration with H_2 antagonists and metoclopramide is strongly advised. Measures to decrease the incidence of deep venous thrombosis, such as subcutaneous heparin, should be considered.

Because of the large size of all the extremities and the extensive subcutaneous fat, peripheral IVs are difficult to start, and blood pressure is hard to monitor noninvasively. Frequently, intra-arterial catheterization is needed for blood pressure monitoring and drawing samples for blood gas analysis. Central catheterization is needed for venous access. Postoperatively, patients must not be extubated until fully awake because of the increased risk of aspiration.

≡ Substance Abuse

Rebekah Wang-Cheng

Drug abuse is a significant medical problem in the United States, and the number of users even among the middle and upper classes of society continues to rise. Addiction can occur with either illicit or prescription drugs. Addiction to a drug is a combination of tolerance, psychological dependence, and physical dependence. The common drugs of abuse are alcohol, barbiturates, benzodiazepines, cocaine, opiates, marijuana, and amphetamines. Cocaine, in particular, has become widely used. The National Institute on Drug Abuse estimated that three million people abused cocaine regularly in 1986, more than five times the number addicted to heroin.

I. DRUGS OTHER THAN ALCOHOL
   A. Preoperative Evaluation
      1. A reliable drug history is difficult to obtain for several reasons, such as fear of legal prosecution, lack of knowledge about the drugs being taken, and exaggeration or denial of habit.

2. Assessment of alcohol and nutritional status is important, because many drug addicts are also alcoholics.

3. The patient should be questioned about a psychiatric history. Depression is a common problem, especially in the patient abusing prescription drugs. The psychiatrist may be able to help identify the drugs ingested.

4. The physical examination may also provide important clues.

    a. If the patient is malnourished, suspect amphetamine use. Most opiate addicts are well nourished.

    b. Injection sites may be recognized by scarring, hyperpigmentation, or phlebitis. Tattoos are often used to mask the sites. Because of ablation of venous return, unilateral edema of the nondominant hand may be present.

    c. Localized urticaria may be seen with recent opiate injection.

    d. Skin abscesses can be the result of "skin popping" (subcutaneous injection of drugs).

    e. Pupils are constricted with opiates and dilated with amphetamines. Spontaneous nystagmus may be from phencyclidine (PCP). Refractile bodies, usually talc from the cutting agent, may be seen in the fundi.

    f. Poor dental hygiene and bruxism may be seen with amphetamine use.

    g. A perforated nasal septum may be seen with cocaine abuse.

    h. Lymphadenopathy is often present, possibly as the result of nonspecific activation of the immune system by repeated injection of impurities.

    i. Amphetamine overdose can cause or mimic subarachnoid bleeding, producing headache, stiff neck, and focal neurologic signs.

    j. Cardiac abnormalities include cardiomyopathy, seen with amphetamine abuse, and infective endocarditis, seen in IV drug abusers. Infective endocarditis is often staphylococcal. Endocarditis may be present without any physical findings of murmur, heart failure, or embolic phenomena.

5. Diagnostic tests
   a. Urine and serum drug screens are helpful in identifying injected or ingested drugs.
   b. Hepatitis, drug-induced or viral, is common. All IV drug users should be screened for HBsAg and have liver enzymes measured. As many as 70% will be antigen positive, and 80% of active addicts will have abnormal liver function tests at one time or another. Many addicts also have alcoholic liver disease.
   c. There is a high incidence of syphilis among IV drug users, so a VDRL test should always be obtained.
   d. A platelet count is important because heroin and quinine can induce thrombocytopenia.
   e. HIV infection is becoming a greater problem with drug abusers and should be tested for.
   f. ECG changes, such as nonspecific T-wave abnormalities and prolonged QT interval, are common in heroin addicts. Arrhythmias, such as atrial fibrillation, are probably secondary to quinine adulterant in heroin.
   g. A chest radiograph may reveal angiothrombotic lung disease, an interstitial lung disease found only in IV drug users that is secondary to cutting agents such as talc or cornstarch. Noncardiogenic pulmonary edema has been seen with use of heroin and methadone and is probably a hypersensitivity alveolitis.
   h. Pulmonary function tests, including diffusion capacity, and arterial blood gases may be helpful in the evaluation of addicts abusing IV narcotics because of the likelihood of pulmonary dysfunction and respiratory depression.
B. Preoperative Care
   1. If the patient is acutely intoxicated, preoperative medications usually are not needed.
   2. In patients who are abusing drugs at the time of hospitalization, withdrawal prior to surgery should not be attempted. Anesthetics will potentiate hemodynamic instability from acute withdrawal.
   3. Preoperative sedatives and narcotics and intraoperative narcotic use should be avoided in the recovering addict.

4. Patients in methadone programs should receive their usual methadone dose preoperatively or an oral methadone equivalent (methadone 3 mg ≈ morphine 10 mg).

C. Intraoperative Considerations
1. Venous access is usually difficult. Even central line placement may be complicated by venous sclerosis.
2. Opiate addicts have a decreased CO_2 drive, and supplemental oxygen can cause respiratory depression. There is often a large alveolar–arterial gradient.
3. Regional anesthetic techniques are useful for the rehabilitated addict. Narcotics should be avoided.
4. Patients who have acutely ingested amphetamines, which cause CNS release of catecholamines, may have increased requirements for volatile anesthetics. Tachycardia, hypertension, and hyperthermia may be present. There will be an increased sensitivity to vasopressor drugs.
5. Patients using IV cocaine or amphetamines usually have an increased requirement for anesthetics because of the increased serum norepinephrine levels secondary to decreased reuptake.
6. Marijuana increases sympathetic nervous system activity and inhibits parasympathetic activity, leading to an increased resting heart rate. In animals, IV administration of tetrahydrocannabinol, the active ingredient of marijuana, decreases anesthetic requirement.
7. Chronic barbiturate use may result in cross-tolerance to the barbiturates used for anesthesia.

D. Postoperative Management
1. Pain control
   a. Postoperative analgesia will usually be satisfactory with average doses of opiates in addition to usual daily intake of methadone for patients in a methadone program. Unrehabilitated opiate abusers may require unusually large amounts of narcotics for postoperative analgesia.
   b. Agonist–antagonist opiates such as pentazocine, nalbuphine, butorphenol, and buprenorphine should be avoided, as they may precipitate withdrawal syndrome in the opiate-dependent patient.

c. One must watch for respiratory depression in excess of what is usually noted for a given amount of prescribed opiate. Addicts are known to supplement their prescribed analgesic medication with narcotics obtained from friends postoperatively or brought in preoperatively.

2. Management of withdrawal syndromes
   a. Narcotics
   Withdrawal from narcotics is usually not life threatening. The onset is about 12 to 16 hours after the last dose. The initial symptoms consist of yawning, crying, piloerection, sweating, rhinorrhea, increased breathing rate, mydriasis, restlessness, and nausea. The worst symptoms occur within 48 to 72 hours and include insomnia, nausea, diarrhea, weakness, abdominal cramps, vomiting, tachycardia, hypertension, involuntary muscle spasms, joint pains, and fever.

   Methadone substitution is approximately milligram for milligram of heroin, with an initial trial dose of about 10 to 20 mg orally three times daily. Clonidine also prevents signs and symptoms of acute withdrawal.

   Narcotic antagonists such as nalorphine, naloxone, or naltrexone will precipitate acute abstinence syndrome in opiate addicts. Agonist–antagonist opiates may also cause acute withdrawal.

   b. Amphetamines
   Abstinence from stimulants produces a three-phase pattern of crash, withdrawal, and extinction. The crash is characterized by extreme exhaustion followed by intense depression and intermittent craving. The depression may be of suicidal degree and last from days to weeks. Physical symptoms include headache, sweating, hot and cold sensations, muscle cramps, and gastrointestinal cramps. Antipsychotic drugs may be needed to control assaultive behavior.

   c. Cocaine
   Cocaine withdrawal symptoms include craving, depression, sleep disorder, and mental ab-

errations. Because depletion of dopamine and norepinephrine may play a role in drug dependence, desipramine has been used to treat cocaine dependence because it blocks norepinephrine uptake. Amantadine, which releases dopamine and norepinephrine from storage sites, or bromocriptine, which acts as a dopamine agonist, have also been effective in treating dependence with minimal side effects.

d. Hallucinogens

With this class of drug, which includes lysergic acid dimethylamide (LSD) and phencyclidine (PCP), aftereffects can be unpredictable. Psychiatric symptoms predominate. Early on, the patient may be restless, hyperactive, and hallucinating. Affect is extremely labile and may shift abruptly from euphoria to severe depression. Antipsychotic drugs may be necessary but must be used with caution, because anticholinergic effects are synergistic.

e. Barbiturates

Barbiturate withdrawal can be life threatening. Anxiety, tremors, hallucinations, and even grand mal seizures may appear 24 to 48 hours after the drug is stopped and may last 1 to 2 weeks. Death may result from status epilepticus. Psychosis occurs between the third and eighth day and may last several weeks. Physical signs include blepharoclonus, tremor, delirium, increased blood pressure with postural hypotension, and hyperthermia.

If the patient has been using more than 600 mg of pentobarbital or its equivalent, the medication should be continued through the perioperative period. Drug withdrawal should not be attempted until the patient is recovered from his or her operative procedure. When the patient is stable, the dosage can be gradually reduced (by no more than 10% per day).

f. Nonbarbiturate sedatives

Patients also develop physical dependence on nonbarbiturate sedatives such as meprobamate, ethchlorvynol, and methaqualone. Sedative-hypnotic withdrawal syndrome usually begins 2 to 7 days after discontinuation and is manifested by restlessness, anxiety, mood swings, tachycardia, and occasionally seizures. Patients should be supported with sedatives during the immediate perioperative period.

g. Benzodiazepines
Benzodiazepine abstinence syndrome may be delayed for several days (diazepam) or occur more acutely (oxazepam), depending on renal clearance rates, buildup in fat stores, and active metabolites. Symptoms are similar to withdrawal from other sedative-hypnotics, and the perioperative precautions are similar to those for other sedatives.

II.   THE ALCOHOLIC PATIENT

A. The health complications of alcohol abuse are numerous and involve almost every system.

1. Excessive alcohol use is directly linked to liver damage, which can lead to fatty liver, hepatitis, and cirrhosis. Less than 10% of alcoholics actually develop Laennec's cirrhosis.

2. Alcoholic cardiomyopathy is associated with conduction defects and, eventually, heart failure. Even in alcoholic patients without clinical evidence of heart disease, left ventricular function is compromised after ingestion of alcohol to blood levels of 150 mg/dl.

3. Both the peripheral nervous system and the CNS are affected by alcohol. The symptoms can also be found in malnourished nonalcoholic individuals. Peripheral neuropathy may be motor and sensory. Wernicke's disease and Krosakoff's psychosis are the CNS disorders that may be seen in chronic alcoholics. Wernicke's disease is characterized by nystagmus, ophthalmoplegia, ataxia, and mental confusion. Loss of memory and inability to learn new material is present in Krosakoff's psychosis.

4. Leukopenia, anemia, and thrombocytopenia may occur, as alcohol directly suppresses bone marrow production. In the presence of cirrhosis, splenic sequestration also occurs.

5. Chronic or recurrent pancreatitis may further complicate the usual poor nutritional status by causing malabsorption.

B. Preoperative Evaluation

1. A drinking history should be obtained that includes the type, amount, and frequency of alcohol intake and any associated drug use. The patient should be specifically questioned about past episodes of withdrawal, seizures, and delirium tremens (DTs).

2. The history and physical examination should address any neurologic, cardiac, hepatic, and gastrointestinal complications.

3. Blood tests should include a complete count with platelets, prothrombin time, partial thromboplastin time, electrolytes, BUN, creatinine, glucose, and liver enzymes. Magnesium and phosphorus are often very low in chronic alcoholics with obvious poor nutrition.

4. Patients who have been drinking excessively and not eating may have profound hypoglycemia, as their liver glycogen stores are often depleted.

5. If the patient appears intoxicated or stuporous, a blood alcohol measurement may be helpful. The legal limit for intoxication is 100 mg/dl. Levels above 400 mg/dl produce stupor, and those above 500 mg/dl may be fatal (Table 13-3).

   a. Although ethanol can be removed by hemodialysis or peritoneal dialysis, usually, supportive care is sufficient until the alcohol is metabolized. Ethanol is eliminated by zero-order kinetics, and serum levels fall by about 15 mg/dl per hour.

   b. Anesthesia should be avoided until the patient is sober if at all possible. One study suggested increased morbidity with blood alcohol levels above 250 mg/dl.

Table 13–3. Correlation of Clinical Effects with Blood Alcohol Percentages

0.05%	Decreased inhibition and impaired judgment
0.10%	Impaired motor functioning and lack of self-criticism
0.15%	Too intoxicated to operate vehicle
0.20%	Motor function grossly impaired
0.30%	Stupor
0.40%	Coma
0.60%	Death

C. Intraoperative Considerations
 1. Alcohol stimulates gastric acid secretion, and patients are at risk for aspiration during induction, especially if they are intoxicated.
 2. Anesthetic requirements are probably increased in the chronic alcoholic, but there are no detailed human studies of the role of alcohol in cross-tolerance with anesthetics. Acute intoxication often reduces the anesthetic requirement.
 3. Hypothermia may be present if the patient has been unprotected in a cold environment. Warmed intravenous fluid and warmed blankets are usually sufficient therapy.
 4. The risk of pulmonary aspiration during induction is very high. Regional anesthesia is a good choice in the quiet acutely intoxicated patient with a full stomach.
 5. In patients with cirrhosis, ascites, and hypoalbuminemia, the amount of active unbound drug may be increased, and drug dosages therefore should be reduced.
 6. The action of succinylcholine may be prolonged in the presence of alcoholic liver disease secondary to decreased production of pseudocholinesterase. In cirrhotic patients, the volume of distribution of pancuronium is increased, necessitating a large initial dose, but the elimination half-life is doubled, resulting in a prolonged duration of action.
 7. Selecting a drug for maintenance of anesthesia may be difficult. Although there is no definite evidence of risk, it probably is best to avoid halothane in the presence of liver disease. All volatile anesthetics have the potential for myocardial depression, especially in cirrhotics with cardiomyopathy. Hepatic perfusion is also decreased by all volatile anesthetics but least with isoflurane.
 8. Fluid balance is often difficult to achieve if ascites is present. Because of low colloid oncotic pressure, the patient may have a contracted intravascular volume and hypotension, leading to secondary hyperaldosteronism. Intravenous administration of sodium-containing fluids may rapidly worsen the ascites.
 9. Invasive monitoring is often necessary in these pa-

tients, because even small changes in their hemodynamic status will compromise hepatic perfusion.

D. Postoperative Care

1. The patient should be observed carefully for withdrawal, which occurs soon after alcohol intake is curtailed. Tremulousness is the earliest sign and is more severe after a night of sleep. It may be accompanied by sweats, nausea, anxiety, fever, and hallucinations. Chlordiazepoxide and most other benzodiazepines are effective for treatment of symptoms and are absorbed less erratically if given orally than if given intramuscularly (exceptions are midazolam and clorazepam). Beta-blockers have also been used, especially if sympathetic overactivity is present.

2. Withdrawal seizures are usually generalized and may be single or multiple. Status epilepticus is rare, and seizures usually respond to diazepam or other benzodiazepines. Seizures may also occur in association with alcohol use rather than after abstinence. Although it is commonly believed that the seizures occur within a few days of abstention, they may take place months after the reported last drink. Sodium thiopental or any of the benzodiazepines will stop withdrawal seizures. Loading with phenytoin and chronic anticonvulsant maintenance is not necessary.

3. DTs occur in about 5% of alcoholics 3 to 5 days after abstinence and carry a mortality rate of 5% to 15%. Symptoms include agitation, disorientation, fever, tachycardia, and autonomic nervous system hyperactivity. Therapy should be initiated with intravenous diazepam 5 mg every 5 minutes or an equivalent dose of chordiazepoxide, midazolam, or lorazepam until the patient is calm. Hypokalemia may precede DTs, so serum potassium should be monitored.

4. Postoperative jaundice is common if a cirrhotic patient has received blood transfusions. This is usually the result of defective hepatic processing of hemolyzed erythrocytes rather than anesthetic toxicity.

III. SUMMARY OF ANESTHETIC CONSIDERATIONS

Preoperative history from drug abusers is usually undependable. Urine or serum drug screens may help in determining the drug(s) being used. Physical examination is usually non-specific. However, cardiac murmurs or S_4 may represent infective endocarditis or cardiomyopathy. In addition to routine electrolytes, blood count, ECG, chest radiograph, and renal panel, these patients should be screened for viral hepatitis, syphilis, and HIV.

Patients acutely intoxicated with alcohol, barbiturates, benzodiazepines, other sedative-hypnotics, or opiates usually require less anesthetic drugs for induction and maintenance. Those acutely intoxicated with marijuana, amphetamines, or cocaine may have higher anesthetic requirements because of generalized increased CNS and sympathetic activity. All acutely intoxicated patients are considered to have full stomachs, and appropriate measures must be taken to prevent aspiration.

Patients in acute withdrawal will have hemodynamic instability and CNS changes. Sedation and stabilization of the blood pressure and pulse rate must be accomplished before surgery.

Chronic abusers of alcohol, sedative-hypnotics, and opiates may require much higher doses of anesthetic agents than expected.

One should be wary of giving sympathomimetics to patients using cocaine or amphetamines, anticholinergics to patients taking hallucinogens, and opiate agonists–antagonists to patients abusing opiate agonists.

Postoperatively, drug abusers should be maintained on whatever medication is needed to prevent withdrawal until they have recovered from their surgical procedures.

Recommended Reading

Arnold DE, Rose RJ, Stoddard P. Intraoperative cardiac dysrhythmias in a patient with bulimic anorexia nervosa. Anesthesiology 1987;67:1003.

Baker TL. Sleep apnea disorders. Introduction to sleep and sleep disorders. Med Clin North Am 1985;69:1123.

Bradley TD, Phillipson ES. Pathogenesis and pathophysiology of the obstructive sleep apnea syndrome. Med Clin North Am 1985;69:1169.

Bruce DL. Alcoholism and anesthesia. Anesth Analg 1983;62:84.

Caroff SN, Rosenberg H, Fletcher JE, Heiman-Patterson TD, Mann SC. Malignant hyperthermia susceptibility in neuroleptic malignant syndrome. Anesthesiology 1987;67:20.

Edwards RP, Miller RD, Roizen MF, Ham J, Way WL, Lake CR, Roderick L. Cardiac responses to imipramine and pancuronium during anesthesia with halothane or enflurane. Anesthesiology 1979;50:421.

Fitzgerald FT. Surgery and the drug dependent patient. In: Bolt RJ, ed. Medical evaluation of surgical patient. Mt. Kisco: Futura Publishing, 1987:117.

Frommer DA, Kulig KW, Marx JA, Rumack B. Tricyclic antidepressant overdose: a review. JAMA 1987;257:521.

Gaines GY, Rees DI. Electroconvulsive therapy and anesthetic considerations. Anesth Analg 1986;65:1345.

Geiduschek J, Cohen SA, Khan A, Cullen BF. Repeated anesthesia for a patient with neuroleptic malignant syndrome. Anesthesiology 1988;68:134.

Hall RCW, Beresford TP, Gardner ER, Popkin MK. The medical care of psychiatric patients. Hosp Commun Psychiatry 1982;33:25.

Herzog DB, Copeland PM. Eating disorders. N Engl J Med 1985; 313:295–303.

Hill GE, Wong KC, Hodges MR. Lithium carbonate and neuromuscular blocking agents. Anesthesiology 1977;46:122.

Khantzian EJ, McKenna GJ. Acute toxic and withdrawal reactions associated with drug use and abuse. Ann Intern Med 1979;90:361.

Kobel M, Creighton RE, Steward DJ. Anaesthetic considerations in Down's syndrome: experience with 100 patients and a review of the literature. Can Anaesth Soc J 1982;29:593.

Koranyi EK. Fatalities in 2070 psychiatric outpatients. Arch Gen Psychiatry 1977;348:1137.

Levy WK. Alcohol and drug abuse in the surgical patient. In: Goldman DR, Brown FH, Levy WK, Slap GB, Sussman EJ, eds. Medical care of the surgical patient: a problem-oriented approach to management. Philadelphia: JB Lippincott, 1982:568.

Martin BA, Kramer PM. Clinical significance of the interaction between lithium and a neuromuscular blocker. Am J Psychiatry 1982;139:1326.

Mitchell JE, Seim HC, Colon E, Pomeroy C. Medical complications and medical management of bulimia. Ann Intern Med 1987;107:71.

Pasulka PS, Bistrian BR, Benotti PN, Blackburn GL. The risks of surgery in obese patients. Ann Intern Med 1986;104:540.

Scheller MS, Sears KL. Postoperative neurologic dysfunction associated with preoperative administration of metoclopramide. Anesth Analg 1987;66:274.

Selvin BL. Electroconvulsive therapy 1987 [review]. Anesthesiology 1987;67:367.

Viegas OJ. Drug abuse and overdose. In: Stoelting RK, Dierdorf SF, eds. Anesthesia and co-existing disease. New York: Churchill Livingstone, 1988:673.

Whittaker M. Plasma cholinesterase variants and the anaesthetist [review]. Anaesthesia 1980;35:174.

Williams JBW, ed. Diagnostic and statistical manual of mental disorders. 3rd rev ed. Washington, DC: American Psychiatric Association, 1987:66.

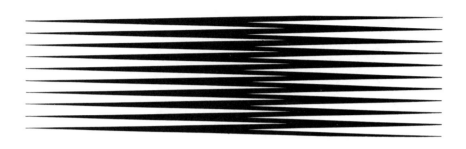

Appendixes

Appendix A

Normal Calculated Cardiovascular Values

Variable	Abbreviation	Formula		Range	Units
Cardiac output	CO	Varies with patient size		4–8	L/min
Cardiac index	CI	$\dfrac{CO}{BSA}$		2.8–4.2	L/min/m^2
Stroke volume	SV	$\dfrac{CO}{\text{heart rate}}$	$\times 1000$	60–90	ml/beat
Stroke index	SVI	$\dfrac{SV}{BSA}$		30–60	ml/beat/ m^2
Left ventricular stroke work index	LVSWI	$\dfrac{1.36 \times (\overline{MAP} - PAOP)}{100}$	$\times SI$	45–65	$\dfrac{g - m/m^2}{beat}$
Right ventricular stroke work index	RVSWI	$\dfrac{1.36 \times (\overline{PAP} - CVP)}{100}$	$\times SI$	5–10	$\dfrac{g - m/m^2}{beat}$
(Total) systemic vascular resistance	SVR (TPR)	$\dfrac{\overline{MAP} - CVP}{CO}$	$\times 80$	800–1200	$\dfrac{\text{dynes-sec}}{cm^5}$
Pulmonary vascular resistance	PVR	$\dfrac{\overline{PAP} - PAOP}{CO}$	$\times 80$	150–250	$\dfrac{\text{dynes-sec}}{cm^5}$

BSA = body surface-area; $\overline{MAP}$ = mean arterial pressure; $\overline{PAP}$ = mean pulmonary artery pressure; PAOP = pulmonary artery occlusion pressure; CVP = central venous pressure.

Appendix B

Normal Measured Cardiovascular Values

Pressure	Abbreviation	Mean (mmHg)	Range (mmHg)
Central venous	CVP	5	2–8
Right atrium	RAP	5	2–8
Right ventricle			
Systolic	–	25	15–30
Diastolic	RVEDP	4	0–8
Pulmonary artery			
Systolic	PAsP	25	15–30
Diastolic	PAdP	12	5–16
Mean	PAP	16	8–18
Pulmonary artery occlusion (pulmonary artery wedge; pulmonary capillary wedge)	PAOP	8	4–12
Left atrium	LAP	8	4–12
Left ventricle			
Systolic	–	120	90–130
End-diastolic	LVEDP	8	4–12

Appendix C

Pulmonary Function Test Values

Measure (abbreviation)	Units	Approximate Values
Ventilatory rate (f)	breath/min	8–18
Tidal volume (V_T)	ml/kg	5–7
Respiratory dead space (V_D)	ml/kg	2–2.2
Minute ventilation (V_E)	L/min	5–10
Forced vital capacity (FVC)	ml/kg	50–70
Forced expiratory volume in 1 sec (FEV_1)	% of FVC	75–80
Maximal expiratory flow rate for 1 L (MEFR)	L/min	>400
Maximal inspiratory flow rate for 1 L (MIFR)	L/min	>300
Maximal inspiratory force (MIF)	mmHg	60–100
Maximal expiratory force (MEF)	mmHg	60–100
Compliance of lungs and thoracic cage (C_T)	L/cm H_2O	0.1
Compliance of lungs (C_L)	L/cm H_2O	0.2
Airway resistance	cmH_2O/L/sec	1.6
Pulmonary resistance	cmH_2O/L/sec	1.9
Work of quiet breathing	kg-M/min	0.5
Maximal work of breathing	kg-M/min	10
Diffusion capacity (steady state)	ml CO/min/mmHg	18
Diffusion capacity (single breath)	ml CO/min/mmHg	31
Diffusion capacity (rebreathing)	ml CO/min/mmHg	27

Appendix D

Respiratory Oxygenation and Ventilation

Values	Abbreviation	Units	Range
O_2 saturation (room air)	SaO_2	%	97–99
O_2 tension (room air)	PaO_2	mmHg	95–99
O_2 tension (100% O_2)	PaO_2	mmHg	640
CO_2 tension	$PaCO_2$	mmHg	35–42
End-tidal CO_2	Pet CO_2	mmHg	2–4 below $PaCO_2$
Alveolar–arterial PO_2 difference (room air)	$P(A\text{-}a)O_2$	mmHg	9
Alveolar–arterial PO_2 difference (100%) O_2	$P(A\text{-}a)O_2$	mmHg	35
Oxygen ratio	PaO_2/FI_{O_2}	mmHg	>300
Venous O_2 saturation	$S\bar{v}O_2$	%	68–77
Mixed venous O_2 tension	$P\bar{v}O_2$	mmHg	35–45
Arterial oxygen content	CaO_2	ml/dl	20
Venous oxygen content	$C\bar{v}O_2$	ml/dl	15
O_2 consumption	$\dot{V}O_2$	ml/min	250
CO_2 production	$\dot{V}CO_2$	ml/min	200

Appendix E

Relative Potency and Equivalent Doses of Commonly Used Glucocorticoids

Steroids	Relative Glucocorticoid Potency	Equivalent Glucocorticoid Dose (mg)	Mineralocorticoid Activity
Short-acting			
Cortisol (hydrocortisone)	1	20	Yes
Cortisone	0.8	25	Yes
Prednisone	4	5	No
Prednisolone	4	5	No
Methylprednisolone	5	4	No
Intermediate-acting			
Triamcinolone	5	4	No
Long-acting			
Betamethasone	25	0.60	No
Dexamethasone	30	0.75	No

INDEX

Entries followed by *f* indicate figures; those followed by *t* indicate tabular material.